MD ANDERSON
CANCER CARE
SERIES

Series Editors

Aman U. Buzdar, MD   **Ralph S. Freedman, MD, PhD**

T0234034

For further volumes:
http://www.springer.com/series/4596

MD ANDERSON CANCER CARE SERIES

Series Editors: Aman U. Buzdar, MD
                     Ralph S. Freedman, MD, PhD

K. K. Hunt, G. L. Robb, E. A. Strom, and N. T. Ueno, Eds., *Breast Cancer*

F. V. Fossella, R. Komaki, and J. B. Putnam, Jr., Eds., *Lung Cancer*

J. A. Ajani, S. A. Curley, N. A. Janjan, and P. M. Lynch, Eds., *Gastrointestinal Cancer*

K. W. Chan and R. B. Raney, Jr., Eds., *Pediatric Oncology*

P. J. Eifel, D. M. Gershenson, J. J. Kavanagh, and E. G. Silva, Eds., *Gynecologic Cancer*

F. DeMonte, M. R. Gilbert, A. Mahajan, and I. E. McCutcheon, Eds., *Tumors of the Brain and Spine*

P. P. Lin and S. Patel, Eds., *Bone Sarcoma*

Lewis E. Foxhall • Maria Alma Rodriguez
Editors

The University of Texas MD Anderson Cancer Center, Houston, Texas

Advances in Cancer Survivorship Management

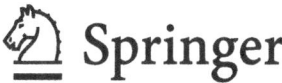

Editors
Lewis E. Foxhall, MD
Department of Clinical Cancer Prevention
Division of Cancer Prevention and
    Population Sciences
The University of Texas MD Anderson
    Cancer Center
Houston, TX
USA

Maria Alma Rodriguez, MD
Department of Lymphoma and Myeloma
Division of Medical Affairs
The University of Texas MD Anderson
    Cancer Center
Houston, TX
USA

Series Editors
Aman U. Buzdar, MD
Department of Breast Medical Oncology
Division of Cancer Medicine
The University of Texas MD Anderson
    Cancer Center
Houston, TX
USA

Ralph S. Freedman, MD, PhD
Department of Gynecologic Oncology
    and Reproductive Medicine
Division of Surgery
The University of Texas MD Anderson
    Cancer Center
Houston, TX
USA

ISBN 978-1-4939-0985-8   ISBN 978-1-4939-0986-5   (eBook)
DOI 10.1007/978-1-4939-0986-5
Springer New York Heidelberg Dordrecht London

Library of Congress Control Number: 2014951825

Printed on acid-free paper

Springer is part of Springer Science+Business Media (www.springer.com)

Foreword

Progress in cancer research, prevention, diagnosis, and treatment during the four decades since the passage of the National Cancer Act of 1971 has been truly remarkable. These advances have made it possible for increasing numbers of people to survive long after a cancer diagnosis. It is estimated that there are now around 12 million cancer survivors in the United States alone and more than 25 million worldwide (Ltekruse et al. 2010; International Agency for Research on Cancer 2008). Although this is cause for celebration, much remains to be done. We are still losing too many lives to this disease, and progress on certain types of cancer has been frustratingly slow. In addition, it is becoming clear that surviving cancer brings with it a whole new set of challenges for these individuals.

In 2003, the President's Cancer Panel heard testimony from more than 200 cancer survivors and caregivers, who described the difficulties involved in living beyond cancer treatment. At that time, there was little recognition of the challenges faced by cancer survivors in trying to reestablish productive lives. The report of the President's Cancer Panel (2004), "Living Beyond Cancer: Finding a New Balance," attempted to describe the sense of abandonment experienced by people who had completed their treatment but now needed a different type of assistance to restore order to their lives. It was clear that information regarding treatments received, follow-up plans, and potential late effects of treatment were not available to most patients; needs for psychological support and financial and legal counseling were not being met; and recognition that life after cancer was dramatically different from life before cancer was lacking in the medical community. These findings were reiterated and amplified in an Institute of Medicine report in 2006, entitled, "From Cancer Patient to Cancer Survivor: Lost in Transition" (Committee on Cancer Survivorship 2010). Both reports made it clear that the end of cancer treatment did not signify the end of the needs of and challenges for cancer survivors. These findings indicated that it was time for a shift in focus from curing the disease to caring for the patient through and beyond the disease.

It is very rewarding to see that cancer care is beginning to be viewed as a continuum from prevention to survivorship care, and that cancer survivorship is emerging as an important aspect of the care of cancer patients. This is evident from the creation of the Office of Cancer Survivorship by the National Cancer Institute in 1996 and in the work of the Lance Armstrong Foundation, which in 2005 created the LIVESTRONG Centers of Excellence Survivorship Network, which seeks to offer "information, care, and services to cancer survivors, their family members, and health care providers" (LIVESTRONG 2011). It is also evident from the work presented in this volume, which describes the MD Anderson experience and models for delivering care and services to cancer survivors. As described here, the needs of patients and models of care may differ depending on the age of the patient at the time of treatment, the type of cancer, the treatment received, and the individual circumstances of each person. Nonetheless, there are common elements to address, regardless of these differences, such as the needs for surveillance for disease recurrence, screening for second primary cancers, education regarding potential late effects of treatment, and access to psychosocial counseling. This book provides an excellent guide to addressing these issues and should be of assistance to community oncologists and physicians and their staffs, all of whom must deal with the ever increasing population of cancer survivors. This is extremely important, because the vast majority of cancer patients are treated in the community, not at comprehensive cancer centers, and long-term follow-up of cancer patients is also largely the province of these health care providers. In my view, this book is important because it will help to disseminate models for the care of cancer survivors to the larger medical community outside the academic medical centers and because it represents a major step forward in helping people live productive lives after cancer treatment.

Margaret L. Kripke, PhD
Vivian L. Smith Chair and Professor of Immunology, Emerita
The University of Texas MD Anderson Cancer Center
Member, President's Cancer Panel
Member, LIVESTRONG Centers of Excellence Network Steering Committee

References

Committee on Cancer Survivorship. Improving care and quality of life. In: Hewitt M, Greenfield S, Stovall E, eds. *From Cancer Patient to Cancer Survivor: Lost in Transition.* Washington, DC: The National Academies Press; 2010.

International Agency for Research on Cancer. World cancer report. Boyle P, Levin B, eds. Lyon, France: IARC; 2008. http://www.iarc.fr/en/publications/pdfs-online/wcr/2008/wcr_2008.pdf. Accessed June 26, 2013.

LIVESTRONG. Defining Survivorship Care: Lessons Learned from the LIVESTRONG Survivorship Center of Excellence Network. LIVESTRONG; 2011. http://www.livestrong.org/pdfs/3-0/COEreport_FINAL. Accessed June 26, 2013.

Ltekruse SF, Kosary CL, Krapcho M, et al. (eds). SEER cancer statistics review, 1975–2007 (based on November 2009 SEER data submission). Bethesda, MD: National Cancer Institute, 2010. http://seer.cancer.gov/csr/1975_2007.

President's Cancer Panel. *Living Beyond Cancer: Finding a New Balance.* Bethesda, MD: National Cancer Institute; 2004.

Contents

Contributors

Shahab U. Ahmed, MD Senior Coordinator of Research Data, Department of Gastrointestinal Medical Oncology, The University of Texas MD Anderson Cancer Center, Houston, TX, USA

Amin Alousi, MD Associate Professor, Department of Stem Cell Transplantation and Cellular Therapy, The University of Texas MD Anderson Cancer Center, Houston, TX, USA

Etsuko Aoki, MD, PhD Assistant Professor, Department of Leukemia, The University of Texas MD Anderson Cancer Center, Houston, TX, USA

Joann L. Ater, MD Professor, Department of Pediatrics, The University of Texas MD Anderson Cancer Center, Houston, TX, USA

Leslie Ballas, MD Radiation Oncologist, Valley Radiotherapy Associates, Los Angeles, CA, USA

Karen Basen-Engquist, PhD, MPH Department of Behavioral Science, Center for Energy Balance in Cancer Prevention and Survivorship, The University of Texas MD Anderson Cancer Center, Houston, TX, USA

Therese B. Bevers, MD Professor and Medical Director, Department of Clinical Cancer Prevention, The University of Texas MD Anderson Cancer Center, Houston, TX, USA

Diane C. Bodurka, MD Professor, Department of Gynecologic Oncology and Reproductive Medicine, The University of Texas MD Anderson Cancer Center, Houston, TX, USA

Genevieve Marie Boland, MD, PhD Fellow, Department of Surgical Oncology, The University of Texas MD Anderson Cancer Center, Houston, TX, USA

Naifa L. Busaidy, MD Associate Professor, Department of Endocrine Neoplasia and Hormonal Disorders, The University of Texas MD Anderson Cancer Center, Houston, TX, USA

Richard Champlin, MD Professor of Medicine and Robert C. Hickey Chair of Clinical Care, Department of Stem Cell Transplantation and Cellular Therapy, The University of Texas MD Anderson Cancer Center, Houston, TX, USA

Alejandro Chaoul, PhD Assistant Professor, Integrative Medicine Program, Department of General Oncology, The University of Texas MD Anderson Cancer Center, Houston, TX, USA

Paul M. Cinciripini, PhD Professor, Department of Behavioral Science, The University of Texas MD Anderson Cancer Center, Houston, TX, USA

Lorenzo Cohen, PhD Professor and Director, Integrative Medicine Program, Department of General Oncology, The University of Texas MD Anderson Cancer Center, Houston, TX, USA

John W. Davis, MD Assistant Professor, Department of Urology, The University of Texas MD Anderson Cancer Center, Houston, TX, USA

Cathy Eng, MD, FACP Associate Professor, Department of Gastrointestinal Medical Oncology, The University of Texas MD Anderson Cancer Center, Houston, TX, USA

Daniel E. Epner, MD, FACP Associate Professor, Department of Palliative Care and Rehabilitation Medicine, The University of Texas MD Anderson Cancer Center, Houston, TX, USA

Carmen P. Escalante, MD Professor and Chair, Department of General Internal Medicine, The University of Texas MD Anderson Cancer Center, Houston, TX, USA

Michael S. Ewer, MD Professor, Department of Cardiology, The University of Texas MD Anderson Cancer Center, Houston, TX, USA

Sherrie L. Flores, RNC, WHCNP-BC, NP-C Advanced Practice Nurse, Department of Endocrine Neoplasia and Hormonal Disorders, The University of Texas MD Anderson Cancer Center, Houston, TX, USA

Lewis E. Foxhall, MD Vice President, Health Policy; Professor, Department of Clinical Cancer Prevention, The University of Texas MD Anderson Cancer Center, Houston, TX, USA

Jack Fu, MD Assistant Professor, Department of Palliative Care and Rehabilitation Medicine, The University of Texas MD Anderson Cancer Center, Houston, TX, USA

M. Kay Garcia, DrPH, MSN, LAc Acupuncturist, Integrative Medicine Program, Department of General Oncology, The University of Texas MD Anderson Cancer Center, Houston, TX, USA

Jeffrey E. Gershenwald, MD Professor, Department of Surgical Oncology, The University of Texas MD Anderson Cancer Center, Houston, TX, USA

Mouhammed Amir Habra, MD Assistant Professor, Department of Endocrine Neoplasia and Hormonal Disorders, The University of Texas MD Anderson Cancer Center, Houston, TX, USA

Karen E. Hoffman, MD, MHSc, MPH Assistant Professor, Department of Radiation Oncology, The University of Texas MD Anderson Cancer Center, Houston, TX, USA

Mimi I. Hu, MD Associate Professor, Department of Endocrine Neoplasia and Hormonal Disorders, The University of Texas MD Anderson Cancer Center, Houston, TX, USA

Katherine A. Hutcheson, PhD Assistant Professor, Department of Head and Neck Surgery, The University of Texas MD Anderson Cancer Center, Houston, TX, USA

Laurel R. Hyle, JD, MPH Associate General Counsel, Office of the General Counsel, Tulane University, New Orleans, LA, USA (formerly Legal Officer, Department of Legal Services, The University of Texas MD Anderson Cancer Center, Houston, TX, USA)

Camilo Jimenez, MD Associate Professor, Department of Endocrine Neoplasia and Hormonal Disorders, The University of Texas MD Anderson Cancer Center, Houston, TX, USA

Maher Karam-Hage, MD Associate Professor, Department of Behavioral Science, The University of Texas MD Anderson Cancer Center, Houston, TX, USA

Jeri Kim, MD Associate Professor, Department of Genitourinary Medical Oncology, The University of Texas MD Anderson Cancer Center, Houston, TX, USA

Deborah A. Kuban, MD Professor, Department of Radiation Oncology, The University of Texas MD Anderson Cancer Center, Houston, TX, USA

Richard Lee, MD Assistant Professor, Integrative Medicine Program, Department of General Oncology, The University of Texas MD Anderson Cancer Center, Houston, TX, USA

Carol M. Lewis, MD, MPH Assistant Professor, Department of Head and Neck Surgery, The University of Texas MD Anderson Cancer Center, Houston, TX, USA

Gabriel Lopez, MD Assistant Professor, Integrative Medicine Program, Department of General Oncology, The University of Texas MD Anderson Cancer Center, Houston, TX, USA

Ellen F. Manzullo, MD Professor, Department of General Internal Medicine, The University of Texas MD Anderson Cancer Center, Houston, TX, USA

Clare McKindley, RD, LD Clinical Dietitian, Department of Clinical Nutrition, The University of Texas MD Anderson Cancer Center, Houston, TX, USA

Christina A. Meyers, PhD, ABPP Professor and Chief (retired), Section of Neuropsychology, Department of Neuropsychology, The University of Texas MD Anderson Cancer Center, Houston, TX, USA

Phuong Khanh Morrow, MD Global Development, Amgen, Thousand Oaks, CA, USA (formerly Assistant Professor, Department of Breast Medical Oncology, The University of Texas MD Anderson Cancer Center, Houston, TX, USA)

Joyce Neumann, MSN, RN, AOCN Advanced Practice Nurse and Program Director, Department of Stem Cell Transplantation and Cellular Therapy, The University of Texas MD Anderson Cancer Center, Houston, TX, USA

William E. Osai, MSN, FNP, MBA Advanced Practice Nurse, Department of Genitourinary Medical Oncology, The University of Texas MD Anderson Cancer Center, Houston, TX, USA

Marcia L. Patterson, MSN, RN, NP-C Nurse Practitioner (retired), Department of Genitourinary Medical Oncology, The University of Texas MD Anderson Cancer Center, Houston, TX, USA

Maria Alma Rodriguez, MD Vice President of Medical Affairs; Professor, Department of Lymphoma and Myeloma, The University of Texas MD Anderson Cancer Center, Houston, TX, USA

Kenneth V.I. Rolston, MD Professor of Medicine, Department of Infectious Diseases, Infection Control and Employee Health, The University of Texas MD Anderson Cancer Center, Houston, TX, USA

Leslie R. Schover, PhD Professor, Department of Behavioral Science, The University of Texas MD Anderson Cancer Center, Houston, TX, USA

Sally Scroggs, MS, RD, LD Clinical Manager of Integrative Health, Cancer Prevention Center, The University of Texas MD Anderson Cancer Center, Houston, TX, USA

Kristin Simar, APN Advanced Practice Nurse, Department of Lymphoma and Myeloma, The University of Texas MD Anderson Cancer Center, Houston, TX, USA

Karen Stolar, MS, FNP-BC, AOCN Advanced Practice Nurse, Department of Stem Cell Transplantation and Cellular Therapy, The University of Texas MD Anderson Cancer Center, Houston, TX, USA

Charlotte C. Sun, DrPH, MPH Associate Professor, Department of Gynecologic Oncology and Reproductive Medicine, The University of Texas MD Anderson Cancer Center, Houston, TX, USA

Shannon N. Westin, MD, MPH Assistant Professor, Department of Gynecologic Oncology and Reproductive Medicine, The University of Texas MD Anderson Cancer Center, Houston, TX, USA

Frances Zandstra, RN Executive Director, Office of Cancer Survivorship, The University of Texas MD Anderson Cancer Center, Houston, TX, USA

Chapter 1
Introduction

Maria Alma Rodriguez

The latter part of the twentieth century brought forth many new discoveries and innovations in cancer therapeutics, diagnostics, and prevention that significantly improved the management of cancer. Together, these new strategies for treatment, detection, and prevention of cancer have led to a progressive decline in cancer-related mortality over the past three decades. This has in turn led to an increasing number of individuals who have completed their cancer treatment and are considered long-term survivors. The number of cancer survivors in the United States is now estimated to be nearly 13 million (approximately 4% of the population), and the number is continually growing.

In 2006, the Institute of Medicine published a report entitled *From Cancer Patient to Cancer Survivor: Lost in Transition* (Hewitt et al. 2006). This report revealed that once patients had completed treatment for their malignancy and had become long-term survivors, the quality and oversight of their health care radically diminished. In a sense, they were lost in the shuffle of transitioning from one clinical provider to another. To resolve this problem, the report called for a national movement, among both those who deliver cancer care to patients and those who set national policy, to increase access to care for cancer survivors, facilitate cancer survivors' transition to community physicians, and increase research funding to address the health concerns of cancer survivors. Five of the report's ten recommendations, with specific strategic areas of focus, were addressed to cancer care providers:

1. Increase awareness and delivery of survivorship care.
2. Provide a survivorship care plan upon completion of treatment (i.e., a detailed treatment summary and follow-up plan).
3. Practice evidence-based medicine (i.e., apply evidence when available or seek evidence when none is available).
4. Develop and monitor quality-of-care measures.
5. Design educational programs for health care providers to address the health care needs of survivors.

L.E. Foxhall, M.A. Rodriguez (eds.), *Advances in Cancer Survivorship Management*, MD Anderson Cancer Care Series, DOI 10.1007/978-1-4939-0986-5_1,

The remaining five recommendations were addressed to law-making bodies of government and research agencies (i.e., National Cancer Institute and Agency for Healthcare Research and Quality):

6. Eliminate employment discrimination against cancer survivors.
7. Ensure that cancer survivors have access to affordable and adequate insurance.
8. Support the Centers for Disease Control and Prevention comprehensive cancer control plans for survivors.
9. Support demonstration projects for survivorship care.
10. Increase funding for survivorship research.

In response to this report, our institution created a task force in 2006 to perform an internal analysis of what we were doing at that time for survivor care planning. At the recommendation of the task force, a steering committee was created, charged with developing a strategic plan to implement a comprehensive survivorship program encompassing clinical, research, educational, and outreach plans: in essence, to address the full spectrum of services related to cancer survivorship.

This book is one of the elements of our strategic plan for education of health care professionals, at multiple levels and of various disciplines. A more recently updated set of recommendations by a workgroup of the Institute of Medicine includes a call for survivorship care that is coordinated and team-based (Levit et al. 2013). In this book, we describe our multidisciplinary care models that align with this recommendation. We hope to share with you our experience as providers of oncology-centered care in a long-standing specialty facility. Over the past 70 years, our institution has served nearly 900,000 patients across the cancer care continuum. We hope to provide meaningful information to help you manage the care of patients who have lived with and through cancer treatment, and to help address another recommendation of the workgroup: to build a workforce with competence in survivorship care.

To help you navigate the information in the book, we have divided the book into five major sections. The first section is focused on *clinical care delivery*, including models of survivorship care and methods for integrating these models into community care.

The second section is *disease-focused*, with each chapter addressing indicated treatment(s) for specific malignant disorders and the overall consequences of those treatments. A common misconception among the general public is that cancer is a single disease; in fact, biologically, each malignancy category is a unique illness. For example, acute leukemia of myeloid origin is not the same disease as acute leukemia of lymphoid origin. Over the past few decades we have learned a great deal about the complex biologic and genetic variations of each malignancy, which can lead to differences even within a common histologic diagnosis. For example, within the category of adenocarcinoma of the breast, further subcategories of breast adenocarcinoma are defined on the basis of unique genetic characteristics. Furthermore, the treatment for one subcategory of malignancy may differ from treatments for other malignancies fitting into different subcategories within the same overall category of malignancy. Hence, the downstream consequences or toxic effects of treatment are widely disparate depending on the specific disease type and its relevant treatment. This section will include clinical practice algorithms developed for specific disease categories. In addition to the printed versions in this book, the reader may access the full content of our algorithms online: http://www. mdanderson.org/education-and-research/resources-for-professionals/clinical-tools-and-resources/practice-algorithms/index.html.

The third section is devoted to *cancer prevention and early detection strategies*. Survivors of one malignancy unfortunately may be at risk for other malignancies, depending on a host of risk factors. This section of the book reviews the ways in which genetics and environment influence such risks, as well as current evidence for lifestyle changes that may decrease risks of malignancy and recommendations for cancer screening and early detection.

The fourth section is focused on *organs and systems*, with each chapter addressing complications of treatment that may occur in specific organs or systems. These chapters also discuss the ways in which certain illnesses or comorbid conditions can predispose the patient to toxic events related to treatment. The cardiovascular system, for example, is affected in various ways by different treatment modalities. In turn, illnesses of the cardiovascular system may limit or inhibit the use of certain therapeutic modalities for cancer. Some organ system concerns may be unique to young individuals. Fertility, for example, is very important in treatment planning and follow-up for patients who are in their reproductive years. Toxic events in the central nervous system, on the other hand, are more common and serious in elderly individuals who may be predisposed to them because of, for example, underlying hypertension or diabetes. This section is meant to be complementary to the second section, with a more detailed and focused description of toxic effects in each organ or system and the relationship between these toxic effects and other health conditions.

The fifth section is devoted to *psychosocial health and recovery*, as well as integrative medicine strategies for recovery of well-being. Survivors of cancer unfortunately suffer from not only physical side effects of their illness and treatment, but also emotional and spiritual traumas. In addition, survivors are at risk of losing their employment, health insurance, relationships, and social support networks. Divorce and unemployment are common downstream events in the lives of individuals who develop malignancies. The economic, social, and legal difficulties many patients face are addressed in this section.

As the lifespan of the population in the United States has lengthened, the number of individuals who develop malignancies has grown and will continue to grow. At the same time, cancer treatment strategies have become more successful, in turn leading to increased survival durations. Thus, the number of long-term cancer survivors is anticipated to increase as well. We therefore recognize that we must facilitate and participate actively in the transition of the cancer patient to community health care providers. One way to start this process is to share our experience with cancer care with others. We hope that this book will serve as an informational reference and resource for you in your practice, and that it will help you as you deliver care that addresses the physical and emotional health needs of cancer survivors.

Suggested Readings

Hewitt M, Greenfield S, Stovall E, eds. *From Cancer Patient to Cancer Survivor: Lost in Transition.* Washington, DC: Institute of Medicine and National Research Council of the National Academies (The National Academies Press); 2006

Levit L, Balogh E, Nass S, Gang PA, eds. Delivering high-quality cancer care: charting a new course for a system in crisis. Washington, DC: Institute of Medicine and National Research Council of the National Academics (The National Academics Press); 2013.

Part I
Clinical Care Delivery

Chapter 2
Models of Survivorship Care

Maria Alma Rodriguez and Frances Zandstra

Contents

L.E. Foxhall, M.A. Rodriguez (eds.), *Advances in Cancer Survivorship Management*,
MD Anderson Cancer Care Series, DOI 10.1007/978-1-4939-0986-5_2,
© The University of Texas M.D. Anderson Cancer Center 2015

Chapter Overview The official definition of a cancer survivor encompasses those experiencing the entire trajectory of cancer care, including diagnosis, treatment, and beyond treatment. For each of these three phases, survivors have different health care needs. A report issued in 2005 by the Institute of Medicine, entitled "From Cancer Patient to Cancer Survivor: Lost in Transition," brought to light the problems that many cancer survivors face once they are past the phase of cancer treatment. Survivors reported they struggled to find health care services and providers in their communities to address their persistent or late-emerging health problems that were secondary to their former cancer diagnosis or effects of treatment. This chapter will describe the process within our institution for developing a multidisciplinary care delivery model, as well as the components of care in the model. The domains of health care that address known and anticipated "after cancer" health care needs of survivors are as follows: surveillance for possible late recurrence of the primary cancer; screening and early detection, as well as prevention, of additional primary cancers; monitoring for and management of persistent or late effects of treatment; and psychosocial health. Communication between the primary oncology teams and community physicians is very important for continuity of care. It is recommended that a summary document be prepared as a care plan for each survivor, detailing the following: type of treatments received; residual and possible future late effects or complications; indicated evaluations for health maintenance; and cancer surveillance/screening.

Introduction: The Cancer Problem

The most current Surveillance Epidemiology and End Results (SEER) projections indicate high lifetime cancer risks for both men and women: 1 in 2 for men and 1 in 3 for women (Howlader et al. 2011). The malignancies for which both men and women are most at risk originate in organs influenced by sex hormones: prostrate carcinoma is the most common cancer in men and breast cancer is the most common cancer in women (Table 2.1). The second most common malignancy is lung cancer, followed by colorectal cancer, in both men and women. These four malignancies ("the big four") constitute the highest solid tumor burden in the US population. Among hematologic malignancies, lymphomas are the most common, ranking seventh in frequency for both men and women.

Why is cancer survivorship a big concern? Paradoxically, while the total number of cancer-related deaths has increased, so has the number of cancer survivors. A great deal of progress has been made in the treatment of malignant diseases. Among the big four cancers (prostrate, breast, colorectal, and lung carcinomas), the only disease for which significant survival progress has not been made is carcinoma of the lung and bronchus. For the other three malignancies, 5-year survival rates have been increasing since the 1970s (Table 2.2; American Cancer Society 2012).

Table 2.1 Cancers occurring most often in men and women in the United States in 2012[a]

Men (848,170 cases); cancer lifetime risk: 1 in 2		Women (790,740 cases); cancer lifetime risk: 1 in 3	
Cancer site	Percentage of cases	Cancer site	Percentage of cases
Prostate	29	Breast	29
Lung and bronchus	14	Lung and bronchus	14
Colon and rectum	9	Colon and rectum	9
Urinary bladder	7	Uterine corpus	6
Melanoma (skin)	5	Thyroid	5
Kidney and renal, pelvic	5	Melanoma (skin)	4
Non-Hodgkin lymphoma	4	Non-Hodgkin lymphoma	4
Leukemia	3	Kidney and renal, pelvic	3
Oral cavity	3	Ovary	3
Pancreas	3	Pancreas	3
All other sites	19	All other sites	23

Source: American Cancer Society (2012)
[a]Excludes basal and squamous cell skin cancers and in situ carcinomas except urinary bladder

Table 2.2 Five-year relative overall survival rates[a] (%) in the United States, 1975–2007

Site	1975–1977	1984–1986	1999–2007
All sites	50	54	68
Breast (women only)	75	79	90
Colon	52	59	66
Leukemia	35	42	55
Lung and bronchus	13	13	16
Melanoma	82	87	93
Non-Hodgkin lymphoma	48	53	69
Ovary	37	40	45
Pancreas	3	3	6
Prostate	69	76	100
Rectum	49	57	69
Urinary bladder	74	78	81

Source: Howlader et al. (2011)
[a]Based on follow-up of patients through 2007

From Cancer Patient to Cancer Survivor

The SEER survival data show that among long-term cancer survivors (those living 5 years or longer beyond the date of their cancer diagnosis), 60% are older than 64 years and approximately 40% are in the working adult age bracket (20–64 years), or those in their productive years of life who are concerned about maintaining employment. It is projected that within the next 40 years the population of long-term cancer survivors aged 65 years or older will double compared with today's numbers. This is very important because a higher frequency of concurrent illness occurs among survivors aged 65 years or older than among other age groups, and this can significantly influence both the management of cancer and the long-term complications of treatment. Therefore, managing the concurrent health problems of cancer patients and survivors is equally as important as managing the cancer itself.

Patients who reach long-term survivorship status can be well and reintegrate into a normal life. Unfortunately, many cancer survivors do not recover their health and do not receive adequate health care. The Institute of Medicine published a comprehensive assessment of the status of cancer survivors in the United States in 2005. This assessment noted that a significant proportion of survivors suffered from chronic, long-term physical, social, or emotional distress. The study, entitled *From Cancer Patient to Cancer Survivor: Lost in Transition*, found that a critical issue for many patients was limited access to health care and lack of coordination of their health care once the cancer treatment and intermediate surveillance was concluded (Hewitt et al. 2006). The study made several recommendations for health care providers, as well as for policy-makers and government bodies, to improve the care of survivors. A more recent updated report emphasizes ten additional recommendations (Levit et al. 2013). One of these recommendations is that care must be coordinated and integrate multidisciplinary expertise. At our own institution, we have developed a multidisciplinary care delivery model that incorporates the elements of care outlined in this chapter.

Surviving Cancer

The development of chemotherapeutic regimens as primary or adjunctive treatment for various cancers evolved rapidly in the 1960s and 1970s, as did the application and awareness of early cancer screening. In 1986, the founders of National Coalition for Cancer Survivorship set out to establish an organization that would change the phrase "cancer victim" to "cancer survivor." To this end, the National Coalition for Cancer Survivorship crafted the definition of a survivor: from the time of diagnosis and for the balance of life. By the early 1990s, there was evidence of a sustained increase in the number of persons diagnosed with cancer who were living 5 years or longer beyond their diagnosis (Fig. 2.1). In 1996, the National Cancer Institute established an Office of Cancer Survivorship (OCS) in response to this trend, as well as in response to the concern that knowledge about the health of cancer survivors and the long-term effects of cancer treatment was significantly lacking. The OCS's first challenge was answering the question: who is a cancer survivor? The OCS adapted the National Coalition for Cancer Survivorship's definition of a survivor: "An individual is considered a cancer survivor from the time of diagnosis through the balance of his or her life" (National Cancer Institute 2012). OCS also expanded that definition to include the family and primary caregivers of the patient, because they all are influenced by the experience of cancer. Given the OCS's very broad definition of who is a cancer survivor, when we speak of survivors' health care needs we are speaking of a large and changing landscape; the cancer survivor's journey today can cover a long chronologic trajectory.

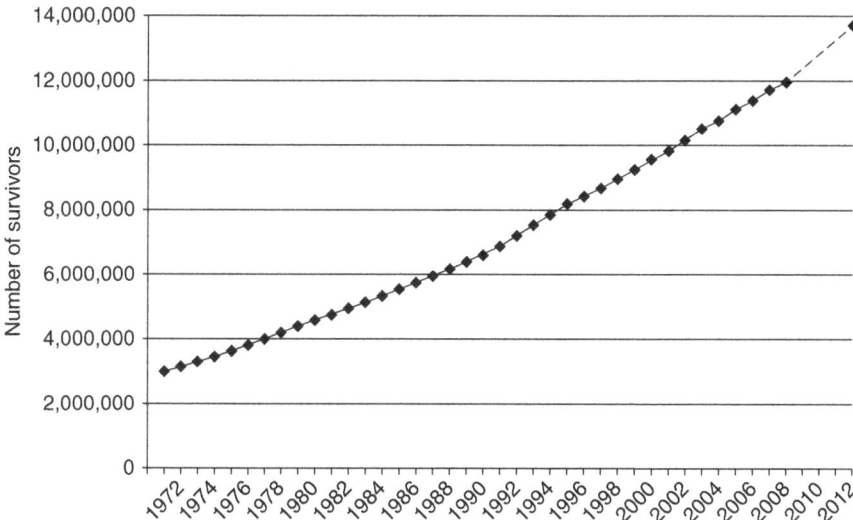

Fig. 2.1 Estimated number of cancer survivors in the United States between 1971 and 2012 (Source: American Cancer Society 2012)

Phases of Survivorship

The health care needs of cancer survivors, then, do not remain the same in later phases of survivorship as they were in the early phases of survivorship. The concept of "seasons of survival" was described in 1985 by Fitzhugh Mullan in an article in which he described his personal experience as a physician and a cancer survivor (Mullan 1985). Dr. Mullan described three principally different cancer survival phases, distinct from each other both on an experiential level and from a clinical perspective.

The *acute phase* begins with the diagnosis of cancer and includes testing for and treatment of the malignancy. Clinical care at this point is principally oncologic (i.e., administered by surgical, radiation, and medical oncologists), with a focus on eradication of the malignancy and management of any acute complications of treatment. From the patient's perspective, the primary experience is one of illness, treatment side effects, anxiety about the treatment, and fear of the cancer, as well as hope of reaching a remission.

The *intermediate phase* of survivorship begins upon reaching remission or concluding the primary treatment. This phase could include maintenance treatment or consolidation therapies for some patients. For example, in some stages of Hodgkin lymphoma, a primary treatment with chemotherapy could be followed by a course of radiation. Another example is breast cancer, which in many cases requires primary treatment with a combination of chemotherapy, radiation, and surgery, followed by hormonal maintenance for several years. In the intermediate phase of survivorship, the primary focus is watchful monitoring with examinations and appropriate studies to determine whether an early relapse will occur. Patients often experience anxiety and fear of recurrence, and recovery from the acute phase of treatment may be prolonged.

The *long-term phase* of survivorship, according to Dr. Mullan, begins when the period of highest risk for recurrence of the disease has passed and patients are considered well from that episode of cancer. The focus of clinical care in long-term survivorship should turn to maintenance of health, management of latent complications of the cancer treatment, reduction of risks of second malignancies, and cancer screening as appropriate. Since 1985, however, a new category of long-term survivorship has also emerged, in which patients live with chronic active cancer in a smoldering phase or with intermittent periods of remission broken by expected continual relapses that may need to be treated repeatedly. In today's reality, these patients are also long-term survivors. The goals of clinical care for these patients are the same as for cancer-free survivors, but in addition they must maintain very close surveillance and undergo intermittent treatment for their primary cancer as appropriate, repeating their trajectory through the earlier phases of survivorship at intermittent times.

Medical and psychosocial concerns therefore differ in each phase of survivorship, because patients' experiences and medical management objectives differ in each phase. The acute phase is obviously focused on effective cancer treatment and medical management of the side effects of the treatment, whether physical or psychological or both. In the intermediate phase, the principal concerns are monitoring for disease recurrence, allowing the patient to rehabilitate and recover from side effects, and managing fear and anxiety about recurrence. In the long-term phase, the main concerns are monitoring for long-term side effects of treatment and prevention and early diagnosis of possible subsequent malignancies. During the long-term phase, patients face issues of social and psychological health, reassessment of relationships, and spiritual and self-image crises. Equally important are pragmatic concerns about the economic consequences of survivorship. Employment discrimination is a reality for some cancer survivors, as is loss of health insurance. Cancer as a precondition excludes some patients from coverage or may exclude them from subsequent insurance coverage, especially if they change employment. These are serious and real concerns that will hopefully be addressed in the future by the newly formulated health care law.

The Uniqueness of Survivors

The most common cancer diagnoses among long-term survivors are breast, prostate, and colorectal cancer, followed by gynecologic malignancies and hematologic cancers. The groups of survivors affected by each of these diseases are distinct in terms of their medical care needs and the consequences of their treatment. These diseases require different therapeutic approaches: different possible surgical interventions, different possible radiation port sites and doses, and very different families of chemotherapeutic agents that in turn have different side effects. In addition, inherent biological differences within each of these malignancies may influence the risk of late recurrences or other second malignancies. Lastly, the anticipated or potential side effects in both the short and the long term are unique to each initial presentation by stage and organ site within each disease category. Therefore, although some health concerns can be generalized to apply to all long-term survivors, each survivor's diagnosis and treatment combination results in specific long-term potential risks and complications.

Survivor Risk Stratification

We conducted a survey of the oncology specialists in our institution (surgical, radiation, and medical oncologists) and asked them to describe the health care services that their long-term survivor patients would need. The consensus was that, on the basis of the factors described above that make different groups unique, not all survivors need the same level of care because they are not all at the same risk of relapse or secondary consequences of their treatment. The 3-tiered model of risk stratification that was proposed is simple, based on broad treatment risk categories and inherent cancer recurrence risks.

Tier 1

These patients have a very low risk of complications from their treatment and a low risk of relapse. This category includes patients presenting with localized malignancies that may require only surgical resection that results in minimal secondary physiologic deformities, and these patients have a high probability of cure from that intervention (for example, patients with localized noninvasive colorectal adenocarcinomas that require only localized bowel resection).

Tier 2

This category includes patients whose malignancies must be treated intensively with multimodal therapy to achieve a favorable outcome. These patients are often exposed to radiation or chemotherapy in addition to surgery. They may experience significant organ- or system-specific complications during treatment or may be at risk for second late malignancies, latent specific organ dysfunction, or other unknown consequences that may remain a concern for the rest of their lives. Tier 2 patients constitute a large group of individuals (the majority of the long-term survivors at our institution, for example, are in this risk group).

Tier 3

Patients in this category have a malignancy with a high risk of relapse or have chronic cancer. They may have active indolent or controlled disease or they may undergo dose-intense treatment, such as a stem cell transplantation or other uniquely toxic therapy, that has known or expected long-term active secondary negative effects.

Stratification of Health Care Needs on the Basis of Risk

The components of health care needed by persons who have survived cancer are therefore quite varied in their complexity, cutting across various specialties and encompassing several domains. The primary concern for survivors when they have their yearly examination is whether their primary cancer has recurred. This requires surveillance studies and careful physical examination. Secondly, survivors are at risk for and fear developing other cancers. Early cancer screening, as appropriate for their age, prior diagnoses, and other risk factors, is therefore a second important component of their care. An additional health care need is cancer prevention and counseling for lifestyle changes to prevent cancer, as well as risk assessment in certain populations for whom genetic counseling may be appropriate. Side effect management, including health maintenance and observation of vital organ function, is important particularly for those who may have already suffered from toxic effects in vital organs or are vulnerable to specific latent toxicities related to the treatment they received. Lastly, quality of life and social health issues are important to address to help the patients maintain healthy relationships with their families, communities, and employers, and to help restore functionality in their lives.

However, the categories of medical care and psychosocial support services that long-term survivors may need can also be stratified by the risk categories noted above. The continuum of multidisciplinary care according to risk tiers is diagrammed in Fig. 2.2 and can be summarized as follows.

Tier 1 Patients

Care should focus on cancer prevention and, when appropriate, psychosocial support. Patients may be anxious about the possibility of getting a second cancer, which can be addressed by encouragement to maintain a healthy lifestyle and conscientiously follow the recommended cancer screening guidelines.

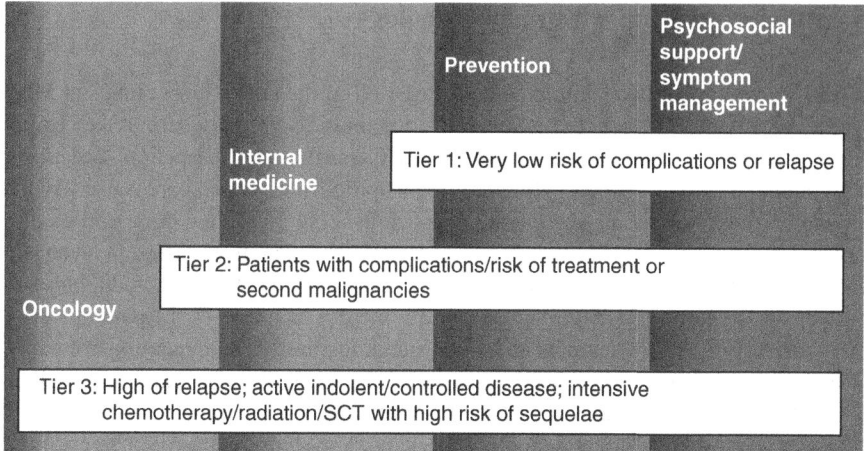

Fig. 2.2 Continuum of care for each risk tier (*SCT* indicates stem cell transplantation)

Tier 2 Patients

Patients may require support across the full spectrum of health care, including psychosocial support, if they suffer from chronic fatigue or ongoing organ dysfunction secondary to treatment toxicity. These patients may also require support from internists or other specialists for treatment-related late or persistent side effects; cancer prevention and screening; management of comorbid conditions to ameliorate risks of organ dysfunction; and, in many cases, ongoing oncologic surveillance because of the long-term risk of secondary malignancies.

Tier 3 Patients

For the rest of their lives, patients in this category need to be monitored for recurrence or new malignancies, as well as for persistent or latent consequences of the treatment itself. These patients remain under the care of their oncologist but also require the care of an internist to monitor their overall health and manage complications. In addition, cancer prevention, secondary cancer screening, and psychosocial support remain important and necessary throughout the rest of their lives.

A Model of Multidisciplinary Oncology

In 1997, a new model was implemented across all of the ambulatory clinics at MD Anderson, intended to deliver on-site, real-time multidisciplinary care. A key principle of the multidisciplinary care centers (MCCs) is that they are patient-centered, tailored to the patient's specific illness. A team approach to patient care is used, with on-site participation by all key oncology specialists (surgical, radiation, and medical oncologists), and a partnership is formed within the team from different levels of providers, including physicians, mid-level providers, nurses, trainees, and administrative support staff. These individuals are all integral members of the patient's primary team (Fig. 2.3). Treatment planning integrates the recommendations of each of the essential treatment specialist groups. Furthermore, decisions are made at the point of service, as the patient comes to the clinic.

There are several benefits with this care delivery system. First, expertise encompassing all of the major oncologic specialties is focused around a specific disease or disease category. Second, having all specialists centrally located in one site decreases the time and energy that patients previously spent coordinating appointments in various centers. Third, timely on-site interaction, discussion, and planning of care among the clinicians can expedite the initiation of appropriate therapy. The proximity of all of the necessary specialists also facilitates collaboration in clinical research protocols across the specialties. Finally, the patients have a "home" they identify as their resource base.

Each MCC also integrates care from specialists in supportive care disciplines, such as social services, patient advocacy, and nutrition. In addition, MCCs have access to and coordinate consultations as needed with specialists in areas that reside outside of the MCC's disease focus, such as physical medicine and rehabilitation and diagnostic services. Within each of these MCCs, we integrate not only clinical service, but also research programs, both clinical and translational, that require the coordination and participation of specialists in multiple disciplines. In addition,

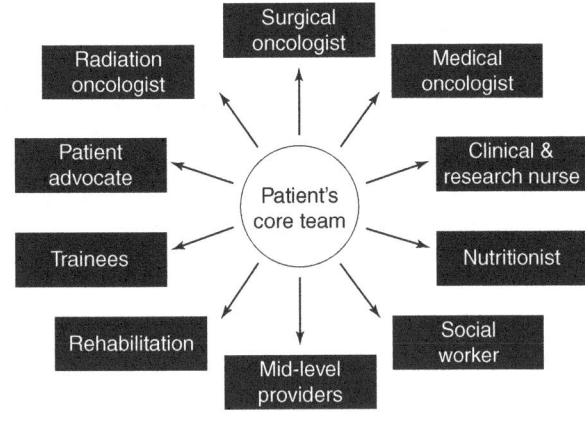

Fig. 2.3 Multidisciplinary care center model used at MD Anderson

medical fellows, residents, and other clinical trainees such as physician assistant students and residents rotate through the MCCs to learn about the management of specific malignant disorders in that setting. Hence, this model also serves as a focused experience and teaching resource for clinical trainees.

The MCC model encompasses multiple levels of service and patient care objectives. It has served very well, in our experience, to meet the needs of cancer care planning during the acute and intermediate phases of survivorship. We have applied this model across all of the major malignancy categories. For example, the oncologic care of all patients with breast cancer resides in one location, the Nellie B. Connally Breast Center. Similarly, the Leukemia Center has a specific disease focus, and all patients undergoing treatment for leukemia are cared for in this center.

Given the success of the MCC model for care delivery during the first two stages of survivorship, we have chosen to extend the application of this model into long-term survivorship. However, the unique clinical needs of long-term survivors are not necessarily focused on oncologic care, but rather on reintegration to wellness. The patient's clinical team therefore changes from principal oncologic specialists (surgeons, radiation oncologists, and medical oncologists) to specialists in cancer prevention, psychosocial issues, and internal medicine, with the continued engagement of oncologists as appropriate depending on the risk tier level of the patient.

Multidisciplinary Survivorship Care

We have launched a pilot program (Fig. 2.4), similar to the MCCs, to test models of multidisciplinary long-term survivor care, which are specific to each malignancy. We designed a process road map to define the scope of the project and defined basic core principles of the project.

The first principle is that survivorship requires tiers of care based on the tiered-risk model described above. The second principle is that the amount of time between diagnosis and long-term survivor status varies by disease type, risk of recurrence, treatment duration, and surveillance guidelines. Although we acknowledge that the endpoint of 5 years of survival beyond the cancer diagnosis (used in the SEER database) is very valid, some patients may be appropriately transitioned to the long-term survivor clinic in less than 5 years if their risk of recurrence is low. Determination of the tiers of care and appropriate time to transition to long-term survivor care for each disease must be defined by the disease experts (i.e., the clinicians in each MCC) who are most qualified to identify the risk factors that are relevant to the disease they treat. A third principle is that an adequate infrastructure to deliver care must be provided, and this needs to be based on metrics to better understand practical logistic limitations and the populations being served. Lastly, a fourth key principle is that the integration of research into the framework of long-term survivor care is as important for survivorship care as it is for acute cancer care.

Fig. 2.4 Important aspects of the multidisciplinary survivorship care model used at MD Anderson (*IS* indicates information services)

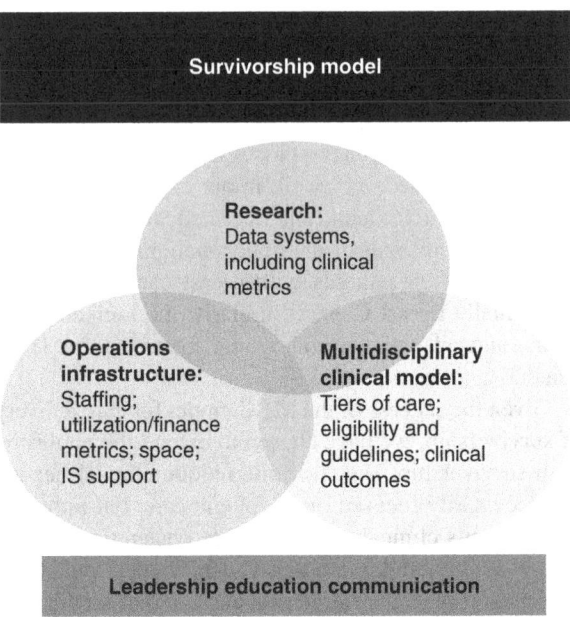

Process of Team Development

The process of developing each pilot clinic began with engagement of the clinical leadership of each MCC. A steering team was formed that included leaders from the corresponding MCC, and these steering teams led the clinical development process. Each steering team first defined criteria of eligibility for patients to transition to the long-term survivorship clinic. To assist the clinicians in this process, we performed an extensive literature review of late effects specific to that disease and its treatment, so that final recommendations were evidence-based as much as possible. The recommendations for care were outlined in clinical practice algorithms, which were standardized across all diseases to address four key domains or categories of care: (1) surveillance of the primary malignancy, (2) cancer prevention and early screening, (3) management of secondary effects of treatment, and (4) psychosocial functioning. For each disease category, however, the content within these domains varied as appropriate to that disease. The algorithm framework is illustrated in Fig. 2.5. The algorithms that appear at the end of the chapters throughout this book follow this general framework.

Each team identified its own multidisciplinary partners. For example, in the pilot Gynecologic Oncology Survivorship Clinic, sex counselors and bone health experts were deemed necessary team members. The multidisciplinary partners then worked together to design the practice algorithms and a transitional plan to address health care needs (which we called a "passport"; see below), as well as patient educational materials relevant to their own disease discipline. Although these processes occurred

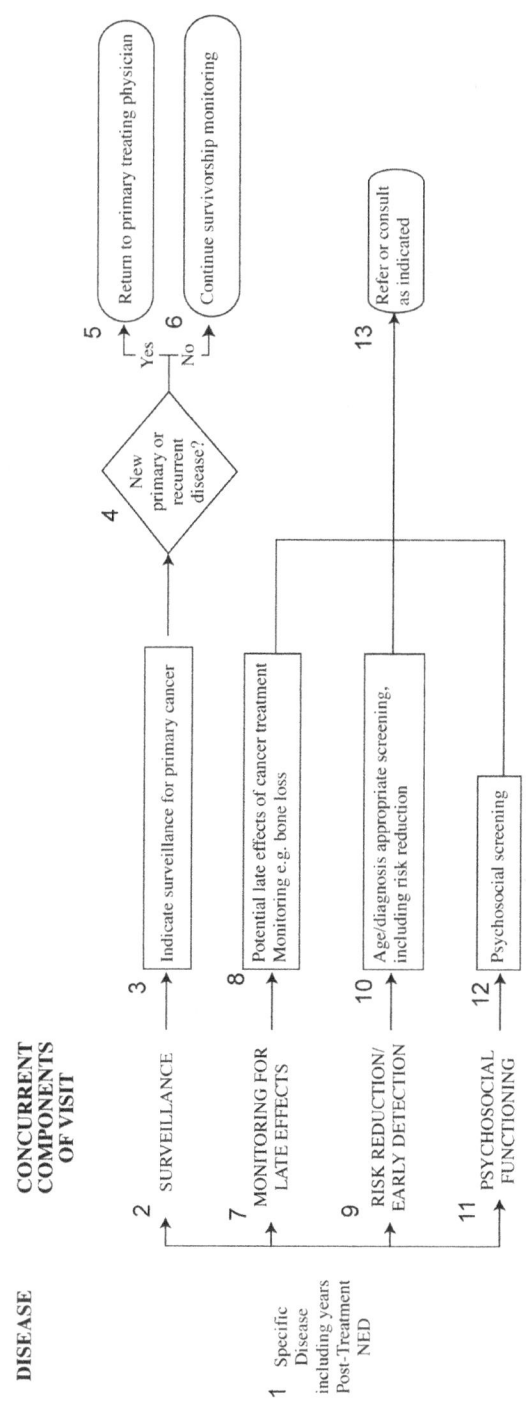

Fig. 2.5 Survivorship clinical practice algorithm standardized template (algorithms for specific malignancies are available online; see Suggested Readings)

in tandem, or in close sequence, a significant amount of time and dedicated support staff was required to help the team stay on task and moving toward the goal and to maintain engagement of the clinicians.

Patients' Point of View

We received support for the overall concept of multidisciplinary care from patients through a series of surveys and focus groups conducted at the beginning of the process. Patients stated that they wanted to have their oncologists direct their survivorship care. However, if the patients' oncologists considered them well enough to go to the survivorship clinic, they were willing to be transitioned to other providers as long as this care remained close to the oncologist or was in some way linked to the primary MCC. The patients did not want the oncologists to lose track of information pertinent to their care.

Patients also told us that they were delighted to have a single place to go to address their side effects of treatment and cancer surveillance and early detection tests at the same time, because many of them did not have adequate and consistent cancer screening and testing available in their communities. Patients who lived far from our institution (defined as those living more than approximately 200 miles away) told us they still wanted us to direct their long-term survivorship care by advising their community physicians about appropriate follow-up evaluations. This feedback aligned with our design of the "passport" document.

Passport Plan for Health

Some patients stated that they would feel abandoned if they were denied long-term follow-up at our facility, whereas others felt that the burden of travel was too much for them to continue coming to our institution for life. Physicians in the community told us that they also feel frustrated if they cannot get timely support or advice on management of patients who have survived cancer. Addressing the expectations of both the patients and the primary care providers is therefore a challenge, and we acknowledged the need to create possible solutions to the problem as the population of survivors grows larger. The Passport Plan for Health document was designed to be one such solution (Fig. 2.6). It is a summary of each individual patient's cancer treatment history, and it includes known and anticipated complications that the patient might experience. The document is HIPAA compliant; patients and their primary care physicians at this time can access this information through a password-protected website.

The Passport Plan for Health also lists for the community physician recommendations for testing and possible consultations that we consider indicated.

MD Anderson Cancer Center

Passport Plan for Health: Breast Cancer

Date Printed: _____
Pt Name: _____
MRN: _____

Healthcare Provider: _____

Allergies:

Cancer Diagnosis: _____ Stage: Left Breast: _____ Right Breast: _____

Histology - Left: _____ Right: _____

Estrogen Receptor: _____ Progesterone Receptor: _____ Her2/neu: _____

Positive genetic findings: _____

Additional Cancer Diagnosis

Past medical history:

CANCER TREATMENT HISTORY:

Surgery   ☐ Yes (indicate date, site and procedure)   ☐ No

Year	Procedure	Site
	Final breast surgery:	
	Final axillary surgery:	
	Breast reconstruction:	
	Other:	

Chemotherapy   ☐ Yes (indicate date, site and procedure)   ☐ No

Drug Name	Cycles/Year	Current Medication	Year Completed

Radiation Therapy   ☐ Yes (indicate date, site and procedure)   ☐ No

Year Completed	Side	Site	Total Dose	Number of Fractions

MD Anderson Cancer Center

Passport Plan for Health: Breast Cancer

Allergies:

Late Effects of Treatment/Signs and Symptoms to Report	Active	Potential	Recommended Consults/Monitoring
	☐	☐	
	☐	☐	
	☐	☐	
	☐	☐	

Recommended surveillance/prevention

Diagnostic Tests / Procedures	Last Performed Year	Location	Counseled Recommendations	Future Date/Location Year	Location
Bone Density (Osteoporosis)					
Gyn Cervical Screening					
Colonoscopy					
Breast Exam; Mammogram					
Skin Exam					
Genetic Counseling					

General Preventive Health Care and Personal Health Behaviors Recommendations

General Recommendations	Specific Recommendations
See primary care provider at least once a year	
Maintain adult vaccinations (per CDC recommendations)	
Maintain a healthy weight through diet and exercise	
Maintain a tobacco-free lifestyle	
Limit alcohol intake	
Use sunscreen and limit time spent in sun	
If distressed, seek support	Review patient education handouts

Other Instructions/ Information:

For questions regarding this patient's care, please notify: _____

Signature/Credentials/ID Code: _____

Telephone: _____
Fax: _____

Fig. 2.6 Passport Plan for Health document template

Recommendations must be tailored to the patient's specific malignancy and treatment, including the risk tier. For tier 1 patients, prevention and cancer screening care can usually be done most conveniently in the patient's community. For tier 2 patients, on the other hand, we generally recommend continued follow-up at our institution, if at all possible, for monitoring the late consequences of treatment. If this is not feasible, the primary care physician can be advised on the appropriate monitoring indicated. Tier 3 patients, on the other hand, must continue to be monitored in our clinics.

Value in Care Delivery

Looming large in our future is health care reform, which purports to follow principles of value-based health care delivery. The concept of value-based health care delivery has been postulated by Michael Porter and Elizabeth Teisburg in their book, *Redefining Health Care: Creating Value-based Competition on Results* (2006). The premise is that compensation for health care is currently based on quantity (of tests or exams) but should be based on the value derived by the patients. Porter and Teisburg define value as health *outcomes* divided by the *cost* of delivering care. Hence if the outcomes of care delivery by system "A" are superior to those of system "B" but the costs are the same in both systems, then the value of system "A" is higher. Porter and Teisburg propose that to maximize value, care delivery must be organized around medical conditions. Medical conditions in turn are defined as interrelated circumstances that must be addressed in an integrated way by multiple specialists and units of service. Systems of care are designed to include all units that address the full cycle of that medical condition. This is intended to optimize the use of expertise for that medical condition in a timely and efficient process. Cancer is an example of a medical condition with a long cycle of care, from early detection to long-term survival.

The value-based model also identifies a *hierarchy of health care outcomes*, with the most important (first tier) outcomes being survival and recovery. In cancer care, recovery equates to complete remission. The second tier in the hierarchy of outcomes as it relates to cancer is time to recovery or return to normal activities, and the third tier is sustainability of health. In cancer care, we and others have focused on diagnosis, treatment, and surveillance for recurrence, and these three steps have always been the key delivery elements in the care models that we have built. However, we must acknowledge that beyond these steps lies long-term survivorship, and that patients will face other health problems besides cancer recurrence, including latent side effects of treatment and exacerbation of other health conditions. Sustainability of health is very important for the patients who have survived the acute treatment of their cancer and remain free of their primary cancer.

Survivorship Research

Research should also be an integral part of the cycle of cancer care delivery; research should optimize the efficiency of research efforts and serve all levels of the cancer cycle: prevention and early detection, treatment, surveillance, and survivorship. Epidemiology, genetics, molecular genetics, and clinical studies on treatment-related morbidities and the impact of comorbidities on outcomes are all important research topics that are relevant from cancer diagnosis to long-term survivorship (Fig. 2.7).

Because many curative strategies have been developed for childhood malignancies, the concept of monitoring pediatric cancer survivors for the long term has been in existence for several decades. As a result, there is a significant body of data on the long-term outcomes of childhood cancer therapies, and these data have led to significant changes in the treatment intervention phase of the cancer care cycle. For example, treatment protocols for childhood lymphoma and leukemia have evolved significantly toward elimination of radiation to prevent cognitive and neurologic developmental toxic effects, as well as musculoskeletal developmental toxic effects. Treatment regimens also have been progressively altered to prevent other late effects of treatment that influence normalcy and quality of life, such as sterility. A great deal of research has been done regarding fertility preservation or conservation

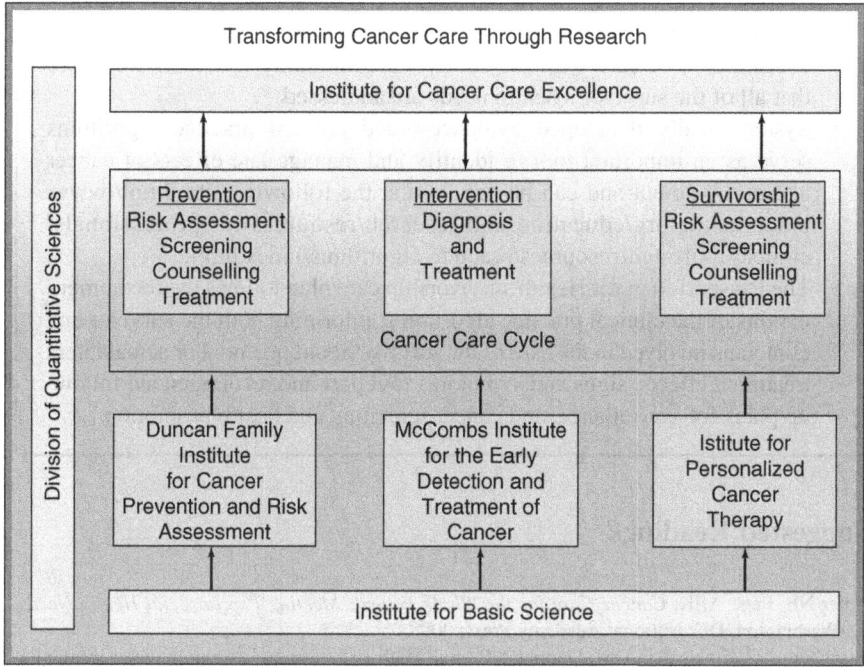

Fig. 2.7 Cancer research focus at MD Anderson

in pediatric cancer patients (Lee et al. 2006). More recently, attention has been focused on the early detection and prevention of breast cancer in girls and young women treated with radiation to the mediastinum, as well as the use of magnetic resonance imaging as a surveillance tool rather than standard mammography for secondary breast cancers (Aisenburg et al. 1997). Hence, significant changes have been made to the treatment strategies for childhood cancer as a consequence of long-term survivorship research. The same level of focus on long-term survivorship outcomes in adults has not yet taken place, but we hope to change that.

Key Practice Points

- Both cancer survivors whose highest risk of cancer recurrence has passed and those living with chronic active disease are considered to be in the long-term survivorship phase.
- Survivors' needs vary in terms of medical care and consequences of their treatment depending on the malignancy they have survived.
- The multidisciplinary care model is an effective way to meet the needs of cancer care planning for patients who have entered the long-term phase of survivorship.
- The essential components of care in the long-term phase of survivorship are surveillance of the primary malignancy, management of latent complications of cancer treatment, reduction of risks for second malignancies (including cancer screening), assessment of psychosocial functioning, and coordination of care with the survivor's community providers to ensure that all of the survivor's health needs are addressed.
- Systematically developed evidence-based clinical practice algorithms serve as an important tool to identify and manage late effects of cancer and its treatment and can be accessed at the following site: http://www.mdanderson.org/education-and-research/resources-for-professionals/clinical-tools-and-resources/practice-algorithms/index.html.
- The Passport Plan for Health survivorship care plan follows the recommendations of the clinical practice algorithms, informing both the survivor and clinicians involved in the care of the survivor about potential or actual latent treatment effects, signs and symptoms to report and recommended follow-up plans for surveillance, and cancer screening and health promotion.

Suggested Readings

Adler NE, Page AEK. *Cancer Care for the Whole Patient: Meeting Psychosocial Health Needs.* Washington, DC: National Academy Press; 2008.

Aisenberg AC, Finklestein DM, Doppke KP, et al. High-risk of breast carcinoma after irradiation of young women with Hodgkin's disease. *Cancer* 1997;79:1203–1210.

American Cancer Society. Cancer facts & figures 2012. http://www.cancer.org/research/cancer-factsfigures/cancerfactsfigures/cancer-facts-figures-2012. Accessed February 14, 2012.

Feeley TW, Fly H, Albright H, Walters R, Burke TW. A method for defining value in healthcare using cancer care as a model. *J Healthc Manage* 2010;55(6):399–411.

Hewitt ME, Greenfield S, Stovall E., eds. *From Cancer Patient to Cancer Survivor: Lost in Transition*. Washington, DC: National Academy Press; 2006.

Howlader N, Noone A, Krapcho M, et al., eds. SEER cancer statistics review, 1975–2008. Bethesda, MD: National Cancer Institute. http://seer.cancer.gov/csr/1975_2008. Based on November 2010 SEER data posted 2011. Accessed December 30, 2011.

Lee SJ, Schover LR, Partridge AH, et al. American Society of Clinical Oncology recommendations on fertility preservation in cancer patients. *J Clin Oncol* 2006;24(18):2917–2931.

Levit L, Balogh E, Nass S, Gang PA, eds. Delivering high-quality cancer care: charting a new course for a system in crisis. Washington, DC: Institute of Medicine and National Research Council of the National Academics (The National Academics Press); 2013.

Mullan F. Seasons of survival: reflections of a physician with cancer. *New Engl J Med* 1985;313:270–273.

National Cancer Institute Office of Cancer Survivorship. About cancer survivorship research: history. http://cancercontrol.cancer.gov/ocs/history.html. Updated July 17, 2011. Accessed November 21, 2012.

National Cancer Institute. Facing forward: life after cancer treatment. http://www.cancer.gov/cancertopics/coping/life-after-treatment. Published July 31, 2012. Accessed December 13, 2012.

Porter ME. A strategy for health care reform—toward a value-based system. *New Engl J Med* 2009;361:109–112.

Porter ME, Teisburg EO. *Redefining Health Care: Creating Value-Based Competition on Results*. Boston, MA: Harvard Business School Press; 2006.

The University of Texas MD Anderson Cancer Center. Clinical practice algorithms. http://www.mdanderson.org/education-and-research/resources-for-professionals/clinical-tools-and-resources/practice-algorithms/index.html. Accessed December 13, 2012.

Chapter 3
Community Care Integration

Lewis E. Foxhall

Contents

Chapter Overview The number of cancer survivors in the United States continues to grow and is approaching 14 million. Cancer survivorship care varies by disease type, but the primary components of care include surveillance for recurrence, screening for second primary cancers, and primary prevention involving lifestyle interventions and improving psychosocial functioning. The goal of survivorship care is to maximize disease-free survival while maintaining optimal quality of life. Optimal care can be provided by primary care physicians in addition to cancer specialists; however, delivery of high-quality care for cancer survivors can be hindered by poor coordination of care, limitations in knowledge and skills related to survivorship care, gaps in evidence-based recommendations for prevention and other areas of survivorship care beyond the first few years, and communication issues. Coordination of care and communication may be improved by the use of a "survivorship care plan" document that provides a concise summary of the patient's treatment and a plan for follow-up care. In addition, variations across ethnic groups in the impact of cancer during the survivorship phase of care have been documented in several areas of study, and cultural, social, and ethnic considerations are important factors in delivering optimal care to cancer survivors.

L.E. Foxhall, M.A. Rodriguez (eds.), *Advances in Cancer Survivorship Management*,
MD Anderson Cancer Care Series, DOI 10.1007/978-1-4939-0986-5_3,
© The University of Texas M.D. Anderson Cancer Center 2015

Number of Cancer Survivors Increasing

The number of cancer survivors has grown steadily from 3.0 million in 1971 to 13.7 million in 2012. As the US population ages and the major risk factors of tobacco exposure and obesity persist, the growth trend is expected to continue. In addition, the effectiveness of cancer treatment has improved dramatically as the products of research and better understanding of disease processes have broadened the armamentarium of oncologists. With improvements in treatment, prevention, and early detection, almost two-thirds of cancer patients are living 5 years or longer after diagnosis. Thus, the number of cancer survivors in primary care as well as in community-based oncology practices will continue to increase.

Despite the progress that has been made, many cancer survivors are not taking advantage of evidence-based strategies that can maximize the duration and quality of life after completion of active treatment. Several barriers to the delivery of high-quality care for cancer survivors were highlighted in the Institute of Medicine report, *From Cancer Patient to Cancer Survivor: Lost in Transition* (Committee on Cancer Survivorship 2005). These include poor coordination of care, limitations in knowledge and skills related to survivorship care, gaps in evidence-based recommendations for prevention and other areas of survivor care beyond the first few years, and challenges related to communication issues. Communication barriers center especially on management of handoffs between cancer treatment specialists and primary care physicians. To highlight this problem area, the Institute of Medicine report is subtitled *Lost in Transition*.

Gaining a thorough understanding of the history of the patient's cancer experience, working together as a coordinated medical team, sharing information among members of the team, and including the patient in a central way in the decision-making process are strategies that can promote the best outcomes for patients. Improving the clinical care of cancer survivors brings the promise of maximizing the benefits of cancer treatment and potentially gaining the longest possible survival duration after diagnosis while optimizing quality of life for each survivor.

Roles of Physicians and Other Health Professionals in Survivorship Care

The roles and responsibilities of physicians and other health care professionals during the patient's long-term survivorship phase, after active treatment is completed, may and often do change. The survivor population is heterogeneous in terms of risk of recurrence and potential complications from treatment. Patients who are free of any evidence of disease after the initial follow-up period and at low risk for recurrence can successfully receive care in the primary care setting alone. Some patients will experience persistent long-term side effects or eventually develop late-onset effects of treatment. However, many of these patients can also receive the majority of their care in the primary care setting alone or in collaboration with oncologists or other specialists. Those who are at high risk for recurrence, have persistent but stable disease, or have substantial treatment-related or other comorbidities should receive follow-up care in a center specializing in care for high-risk patients.

Long-term follow-up care of cancer survivors can be successfully delivered by oncology specialists or by primary care physicians. Several studies have demonstrated the interest and effectiveness of primary care physicians in this role (Earle 2006). Other studies showed no differences in outcome for patients with commonly occurring cancers whether they received care from primary care physicians or cancer specialists. However, primary care physicians have expressed concern about their limited level of training and a perceived lack of adequate office time related to survivorship care, and some have noted problems communicating with oncologists. In addition, oncologists find it difficult to relinquish care of patients with whom they have had long, nurturing relationships.

Multiple models of delivery of survivorship care services have been described and are being implemented (Committee on Cancer Survivorship 2005). Continued follow-up care by the oncology specialists that delivered the patient's initial treatment is common. Oncologists and patients have a high level of trust and familiarity that has made this approach desirable for many patients. Survivors have expressed expectations that oncologists have the best training and skills to provide surveillance for recurrence. Primary care physicians are also willing to take the lead in providing follow-up care and are cited by patients as being able to provide better screening for second primary cancers and delivery of primary preventive services than other types of physicians. However, some patients express concern about primary care physicians' expertise and about whether they have adequate time to address the full range of issues that may arise during follow-up care. This discordance may contribute to a failure in delivery of active follow-up care for cancer survivors. Patients may be hesitant to seek the additional services they need from another clinician. Further discordance is found between opinions of primary care physicians and oncologists concerning their respective knowledge, skills, and practices (Potosky et al. 2011).

A cancer survivor's medical needs may change as the clinical course evolves over time. Some patients will remain disease-free after treatment but others will develop recurrence of the initial cancer. A second primary cancer may be diagnosed and require treatment. The patient may struggle with persistent adverse effects of treatment or complications may develop some time after treatment and require additional management interventions. Psychosocial functioning can be impaired owing to the impact of the disease process on the patient or caregivers and family members. In these various scenarios, patient and physician expectations for survivorship care vary and may at times be discordant. Open discussion of the patient's concerns and the delivery of anticipatory guidance are important at the various junctures in the patient's cancer journey. Clear, proactive communication can result in better alignment of expectations and enhance the likelihood that the patient will receive recommended care in a patient-centered fashion. More research is needed in the techniques and different models of delivering survivorship care and in teaching effective communication skills related to patient preferences and cultural contexts.

Projected shortages in the medical workforce raise concern for the advancement of quality cancer survivorship care. Although the number of survivors is continuing to grow, concerns have also been voiced concerning the projected shortage of both oncologists and primary care physicians.

Risk Assessment and Risk Reduction

Risk assessment and personalized risk reduction interventions through primary and secondary prevention strategies are an important adjunct to surveillance for recurrence of disease in cancer survivors. In addition to implementing active behavioral interventions to reduce major risk factors, survivors must increase screening for second primary cancers because second primary cancers are a substantial proportion of all newly diagnosed cancers (Vogle 2006).

Cancer survivors more often make positive than negative health-related behavioral changes after completion of treatment. Young patients who have attained postsecondary education, have survived several years since the diagnosis, and have expressed spiritual well-being and fear of recurrence are most likely to act in a positive fashion (Hawkins et al. 2010). However, young patients who are young at diagnosis are also more likely to make negative behavioral changes. In addition, increased risk of negative behavioral change is associated with Hispanic origin, African-American origin, non-married status, and reduced self-perceived state of physical and emotional health (Hawkins et al. 2010).

Regardless of the type of clinician delivering the follow-up care, the primary and secondary preventive services must be delivered effectively and all clinicians should be involved in the patient's care. In addition, the patient should understand who is responsible for assuring that the patient is receiving the recommended preventive services. In addition to receiving information about the recommended surveillance measures for recurrent cancer, the patient should understand areas of health risk and be given anticipatory guidance regarding risk reduction strategies. Additional guidance should be given regarding management of long-term and late complications of treatment, as well as psychosocial functioning. Preventive or follow-up services are missed as a result of poor communication between multiple physicians who may have differing understandings of each other's roles (Earle and Neville 2004). Research is needed to elucidate the relationship between the clinical setting used and the optimal delivery of preventive services to and clinical outcomes of survivors.

Coordination of Care for Survivors

Coordination of medical service delivery among health care professionals and patients, their families, and caregivers is a critical component of providing optimal clinical preventive services to cancer survivors, as highlighted in the Institute of

Medicine report (Committee on Cancer Survivorship 2005). Conversely, fragmentation of care and lack of coordination lead to suboptimal quality of care (Earle and Neville 2004). Integration of care for cancer survivors into the practice of primary care physicians and coordination of care among primary care physicians, oncologists, and other specialty clinicians is a key aspect of successful delivery of preventive and treatment services for survivors. The transition from active treatment to survivorship is an important process that appears to benefit greatly from active coordination among service providers and clear communication between patients and health care professionals. Patients with cancer may be cared for by a variety of specialists during the active treatment phase of their disease. The primary care physician may also continue to see the patient during active treatment, but more frequently cancer specialists have the lead responsibility during this phase of the disease process.

Coordination of care and communication may be improved by the use of a "survivorship care plan" document that provides a concise summary of the course of the patient's disease and treatment and a plan for follow-up care, including surveillance and preventive interventions. This is an important recommendation from the Institute of Medicine survivorship report (Committee on Cancer Survivorship 2005). This care plan document is recommended to be used with each cancer survivor.

The survivorship care plan document is intended to serve as a summary of the patient's cancer experience that includes the treatments completed and any adverse effects encountered. Importantly, it should also describe a follow-up care plan that includes surveillance for recurrence of the primary cancer, screening for second primary cancers, preventive services, counseling and immunizations related to general risks to the patient's health, identification and management of long-term persistent adverse effects of the cancer or its treatment, and interventions to support psychosocial functioning. The document should also provide direction to the patient as to which clinician will deliver the various services and interventions needed. Communication between members of the health care team and a focus centered on the patient should lead to a better understanding of the services that are recommended, the schedule for delivery, and the source of care that will be provided.

The survivorship care plan is a resource that is needed but frequently missing from many patients' records. Both those who have provided active treatment and those who will provide long-term follow-up care should understand their respective roles in managing care for cancer survivors. The patient should also be involved in a proactive fashion and needs to understand the plan and the benefits of follow-up, as well as the roles of the health care team members involved in providing that care. Although little evidence currently suggests that regular use of this document will result in improved outcomes for survivors, the Institute of Medicine suggests that use of such a document has "face validity" and should be used until there is evidence to the contrary.

Several versions of care plans have been developed and placed in use, including web-based versions. Locating and abstracting the data necessary to complete a care summary and plan can be time-consuming, and these tasks are not usually covered by health insurance plans. Additionally, the time needed to explain the plan to survivors is not a covered benefit in most health care plans. This may be perceived as a burden by clinicians and serve as a barrier to use.

Communication Skills

Communication among health care professionals related to management of patients is a practice behavior that both primary care and specialty physicians think they do well. However, both primary care and specialty physicians have been shown to have opportunities for improvement in this practice (O'Malley and Reschovsky 2011). Clinicians demonstrate critical elements of communication, including careful listening, providing clear explanations, giving enough time to patients, and behaving respectfully only 60% of the time. Patients report unmet needs for cancer information across many areas of survivorship. In addition to treatment-related concerns, patients have reported information needs in the areas of health promotion, long-term treatment effects, and interpersonal and psychological problems. Communication skills, especially those targeting the most difficult management issues in survivorship, are critical tools for all clinicians. Addressing the difficult transitions of recurrence, diagnosis of a second primary cancer, and end-of-life care are often areas of communication that create anxiety and discomfort for clinicians as well as patients. Resources providing focused training in these areas are available and may be used to improve the quality of communication in these challenging situations. In addition, research regarding the effects of the quality of communication among the members of the medical team on the patient is needed.

Medical and nursing school curricula and postgraduate training traditionally have not included core knowledge elements related to cancer survivorship care that clinicians need. Although the core knowledge elements have been described, curricula delivering this knowledge have only recently been developed. Additionally, training on competencies important to optimal survivorship management may not have been provided through traditional graduate medical education programs in oncology or primary care. Continuing medical education programs for clinicians who have completed training only recently began to address issues in survivorship care. A substantial proportion of primary care physicians have expressed a need for more information on guidelines and decision aids and community resources for survivorship care. Appreciation has increased among cancer specialists and primary care physicians of the value of obtaining education related to clinical and supportive services. Although barriers exist, it is critical that clinicians begin to address attitudinal issues and knowledge gaps and improve their skills related to survivorship care delivery.

Understanding the patient's cancer treatment history, communicating with other physicians in the care team to develop a plan for follow-up care, and actively engaging the patient and caregivers may seem like a straightforward approach, but this is often not accomplished. Patients may feel confused about which steps to take to maintain optimal health and well-being, and health care professionals are responsible for helping them in this continuing phase of care. Some literature suggests that cancer survivors are at risk of not receiving even routine preventive services on par with the most vulnerable populations, including the elderly and those with one or more chronic condition (Earle and Neville 2004). Cancer survivors need particular attention to ensure that they receive recommended preventive services as well as management of other chronic conditions.

Cultural, Social, and Racial and Ethnic Considerations in Survivorship Care

Improved knowledge of the etiology and molecular biology of cancer has led to substantial improvements in the effectiveness of treatment. Reduced use of tobacco and increased use of early detection interventions have produced a decline in mortality rates of about 20% overall over the last 20 years. However, these declines in mortality rates have not been shared equally among all populations (Partridge 2011). Disparities in cancer-related outcomes related to sociodemographic and educational differences have been documented in national studies. Health inequities persist across substantial portions of the US population (Centers for Disease Control and Prevention 2011).

Disparities have also been demonstrated among cancer survivors. Cancer patients with a low socioeconomic status are diagnosed at later stages, are less likely to receive effective treatment, and have higher all-cause mortality rates than patients with a high socioeconomic status. This pattern has been demonstrated in patients with breast, colorectal, and prostate cancer. Limited access to screening and early detection among patients with low socioeconomic status, especially in those with breast and colorectal cancer, is a likely contributor to the diagnosis occurring at a later stage. Limited access to clinical preventive services in areas not related to cancer may also increase all-cause mortality rates. Lack of health insurance or inadequate insurance may hinder access to timely and effective treatment.

Delays in diagnosis and treatment vary somewhat by ethnic group. In patients with breast and cervical cancer, women of Hispanic origin were shown to experience delays in diagnosis more commonly than women of other origins, and African-American women were shown to have greater likelihood of experiencing delays in treatment than were white and Asian women. Significant proportions of cancer survivors find the cost of care to be a barrier and forgo medical and dental care, mental health care, and medications. More than two million US cancer survivors did not receive needed services because of costs, according to a study based on the National Health Interview Survey that was conducted between 2003 and 2006 (Weaver et al. 2010). Because the number of uninsured individuals has risen, this number may be higher today.

Cancer survivors generally are more likely to have fair to poor health, limited functioning, psychological distress, and high body mass indexes than the general population. No differences have been observed between cancer survivors and the general population related to physical activity, tobacco use, or alcohol use. However, estimates of health status and the presence of risk factors related to behaviors among cancer survivors vary across ethnic groups. For example, African-American survivors are more likely to rate themselves as having fair or poor health status compared with white survivors. Clinicians should be aware of these disparities and consider interventions to address the adverse health behaviors in vulnerable survivor populations.

Opportunities to address health disparities are limited by current levels of participation in survivorship programs by diverse and vulnerable populations. Tailoring interventions to diverse demographic and cultural groups is needed to improve delivery of survivorship care to these groups and to reduce outcome gaps in priority populations. Tobacco use, for example, remains a risk for cancer survivors. After declining for several years, the prevalence of cigarette smoking has stabilized. Smoking rates are higher among cancer survivors aged 40 years or older than among non-cancer populations of the same age. Smoking is more common in survivors of cervical cancer and melanoma than in survivors of other cancers. Smoking cessation programs targeting these groups should be prioritized.

Variations across ethnic groups in the impact of cancer during the survivorship phase of care have been documented in several areas of study. Colorectal cancer presents a greater burden to African-American compared with white populations in the United States. Whites are more likely to be screened for colorectal cancer than are African-Americans. Better understanding of the basis of these differences is needed to direct more effective interventions. In patients with cervical cancer, Hispanic women have better outcomes than white women, despite the fact that Hispanic women generally have lower socioeconomic status levels. Variations in comorbid conditions, social support, religion, and culture may affect this paradoxical relationship. African-American women with cervical cancer have higher mortality rates and appear to be treated with surgery less frequently than white and Hispanic women. A study of the prevalence of persistent symptoms in patients with breast cancer at least 3 months after completion of treatment showed that Hispanic women reported more symptoms than did white and African-American women. The most common symptoms were related to depression, treatment-related fatigue and myalgia, hormonal disturbances, and pain.

Information needs of minority survivors should be considered. Information regarding cancer support groups, long-term effects of treatment, and the experiences of other patients with cancer were the three most commonly reported needs in a study of Massachusetts cancer survivors. Survivors who were African-American, had low income levels, or had poor physical or mental health experienced greater difficulty obtaining needed information than did other groups. Similarly, findings from an analysis of HINTS data revealed that almost 40% of respondents rated the quality of information they received as fair or poor (Arora et al. 2008).

Cultural and linguistic barriers, as well as barriers related to access to care, have also been reported as creating information challenges for Hispanic women. These barriers appeared to be mitigated by a searching mechanism involving support networks (Sorensen et al. 2009). Another study of primarily Spanish-speaking survivors revealed concerns related to the risk of feeling worse if they had more information, along with a fatalistic attitude that compounded difficulties in finding information in their preferred language (Davis et al. 2009). A larger study identified information needs related to tests and treatment, health promotion, side effects of treatment, and symptoms and issues related to interpersonal and emotional problems. Survivors who were young at the time of diagnosis and minority patients experienced greater difficulty obtaining needed information than did other demographic groups. Most respondents indicated needs related to health maintenance (Beckjord et al. 2008). The survivorship care plan described above may be a useful tool to facilitate dissemination of this information to these cancer survivors.

Key Practice Points

- The goal of survivorship care is to maximize disease-free survival while maintaining optimal quality of life.
- Primary components of survivorship management include surveillance for recurrence, screening for second primary cancers, and primary prevention involving lifestyle interventions and improving psychosocial functioning.
- Several barriers to the delivery of high-quality care for cancer survivors include poor coordination of care, limitations in knowledge and skills related to survivorship care, gaps in evidence-based recommendations for prevention and other areas of survivorship care beyond the first few years, and communication issues.
- Coordination of care and communication may be improved by the use of treatment summary and survivorship care plan documents that provide a concise summary of the patient's treatment and a plan for follow-up care.
- Variations across ethnic groups in the impact of cancer during the survivorship phase of care have been documented in several areas of study. Cultural, social, and ethnic considerations are important factors in delivering optimal care to cancer survivors.

Suggested Readings

Arora NK, Bradford WH, Rimer BK, Viswanath K, Clayman M, Croyle RT. Frustrated and confused: the American public rates its cancer-related information-seeking experiences. *J Gen Intern Med* 2008;23:223–228.
Ashing-Giwa KT, Gonzalez P, Lim JW, et al. Diagnostic and therapeutic delays among a multiethnic sample of breast and cervical cancer survivors. *Cancer* 2010;116:3195–3204.

Beckjord EB, Arora NK, McLaughlin W, Oakley-Girvan I, Hamilton AS, Hesse BW. Health-related information needs in a large and diverse sample of adult cancer survivors: implications for cancer care. *J Cancer Surviv* 2008;2:179–189.

Bober SL, Recklitis CJ, Campbell EG, et al. Caring for cancer survivors: a survey of primary care physicians. *Cancer* 2009;115:4409–4418.

Byers TE, Wolf HJ, Bauer KR, et al. The impact of socioeconomic status on survival after cancer in the United States: findings from the National Program of Cancer Registries Patterns of Care Study. *Cancer* 2008;113:582–591.

Centers for Disease Control and Prevention. CDC Health Disparities and Inequalities Report—United States, 2011. *Morbidity and Mortality Weekly Report* 2011;60(Suppl):1–114.

Cheung WY, Neville BA, Cameron DB, Cook EF, Earle CC. Comparisons of patient and physician expectations for cancer survivorship care. *J Clin Oncol* 2009;27:2489–2495.

Cheung WY, Neville BA, Earle CC. Associations among cancer survivorship discussions, patient and physician expectations, and receipt of follow-up care regarding the care of cancer survivors. *J Clin Oncol* 2010;28:2577–2583.

Davis SW, Diaz-Mendez M, Garcia MT. Barriers to seeking cancer information among Spanish-speaking cancer survivors. *J Cancer Educ* 2009;24:167–171.

Del Giudice ME, Grunfeld E, Harvey BJ, Piliotis E, Verma S. Primary care physicians' views of routine follow-up care of cancer survivors. *J Clin Oncol* 2009;27:3338–3345.

Dimou A, Syrigos KN, Saif MW. Disparities in colorectal cancer in African-Americans vs whites: before and after diagnosis. *World J Gastroenterol* 2009;15:3734–3743.

Earle CC. Failing to plan is planning to fail: improving the quality of care with survivorship care plans. *J Clin Oncol* 2006;24:5112–5116.

Earle CC, Neville BA. Under use of necessary care among cancer survivors. *Cancer* 2004;101:1712–1719.

Eggly SS, Albrecht TL, Kelly K, Prigerson HG, Sheldon LK, Studts J. The role of the clinician in cancer clinical communication. *J Health Commun* 2009;14:66–75.

Fu OS, Crew KD, Jacobson JS, et al. Ethnicity and persistent symptom burden in breast cancer survivors. *J Cancer Surviv* 2009;3:241–250.

Greenfield DM, Absolom K, Eiser C, et al. Follow-up care for cancer survivors: the views of clinicians. *Br J Cancer* 2009;101:568–574.

Grunfeld E, Earle CC. The interface between primary and oncology specialty care: treatment through survivorship. *J Natl Cancer Inst Monogr* 2010;2010:25–30.

Grunfeld E, Mant D, Yudkin P, et al. Routine follow up of breast cancer in primary care: randomised trial. *BMJ* 1996;313:665–669.

Guidry JJ, Torrence W, Herbelin S. Closing the divide: diverse populations and cancer survivorship. *Cancer* 2005;104:2577–2583.

Hawkins NA, Smith T, Zhao L, Rodriguez J, Berkowitz Z, Stein KD. Health-related behavior change after cancer: results of the American Cancer Society's studies of cancer survivors (SCS). *J Cancer Surviv* 2010;4:20–32.

Hewitt M, Greenfield S, Stovall E, eds. From Cancer Patient to Cancer Survivor: Lost in Transition. Washington, DC: The National Academies Press; 2005.

Hewitt ME, Bamundo A, Day R, Harvey C. Perspectives on post-treatment cancer care: qualitative research with survivors, nurses, and physicians. *J Clin Oncol* 2007;25:2270–2273.

Hill-Kayser CE, Vachani C, Hampshire MK, Jacobs LA, Metz JM. An internet tool for creation of cancer survivorship care plans for survivors and health care providers: design, implementation, use and user satisfaction. *J Med Internet Res* 2009;11:e39.

Kantsiper M, Mcdonald EL, Geller G, Shockney L, Snyder C, Wolff AC. Transitioning to breast cancer survivorship: perspectives of patients, cancer specialists, and primary care providers. *J Intern Med* 2009;24:S459–S466.

Lewis RA, Neal RD, Williams NH, et al. Follow-up of cancer in primary care versus secondary care: systematic review. *Br J Gen Pract* 2009;59:e234–e247.

Mao JJ, Bowman MA, Stricker CT, et al. Delivery of survivorship care by primary care physicians: the perspective of breast cancer patients. *J Clin Oncol* 2009;27:933–938.

McInnes DK, Cleary PD, Stein KD, Ding L, Mehta CC, Ayanian JZ. Perceptions of cancer-related information among cancer survivors: a report from the American Cancer Society's Studies of Cancer Survivors. *Cancer* 2008;113:1471–1479.

Ok H, Marks R, Allegrante JP. Perceptions of health care provider communication activity among American cancer survivors and Adults Without Cancer Histories: an analysis of the 2003 Health Information Trends Survey (HINTS) Data. *J Health Commun* 2008;13:637–653.

O'Malley AS, Reschovsky JD. Referral and consultation communication between primary care and specialist physicians: finding common ground. *Arch Intern Med* 2011;171:56–65.

Partridge EE. Elimination of cancer disparities via organizational transformation and community-driven approaches. *CA Cancer J Clin* 2011;61:5–7.

Pollack LA, Adamache W, Ryerson AB, Eheman CR, Richardson LC. Care of long-term cancer survivors: physicians seen by Medicare enrollees surviving longer than 5 years. *Cancer* 2009;115:5284–5295.

Potosky AL, Han PK, Rowland J, et al. Differences between primary care physicians' and oncologists' knowledge, attitudes and practices. *J Gen Intern Med* 2011;26:1403–1410.

Schootman M, Deshpande AD, Pruitt SL, Aft R, Jeffe DB. National estimates of racial disparities in health status and behavioral risk factors among long-term cancer survivors and non-cancer controls. *Cancer Causes Control* 2010;21:1387–1395.

Shugarman LR, Sorbero ME, Tian H, Jain AK, Ashwood JS. An exploration of urban and rural differences in lung cancer survival among medicare beneficiaries. *Am J Public Health* 2008;98:1280–1287.

Siegel R. Cancer treatment and survivorship statistics, 2012. *CA Cancer J Clin* 2012;62:220–241.

Sorensen L, Gavier M, Helleso R. Latina breast cancer survivors informational needs: information partners. *Stud Health Technol Inform* 2009;146:727.

Tseng TS, Lin HY, Martin MY, Chen T, Partridge EE. Disparities in smoking and cessation status among cancer survivors and non-cancer individuals: a population-based study from National Health and Nutrition Examination Survey. *J Cancer Surviv* 2010;4:313–321.

Vogle VG. Identifying and screening patients at risk of second cancers. *Cancer Epidemiol Biomarkers Prev* 2006;15:2027–2032.

Weaver KE, Rowland JH, Bellizzi KM, Aziz NM. Forgoing medical care because of cost: assessing disparities in healthcare access among cancer survivors living in the United States. *Cancer* 2010;116:3493–3504.

Part II
Surveillance

Chapter 4
Adult Survivorship of Pediatric Cancers

Joann L. Ater

Contents

L.E. Foxhall, M.A. Rodriguez (eds.), *Advances in Cancer Survivorship Management*,
MD Anderson Cancer Care Series, DOI 10.1007/978-1-4939-0986-5_4,
© The University of Texas M.D. Anderson Cancer Center 2015

Chapter Overview Advances in therapies over the past four decades have improved overall survival for children and adolescents with cancer. Currently, 80% of patients diagnosed with cancer before the age of 20 years will survive beyond 5 years from diagnosis. Improved outcomes have resulted in a growing population of adult survivors of childhood cancer. Survival of childhood cancer comes at the price of lifelong chronic health issues in at least 62% of survivors. Radiation therapy, especially at a young age, carries the highest risk of late adverse outcomes. Radiation therapy has been associated with an increased risk for late premature mortality, subsequent neoplasms, obesity, and pulmonary, cardiac, and thyroid dysfunction, as well as an increased overall risk for chronic health conditions. Surgery and chemotherapy also increase the risk for chronic health conditions such as cardiomyopathy, osteoporosis, renal dysfunction, hearing loss, pulmonary dysfunction, and liver dysfunction. Although many survivors are satisfied with their quality of life, long-term follow-up for all adult survivors of childhood cancer is recommended to screen for second malignancies and late effects of therapy, make appropriate referrals for care of treatment-related health conditions, and provide psychosocial support and advice. This chapter will discuss the practices and recommendations for care of adult survivors in the Childhood Cancer Survivor Clinic at MD Anderson.

Introduction

Substantial improvements in treatment effectiveness for childhood cancers have resulted in cure or increased survival times for this population. Current estimates are that 80% of all patients diagnosed with cancer before the age of 20 years will be cured. As a consequence of both improved survival rates and increasing incidence of childhood cancer, the number of long-term survivors of childhood cancer in the United States is rapidly increasing. An estimated 320,000 or more childhood cancer survivors are living in the United States, and at least 75% of these survivors are now adults. Of these, 24% have survived more than 30 years (Mariotto et al. 2009).

These individuals are living long enough to demonstrate the human costs of cure (Diller et al. 2009). Short- and long-term side effects of treatment are common and have the potential to adversely affect the survivor's future physical, cognitive, and psychosocial health. Some problems, such as cognitive deficits from cranial radiation therapy, are apparent within 3–5 years after completion of therapy. However, other problems occur after long latencies. For example, the risk for anthracycline-induced cardiomyopathy can continue for decades after the treatment. In an epidemiologic study of childhood cancer survivors treated between the 1960s and early 1990s, investigators found that 62% of adult survivors of childhood cancer had at least one chronic health condition and 27% had a severe condition (grade 3 or 4) related to the cancer or treatment. The most common severe and life-threatening (grade 3 and 4) chronic health conditions identified in the national Childhood Cancer Survivor Study were as follows, in decreasing order of incidence: major joint replacement, congestive heart failure, second malignant neoplasm, cognitive dysfunction, coronary artery disease, cerebrovascular accident, renal failure, hearing loss, legal blindness or loss of an eye, and ovarian failure (Oeffinger et al. 2006).

There is a growing need to screen for and, if possible, prevent or decrease late-occurring problems such as heart disease, thyroid dysfunction, osteoporosis, and second malignancies to promote and maximize the physical and psychosocial health of long-term cancer survivors and their families. With this in mind, the Children's Oncology Group has developed evidence-based guidelines that recommend follow-up screening and care of childhood cancer survivors who are at risk for late effects (available at http://www.survivorshipguidelines.org). These guidelines for follow-up and surveillance for known late effects of cancer and cancer treatment are quite specific for the exact type of treatments and doses of chemotherapy and radiation that the patient received. They are primarily designed for use in specialized clinics for childhood cancer survivors. However, many adult survivors of childhood cancer, for various reasons, do not attend a specialized clinic for childhood cancer survivors, relying instead on their local physicians for care. This chapter will discuss the main principles of care of adult survivors of childhood cancer that are used in the Childhood Cancer Survivor Clinic at MD Anderson and highlight the most important issues for primary care physicians in the community.

Common Childhood Cancers

Childhood cancers comprise an extensive array of types of cancers, but most childhood cancers fall into categories of disease that are uncommon in adults. Carcinomas are rarely seen in children but can occur in adolescents. The most common types of childhood cancer are leukemia/lymphoma, embryonal cancers such as neuroblastoma, Ewing sarcoma, primitive neuroectodermal tumor/medulloblastoma, Wilms tumor of the kidney, rhabdomyosarcoma, and other central nervous system tumors. Among central nervous system tumors, the most common to appear in children include low-grade astrocytoma, medulloblastoma, and ependymoma; anaplastic astrocytoma and glioblastoma are more commonly seen in adults. Low-grade astrocytoma, medulloblastoma, and ependymoma have higher survival rates than other types of brain tumors; thus, the population of adult survivors of childhood brain tumors is increasing. Germ cell tumors also occur in children. The types of cancer associated with the highest numbers of current living survivors are brain tumors, acute lymphoblastic leukemia, germ cell tumors, and Hodgkin lymphoma. Among adult survivors of childhood cancer who were diagnosed before 1975, the most common sites of the original cancer are germ cells, soft tissue, kidneys, and bones (Mariotto et al. 2009).

Surveillance for Recurrence of Primary Cancer

Children and young adults are eligible for referral to the Childhood Cancer Survivor Clinic at MD Anderson when they are in remission or free of progressive cancer and 2 years have passed since treatment was completed. For most types of childhood cancer, disease surveillance tests are performed until 5 years have passed since treatment was completed. Each type of childhood cancer has specific recommendations for disease surveillance that are based on tumor location, most common site of metastatic disease, and natural history of the primary cancer. Any childhood cancer survivor referred back to the primary physician for continued surveillance should have detailed recommendations from the pediatric oncologist. If recommendations are not provided, it is appropriate to request this information. All patients in our Childhood Cancer Survivor Clinic who are transferred to the community are given a "Passport for Care" (Horowitz et al. 2009) that includes recommendations for both surveillance and monitoring for late effects of therapy. It is beyond the scope of this chapter to provide detailed recommendations for every type of childhood cancer. However, most survivor clinics do not recommend continued disease surveillance for more than 5 years after treatment completion because the risk of recurrence is low.

Some exceptions exist, however. For example, patients who had central nervous system tumors and patients who have already had one recurrence are at increased risk of recurrence beyond 5 years. In our clinic, patients with central nervous system tumors usually undergo routine magnetic resonance imaging of the brain for 10 years after treatment completion and then follow-up imaging for any symptoms or physical findings on a neurologic examination. This recommendation is based on a study of long-term follow-up of childhood brain tumor survivors who had survived for more than 5 years. In these patients, the risk of recurrence or death from the primary tumor continued for up to 30 years. Cumulative all-cause mortality rates were 13.5% at 15 years, 17.1% at 20 years, 21.5% at 25 years, and 25.8% at 30 years. Progression of primary disease was the cause of death in 61% of patients, followed by medical causes, including second neoplasm, in 9% (Armstrong et al. 2009).

Treatment-Related Late Effects

A complete list of late effects of treatment for childhood cancers is available at http://www.survivorshipguidelines.org and in an excellent publication (Dickerman 2007). The following treatment-related late effects are the most common ones that we encounter in the Childhood Cancer Survivor Clinic at MD Anderson.

Surgery

The late effects of cancer surgery are primarily related to the type of surgery and age of the patient at the time of the procedure. The following sections provide brief summaries of the most common surgery-related problems that we see in our adult survivors of childhood cancer.

Neurosurgery

The removal of a brain tumor can sometimes be curative. However, the consequences of neurological deficits that sometimes occur as a consequence of central nervous system surgery can be life-long. The seriousness of the deficit is related to the tumor location in the brain. Childhood brain tumors are most commonly found in the cerebellum and midline of the brain. Cerebellar surgery about 10% of the time can result in transient cerebellar mutism. The mutism usually resolves within 6 months, but patients often have learning and speech problems that are permanent. In addition, cranial nerve deficits caused by surgery can be permanent, resulting in such problems as hearing loss, visual deficit or field cut, or facial weakness. Tumors located in the region of the hypothalamus, such as juvenile pilocytic astrocytoma, germ cell tumors, and craniopharyngioma, are a particular problem. Both the tumor itself and the surgery can result in panhypopituitarism with hormonal deficiencies that can lead to life-threatening long-tern problems, even if hormone replacement therapy is available. For these patients, care by an endocrinologist is essential.

After a craniotomy, patients are also at risk for seizures or headaches. Both can be concerning as a sign of a recurrent or secondary tumor. However, more commonly the seizures are related to the scarring and gliosis at the site of the original surgery. Tumors in the cerebral hemispheres, especially the temporal and frontal lobes, are most often associated with seizures that can begin years after the surgery and other treatments are completed.

Orthopedic Surgery

Bone tumors such as osteosarcoma and Ewing sarcoma most commonly affect the long bones. Patients are treated with either amputation or limb-salvage surgery. Some patients who have undergone amputation and have a well-fitting prosthetic limb can function very well with little limitation to activity. Others experience chronic pain and even phantom pain for decades after the procedure. Limb-salvage surgery, although it spares the limb and is psychologically appealing to patients, requires follow-up by the orthopedic surgeon for years to ensure the integrity of internal hardware and reconstruction. For prepubescent children who have undergone laminectomy to remove a primary spinal cord tumor, kyphosis and scoliosis can occur when the children reach the adolescent growth spurt. Sometimes the curvature is severe enough that orthopedic intervention is necessary during the adolescent or young adult years.

Thoracic and Abdominal Surgery

In patients who undergo abdominal surgery, the risk of bowel obstruction caused by adhesions lasts for as long as 20 years or more after the surgery. Surgical intervention may also be responsible for surgical menopause or sterility. Secondary problems related to oophorectomy and the resulting premature menopause include bone loss, osteopenia and osteoporosis, and loss of fertility. In our clinic, screening for osteoporosis begins during adolescence for patients who have premature menopause.

Patients who have undergone splenectomy or spleen ablative therapy are at particular risk for infections. These patients should be placed on a prophylactic antibiotic, usually penicillin or erythromycin, during childhood. However, regardless of age, anyone who has undergone splenectomy should receive prompt medical attention and antibiotics for suspected bacterial febrile illnesses. Pneumococcal vaccine to prevent pneumococcal pneumonia should also be given routinely: the generally accepted immunization schedule for pneumococcal vaccine is every 5 years. Patients who do not have a functioning spleen should also be vaccinated against hepatitis B.

Chemotherapy

Long-term and late effects of chemotherapy include potential injury to the heart, liver, lungs, gonads, kidneys, and bone marrow. Some of these late effects are increased in prepubescent children who are still growing. Issues specific to this population are discussed here.

Heart

Cardiotoxicity is one of the most serious chronic complications of treatment for cancer, and children are particularly vulnerable. Thirty-year survivors of childhood cancer have been shown to have a 15 times higher rate of heart failure, a 10 times higher rate of other cardiovascular diseases, and a 9 times higher risk of stroke than age-matched sibling controls. Cardiotoxicity may manifest as cardiomyopathy, pericarditis, congestive heart failure, valvular heart disease, or premature coronary artery disease. The most common causes of cardiotoxicity are anthracycline-based chemotherapy and radiation therapy to the neck and mediastinum (Shankar et al. 2008). Anthracyclines are a class of antineoplastic agents that are highly efficacious in the treatment of pediatric and adult hematologic cancers, including acute myeloid leukemia, acute lymphoblastic leukemia, Hodgkin disease, and non-Hodgkin lymphoma, as well as solid tumors, sarcomas, and ovarian cancer. Among children in the United States who are survivors of childhood cancer, approximately 50% have received anthracyclines. Cumulative dose-related cardiac adverse effects may become apparent at the time that the first dose is administered, and clinical data suggest that deterioration of cardiac function is sustained throughout treatment and may continue for many years after treatment is completed. As patients age, other risk factors for cardiovascular disease, such as hypertension, hyperlipidemia, diabetes, and obesity, may contribute to the clinical progression of cardiac damage in adulthood.

Known risk factors for anthracycline-induced cardiac adverse effects include high cumulative doses of anthracycline, high anthracycline dose intensity, female sex, age younger than 5 years at diagnosis, radiation therapy, and combining anthracyclines with other cardiotoxic chemotherapy. Patients who were treated for lymphoma, Hodgkin lymphoma, sarcomas, or myeloid leukemia generally have the highest risk of cardiotoxicity because of the high doses of anthracyclines they usually receive, often accompanied by radiation. Higher than expected occurrences of cardiac adverse effects are observed in patients who receive anthracyclines in combination with new targeted drugs, such as the human epidermal growth factor receptor-2 antibody trastuzumab. These risk factors provide helpful monitoring guidelines, although they do not predict the risk of cardiac adverse effects for all patients.

Both early- and late-onset cardiac adverse effects are characterized by symptomatic or asymptomatic progressive decrease in left ventricular function, often resulting in congestive heart failure. This progressive cardiomyopathy can appear anywhere from 1 to 30 years or more after treatment is completed. The incidence of congestive heart failure has been shown to range from 10% to 26% in cancer patients treated with anthracyclines at doses below the current recommended limits. The incidence of subclinical cardiac adverse effects ranges from 0 to 57%, depending on how cardiac adverse effects are defined and the dose of anthracyclines used (Gianni et al. 2008; Shankar et al. 2008). Overt congestive heart failure can occur in asymptomatic patients who undergo stress such as childbirth.

In 2003, the Children's Oncology Group released risk-based, exposure-related guidelines for children treated with anthracyclines. These guidelines include recommendations for echocardiograms every 1–5 years depending on exposure (see Table 4.1). These recommendations differ substantially from those given for patients treated for cancer during adulthood and should be followed carefully.

Table 4.1 Recommended schedule for echocardiograms or multiple-gated acquisition scans in children treated with anthracyclines

Anthracycline dose[a]	Age at first treatment		
	<1 year	1–4 years	>5 years
With chest radiation			
<300 mg/m^2	Every year	Every year	Every 2 years
>300 mg/m^2	Every year	Every year	Every year
Without chest radiation			
<100 mg/m^2	Every 2 years	Every 5 years	Every 5 years
100–200 mg/m^2	Every 2 years	Every 2 years	Every 5 years
200–300 mg/m^2	Every year	Every 2 years	Every 2 years
>300 mg/m^2	Every year	Every year	Every year

Adapted from the Children's Oncology Group Guidelines, available at http://www.childrens oncologygroup.org

[a]Based on total does of doxorubicin/daunorubicin or equivalent doses of other anthracyclines (doxorubicin: total dose × 1; daunorubicin: total dose × 0.833; epirubicin: total dose × 0.67; idarubicin: total dose × 5; mitoxantrone: total dose × 4). Survivors who received ≥40 Gy radiation to the heart or ≥30 Gy radiation to the heart plus anthracycline-based chemotherapy should be advised to have stress testing by a cardiologist 5–10 years after the radiation, with subsequent stress testing as advised by the cardiologist.

In addition, survivors should be encouraged to have a healthy lifestyle with exercise and a healthy diet to prevent other known risk factors for cardiovascular disease, such as obesity and hyperlipidemia. See Chaps. 15, 16, and 17 for detailed discussion about healthy lifestyles for cancer survivors.

Liver

Many chemotherapeutic agents, such as methotrexate, mercaptopurine, and busulfan, can place the survivor at risk for hepatic damage. Yearly liver function tests and liver biopsies, if indicated, are necessary to assess the integrity of the liver. Because of blood product administration, cancer patients are also at risk for hepatitis C infection; therefore, testing for hepatitis C should be done at some point after blood-product administration is completed. These patients should also be immunized against hepatitis B. Alcohol and large doses of acetaminophen should be avoided.

Lungs

Busulfan may cause diffuse pulmonary fibrosis. A chest X-ray will reveal diffuse interstitial and intraalveolar infiltrates, which may appear at any time after treatment is completed. This late effect is associated with progressive deterioration in lung function.

Pulmonary fibrosis may also occur after treatment with high doses of cyclophosphamide or nitrosourea-based drugs. Pulmonary function studies will reveal a diffuse interstitial fibrosis, restrictive pulmonary disease, and arterial hypoxemia. A chest X-ray will show a pattern of diffuse interstitial fibrosis with patchy basilar infiltrates. In the chronic stage, pulmonary fibrosis associated with treatment with cyclophosphamide or nitrosourea-based drugs also manifests as diffuse interstitial and intraalveolar fibrosis.

Gonads

Many chemotherapeutic drugs have the potential to cause gonadal failure or impairment. Alkylating agents, particularly cyclophosphamide and ifosfamide, can damage the testes, resulting in sterility or lack of testosterone production. The risk is greater in pubescent boys than in younger boys. The ovaries can also be damaged in pubescent girls. This may result in infertility, lack of estrogen production, or premature menopause. Damage to the gonads may manifest as delayed puberty, amenorrhea (in girls), absence of secondary sexual characteristics, growth retardation, or infertility. Levels of follicle-stimulating hormone, luteinizing hormone, and insulin-like growth factor should be determined, semen analysis performed (in boys), and testosterone or estrogen levels checked. A referral to a fertility expert is always indicated if pregnancy is desired. Conceptions achieved by "infertile" long-term survivors, both male and female, have been reported. See also Chap. 25 on sexuality.

Kidneys

Cisplatin is toxic to the kidneys and may cause lifelong renal insufficiency or failure. Assessment of renal function should be routine in patients who have received cisplatin. (It may also cause hearing impairment.)

Radiation

The younger the patient when the radiation is administered, the greater the damage that can occur (Bhatia and Constine 2009; Armstrong et al. 2010). The following sections summarize the most substantial radiation-induced sequelae, which may affect various organs and systems.

Head and Neck

Radiation to the head and neck causes growth retardation of the involved area. If radiation is administered to the eyes, the bitemporal diameter will be reduced. Radiation administered to the brain may result in a small head. If the pituitary gland is involved, side effects may include absent or delayed sexual maturity, thyroid insufficiency, hypopituitary dwarfism, or diabetes insipidus. Care for patients who have undergone radiation therapy involving the pituitary gland preferably should include the assistance of an endocrinologist.

With nasopharyngeal radiation, extensive damage to the teeth, mandible and maxillary ridge, sinus cavities, and structures of the mouth and nasopharynx may occur. Vision and hearing may also be affected, dry eyes and skin damage may occur, and sinus infections may be a serious problem. Dental radiation predisposes the patient to caries, abnormal tooth growth, and destruction of the hard and soft palates. Care must be taken with all dental procedures: hyperbaric oxygen before and after treatment may be required.

Radiation involving the neck affects the thyroid. Careful attention must be paid to the thyroid gland throughout the patient's lifespan to monitor for a secondary cancer and for hypothyroidism or hyperthyroidism. Damage to the muscles and vascular structures of the neck may also occur, and patency of the carotid arteries may increase the risk of stroke.

Musculoskeletal

Skeletal growth abnormalities are common and can occur in patients who have received >15 Gy radiation to the growth plates. This can result in decreased height (with spinal radiation), decreased long-bone length, and chest growth disturbances. Significant scoliosis is uncommon in patients who have received <35 Gy radiation to the spine. In addition to bone growth impairment, muscular hypoplasia in the irradiated field is common.

Table 4.2 Recommendations for surveillance of late effects in survivors of childhood cancer

Cancer diagnosis	Site of primary cancer	Laboratory tests	Diagnostic tests and frequency
General recommendations for all survivors of childhood cancer	All	Complete blood count, urinalysis, electrolytes, magnesium, calcium, phosphorus, blood urea nitrogen, creatinine, fasting glucose, liver function tests	Annual history and physical examination with blood pressure, height, weight, and body mass index (monitor for obesity)
Acute lymphoblastic leukemia/acute myeloid leukemia (ALL/AML)	Bone marrow, central nervous system, testes, ovary	Thyroxine, thyroid-stimulating hormone, follicle-stimulating hormone, luteinizing hormone, estrogen/testosterone, sperm count if patient wishes, fasting lipid panel	Annual neurologic examination if cranial radiation; eye examination for cataracts; echocardiogram or electrocardiogram following guidelines; bone density at 18 years and 2–3 years after if abnormal; neuropsychological evaluation if clinically indicated
Central nervous system	Brain and spinal cord	Same as ALL/AML	Same as ALL/AML; neuropsychological evaluation repeated every 3–5 years after treatment completion or if school or employment issues; audiogram at baseline and every 5 years thereafter
Hodgkin/non-Hodgkin lymphoma	Neck/chest	Same as ALL/AML	Chest X-ray, pulmonary function tests at baseline and every 3 years thereafter, more often if received carmustine, lomustine, or bleomycin; echocardiogram or electrocardiogram per guidelines; breast screening per Table 4.3
	Abdomen/pelvis	Same as ALL/AML, plus stool hemoccult	Colonoscopy per Table 4.3

Table 4.2 (continued)

Cancer diagnosis	Site of primary cancer	Laboratory tests	Diagnostic tests and frequency
Wilms tumor, neuroblastoma, rhabdomyosarcoma, germ cell tumors, other solid tumors	Head, neck, chest	Same as ALL/AML	Same as Hodgkin disease for neck/chest, plus audiogram 5 years after treatment completion and as necessary if received cisplatin
	Abdomen	Same as ALL/AML, plus stool hemoccult	Same as chest, plus colonoscopy per Table 4.3
Ewing sarcoma and osteosarcoma	Long bones	Same as ALL/AML	X-ray of limb yearly
	Chest, pelvis	Same as ALL/AML	Same as Hodgkin disease for neck/chest

Radiation to the chest may damage the heart, large vessels, and lung. Careful attention must be paid to lung function and cardiac output and electrical activity. An echocardiogram, electrocardiogram, and occasionally pulmonary function testing should be performed as follow-up for such patients. See Tables 4.1 and 4.2 for follow-up recommendations.

Central Nervous System

Central nervous system irradiation, especially whole-brain irradiation, increases the risk of learning disabilities, late-onset seizures, hearing loss, and cognitive dysfunction (Armstrong et al. 2009). Radiation to the hypothalamic/pituitary axis can also lead to hormonal deficiencies, especially growth, thyroid-stimulating, adrenocorticotropic, and follicle-stimulating/luteinizing hormones (in order from most to least common; Nandagopal et al. 2008).

Abdomen or Pelvis

Radiation involving the abdomen or pelvis may damage organs within the radiation field. Radiation of >8 Gy to the ovary can result in sterility, especially in girls in their teens or early 20s. In boys, 4–6 Gy radiation to the abdomen or pelvis can result in aspermia and 24 Gy can result in decreased testosterone. Boys are more sensitive than men to these late effects. Secondary damage may occur from malfunctioning or nonfunctioning organs. If the ovaries are damaged, in addition to infertility, estrogen deficiency can occur, leading to osteopenia or osteoporosis. Fibrosis of the genitourinary tract may also occur, which may cause hydronephrosis, small urinary bladder, and kidney damage. If the radiation port involved the femoral arteries, stenosis may develop. Patients who have undergone radiation to the spleen must be treated similarly to those who have undergone surgical splenectomy.

Risk-Based Surveillance for Treatment-Related Late Effects

A description of potential late effects of cancer therapy and recommendations for managing these effects is available from the Children's Oncology Group (http://www.childrensoncologygroup.org/index.php/lateeffectsoftreatment). Specific recommendations for patient monitoring related to every aspect of treatment are available at http://www.survivorshipguidelines.org.

The survivorship guidelines note that all adult survivors of childhood cancer should have an annual history and physical examination. When a physician is seeing the patient for the first time, the physician should gather information about the patient's cancer diagnosis, age at treatment, complications of treatment, any recurrences and subsequent treatment, and known problems related to the treatment. In addition, a review of organ systems is indicated to identify symptoms that may be related to previous treatments. The patient should have a complete physical examination that includes blood pressure and body mass index screening and examination of all organ systems. Women should have regular breast and gynecologic examinations by family physicians or their own obstetrician/gynecologist. Table 4.2 shows guidelines for additional studies, based on the most common diagnoses and the treatments usually given for these diagnoses.

Prevention of Second Primary Cancers and Late Effects

All childhood cancer survivors should receive the same general advice about sun exposure, diet, smoking cessation, and Pap smears and other preventive screenings that are advised for the general adult population. In addition, the risk of developing a subsequent neoplasm is more than 19 times higher for childhood cancer survivors than for age-matched siblings because of the survivors' potential exposure to radiation or certain agents and because the survivors may have a somewhat increased genetic risk. Therefore, screening for certain types of cancers is recommended to begin earlier in survivors than in the general population, as shown in Table 4.3. The most common types of second malignant neoplasms are skin cancer, breast cancer, and thyroid cancer. In addition, survivors are at increased risk for other cancers such

Table 4.3 Cancer screening recommendations for survivors of childhood cancer

Second malignant neoplasm	Risk factors	Screening recommendations
Skin cancer	10–20% of patients; increased risk in irradiated skin	Annual skin exams by dermatologist; close monitoring of irradiated skin and palms and soles
Breast cancer	Risk in women younger than 30 years is elevated 5–54 times depending on radiation dose to thorax	Yearly mammograms or magnetic resonance imaging of breasts beginning 8 years after radiation or at age 25 years, whichever occurs later, for women who had chest radiation
Thyroid cancer	Increased risk with radiation to head, neck, or chest	Annual history and physical examination; free thyroxine, thyroid-stimulating hormone tested yearly; thyroid ultrasound every 3–4 years after treatment completion or sooner if nodule is found
Leukemia (acute myeloid leukemia/ myelodysplastic syndrome)	Increased risk with exposure to alkylating agents, topoisomerase inhibitors	Annual history and physical examination, including complete blood count with differential and platelet count (highest risk, first 5 years after exposure)
Brain tumors	Increased risk with cranial radiation for brain tumor, acute lymphoblastic leukemia, some head and neck cancers; the younger the age at primary diagnosis, the greater the risk	Latency period 9–10 years after radiation; monitor with annual history and physical examination, including yearly neurological exam (more often if indicated by examination or symptoms)
Other carcinomas	Can occur in patients who have or have not undergone radiation therapy	Latency period 5–30 years, median 15 years; yearly history and physical examination; if abdominal radiation: colon cancer screening with colonoscopy every 10 years beginning 15 years after completion of treatment or at age 35 years, whichever is later

as head and neck, kidney, bladder, lung, gastrointestinal and colon, and genitourinary cancers. In the Childhood Cancer Survivor Study, patients with second cancers were more likely to have been diagnosed with cancer in early childhood, with a primary diagnosis of Hodgkin lymphoma, soft tissue sarcoma, or neuroblastoma, as well as more likely to have a first-degree relative with a history of cancer and a personal history of alcohol use. Survivors of Wilms tumor also had an increased risk of developing colorectal and other gastrointestinal carcinomas (Bhatia and Sklar 2002).

In addition to altered screening recommendations for survivors of childhood cancers, increased emphasis should be made on a healthy lifestyle and diet, both to decrease the risk of some adult cancers and to decrease the risk of cardiovascular disease, especially in patients exposed to anthracyclines (see Chap. 19 on cardiovascular issues). Children and adults with a genetic predisposition to a second malignancy, such as those with neurofibromatosis, Li-Fraumeni syndrome, Beckwith-Wiedemann syndrome, familial polyposis, or multiple endocrine neoplasia syndromes, should be followed in specialty clinics for these disorders or in the Childhood Cancer Survivor Clinic. Such clinics are available at MD Anderson.

Psychosocial Functioning

Although many childhood cancer survivors show tremendous resilience and strength in overcoming the trauma of cancer at a young age, a significant proportion report more symptoms of global distress and poorer physical function than controls. Other reported late effects include anxiety, depression, and posttraumatic stress. These factors can significantly hinder attainment of lifetime educational, social, and vocational goals. As a result, survivors are less likely to be married, have a higher risk of experiencing unemployment and legal difficulties, and are likely to attain lower educational achievements than other adults. Survivors who have had cranial radiation or surgery are at the highest risk of experiencing psychosocial problems. In addition, survivors who experienced psychological problems as adolescents have an increased risk of developing poor health behaviors in adulthood. In our clinic, we frequently refer patients to our vocational councilors, psychologists, and psychiatrists for psychosocial support and advice about school and careers (Zeltzer et al. 2009; Krull et al. 2010).

Key Practice Points

- Although the patient may be cured of the primary tumor, the patient may have an increased risk of developing second or multiple subsequent neoplasms at a younger age than expected in the general population because of treatment exposures and genetic predisposition.

- The risk for late cardiac adverse effects from exposure to anthracyclines and radiation to the heart can continue for many years after treatment, but treatment for these adverse effects is available if they are found early.
- Stress, such as childbirth, can precipitate heart failure in young women who received treatment with anthracyclines. Young women who received more than a 200-mg/m^2 cumulative dose of anthracyclines should be monitored by a cardiologist during pregnancy.
- Cranial radiation increases the risk of mental impairment, difficulty with executive functioning, stroke, endocrine deficits, and secondary neoplasms, and these increased risks continue throughout life.
- Central nervous system tumors can recur many years after diagnosis, so an annual history and physical examination, including a neurological examination and magnetic resonance imaging of the brain, are warranted for at least 10 years after diagnosis, and longer if symptoms or residual tumor tissue is present.
- Every adult survivor of childhood cancer should have a summary of their treatment history and recommendations for future care and monitoring provided by the treating center. Survivorship clinics throughout the United States can provide this information. For a directory of childhood survivorship services and recommendations for monitoring for late effects, see http://www.survivorshipguidelines.org.

Suggested Readings

Armstrong GT, Liu Q, Yasui Y, et al. Long-term outcomes among adult survivors of childhood central nervous system malignancies in the Childhood Cancer Survivor Study. *J Natl Cancer Inst* 2009;101:946–958.

Armstrong GT, Stovall M, Robison LL. Long-term effects of radiation exposure among adult survivors of childhood cancer: results from the childhood cancer survivor study. *J Radiat Res* 2010;174:840–850.

Bhatia S, Constine LS. Late morbidity after successful treatment of children with cancer. *Cancer J* 2009;15(3):174–180.

Bhatia S, Sklar C. Second cancers in survivors of childhood cancer. *Nat Rev Cancer* 2002;2: 124–132.

Dickerman JD. The late effects of childhood cancer therapy. *Pediatrics* 2007;119(3):554–568.

Diller L, Chow EJ, Gurney JG, et al. Chronic disease in the Childhood Cancer Survivor Study cohort: a review of published findings. *J Clin Oncol* 2009;27:2339–2355.

Gianni L, Herman E, Lipshultz S, Minotti G, Sarvazyan N, Sawyer D. Anthracycline cardiotoxicity: from bench to bedside. *J Clin Oncol* 2008;26:3777–3784.

Horowitz ME, Fordis M, Krause S, McKellar J, Poplack DG. Passport for care: implementing the survivorship care plan. *J Oncol Practice* 2009;5:110–112.

Hudson MM. Reproductive outcomes for survivors of childhood cancer. *Obstet Gynecol* 2010;116: 1171–1183.

Krull KR, Huang S, Gurney JG, et al. Adolescent behavior and adult health status in childhood cancer survivors. *J Cancer Survivorship* 2010;4(3):210–217.

Mariotto AB, Rowland JH, Yabroff KR, et al. Long-term survivors of childhood cancers in the United States. *Cancer Epidemiol Biomarkers Prev* 2009;18:1033–1040.

Nandagopal R, Laverdiere C, Mulrooney D, Hudson MM, Meacham L. Endocrine late effects of childhood cancer therapy: a report from the Children's Oncology Group. *Horm Res* 2008; 69(2):65–74.

Oeffinger KC, Mertens AC, Sklar CA, et al. Chronic health conditions in adult survivors of childhood cancer. *N Engl J Med* 2006;355:1572–1582.

Shankar SM, Marina N, Hudson MM, et al. Monitoring for cardiovascular disease in survivors of childhood cancer: report from the Cardiovascular Disease Task Force of the Children's Oncology Group. *Pediatrics* 2008;121:e387–e396.

Zeltzer LK, Recklitis C, Buchbinder D, et al. Psychological status in childhood cancer survivors: a report from the Childhood Cancer Survivor Study. *J Clin Oncol* 2009;27(14):2396–2404.

Chapter 5
Breast Cancer Survivorship Management

Phuong Khanh Morrow

Contents

Chapter Overview Owing to improvements in screening and adjuvant therapy, survival following the diagnosis of breast cancer has improved markedly over the past three decades. This chapter will focus on MD Anderson's recommendations for surveillance and treatment in breast cancer survivors. Because randomized trials have not demonstrated a survival benefit with intensive monitoring, current guidelines support the use of medical history review, physical examination, and annual mammograms as the bedrock of breast cancer surveillance. In addition, given the multidisciplinary approach to breast cancer treatment and surveillance, it is essential to monitor for and

L.E. Foxhall, M.A. Rodriguez (eds.), *Advances in Cancer Survivorship Management*,
MD Anderson Cancer Care Series, DOI 10.1007/978-1-4939-0986-5_5,
© The University of Texas M.D. Anderson Cancer Center 2015

treat long-term effects of breast cancer treatment, including lymphedema, cardiac toxicity, ovarian failure, bone disorders, and secondary malignancies.

Introduction

Owing to improvements in screening and adjuvant therapy, survival following the diagnosis of breast cancer has improved markedly over the past three decades (Berry et al. 2005). As a result, an increasing number of breast cancer survivors are requiring evaluation and treatment after the diagnosis of breast cancer. This chapter will focus on MD Anderson's recommendations for surveillance and treatment in breast cancer survivors.

Surveillance

Type of Monitoring

A great concern for breast cancer survivors is the need for close monitoring for recurrent or metastatic disease. However, two large Italian trials, involving an aggregate of more than 2,500 patients with breast cancer, found no improvement in overall survival in patients who underwent intensive surveillance, including physical examination, mammogram, and rigorous tests such as bone scans and chest x-rays, compared with patients who received routine physical examinations and mammograms only (GIVIO Investigators 1994). As a result, current National Comprehensive Cancer Network (NCCN), American Society of Clinical Oncology (ASCO), and MD Anderson guidelines support surveillance of breast cancer survivors with physical examinations and mammograms; the use of more intensive monitoring is not recommended (see survivorship algorithms for invasive and noninvasive breast cancer, presented at the end of this chapter).

Interval for Monitoring

ASCO recommends that patients undergo a medical history review and physical examination every 3–6 months for the first 3 years following completion of primary therapy; this interval increases to 6–12 months at years 4 and 5 (Khatcheressian et al. 2006). After year 5, patients should undergo the medical history review and physical examination annually, unless earlier evaluation is clinically warranted. NCCN guidelines recommend similar intervals. The surveillance interval pattern used at MD Anderson is similar to that of the ASCO and NCCN guidelines; patients undergo a medical history review and physical examination every

3–6 months for 3 years, every 6–12 months for the next 2 years, and then annually after year 5.

History and Physical Examination

The medical history review and physical examination serve as the primary mechanism for detection of breast cancer recurrence (Lu et al. 2011). The medical history review should include questions that facilitate the detection of local recurrence or metastatic disease, covering the following:

- Lumps, nodules, fullness, or skin changes (to detect local recurrence)
- Persistent or worsening bone pain (to detect bone metastases)
- Abdominal pain, increased abdominal girth, anorexia, or jaundice (to detect liver metastases)
- Persistent cough, pleuritic chest pain, or shortness of breath (to detect pulmonary metastases)
- New onset or worsening headache, visual changes, nausea, vomiting, dizziness, weakness, bowel or bladder incontinence, or changes in sensation (to detect metastases in the brain or spinal cord)
- Changes in bowel habits or alteration in consistency or color of the stool (to detect gastrointestinal metastases)
- Pelvic pain or discomfort or new-onset vaginal bleeding or spotting (to detect genitourinary metastases)

Physical examination should involve a complete examination of the patient from head to toe, including a neurologic examination, cardiac examination, pulmonary examination, abdominal evaluation, and evaluation of the breasts and lymph node basins.

Breast Imaging

Mammography remains the primary imaging technique for breast cancer, because it is the only imaging method that has consistently been found to reduce breast cancer–related mortality (Tabar et al. 2001). MD Anderson recommends obtaining a mammogram of a breast treated with breast-conserving therapy after 6 months, and then obtaining a bilateral mammogram annually. For patients who have undergone mastectomy, a mammogram of the contralateral breast should be obtained annually. For patients who have undergone mastectomy and reconstruction, a mammogram is not obtained for the reconstructed breast because mammography of the reconstructed breast has not been shown to increase detection of local recurrence (Fajardo et al. 1993).

Ultrasound is not currently recommended as a primary imaging technique for breast cancer. Instead, it is primarily used as an adjunct to mammography to further evaluate architectural distortion detected by the mammogram, distinguish between a solid mass and a cyst, and assist in localization of a mass or nodule to facilitate biopsy.

The use of magnetic resonance imaging (MRI) of the breast is also increasing. MRI has been found to have greater sensitivity for detection of breast malignancies than mammography, but no current evidence indicates that use of breast MRI improves outcomes when used as a breast surveillance technique (Kuhl et al. 2005). Thus, breast MRI is not routinely recommended for breast cancer surveillance, although it may be used as an adjunct to mammography in patients who have unique characteristics, such as BRCA1/2 mutation carrier status.

Screening for Second Primary Breast Cancers

Breast cancer survivors have a markedly higher risk of developing a second primary breast cancer, compared with the risk of developing primary breast cancer in the general population (Chaudary et al. 1984). Techniques for monitoring for a second primary breast cancer include mammography, ultrasonography, and MRI, as previously described.

Late Effects of Treatment

Surgery and Lymphedema

Mastectomy and axillary lymph node dissection increase the risk of developing lymphedema, which is associated with limb discomfort and decreased quality of life (Beaulac et al. 2002). Furthermore, chronic massive lymphedema may lead to Stewart-Treves syndrome, a rare disease that is associated with the development of lymphangiosarcoma of the involved extremity (Cozen et al. 1999). More commonly, lymphedema of the arm increases the likelihood of skin infections, such as cellulitis, for which close monitoring should be performed.

Chemotherapy

Cardiac Toxicity

Compared with first-generation regimens such as CMF (cyclophosphamide, methotrexate, and 5-fluorouracil), treatment with anthracyclines has been associated with a significant reduction in breast cancer–related mortality and overall mortality (Early Breast Cancer Trialists' Collaborative Group 2012). However, anthracycline use increases the risk of congestive heart failure in a dose-dependent fashion (Bristow et al. 1981). The risk of anthracycline-related cardiomyopathy increases with age, combination with trastuzumab, and combination with mediastinal radiation therapy (Pinder et al. 2007).

In contrast with anthracycline-related cardiomyopathy, trastuzumab-related cardiotoxicity is often reversible with treatment discontinuation and is not dose-dependent (Keefe 2002). Most often, trastuzumab-related cardiomyopathy is detected by echocardiogram or multigated acquisition scan and is not clinically apparent at the time of diagnosis. Monitoring for cardiac complications from each regimen requires a multidisciplinary approach, with input from each patient's primary care physician, oncologist, and cardiologist.

Neurologic Toxicity

Review of cross-sectional cognitive outcome studies reveals that the prevalence of chemotherapy-associated cognitive decline ranges from 17% to 75% (Correa and Ahles 2008). Prospective studies of breast cancer survivors undergoing chemotherapy have generated conflicting results, with some studies noting a significant decline in cognitive function and others finding no difference compared with baseline (Wefel et al. 2004b; Shilling et al. 2005; Bender et al. 2006; Hurria et al. 2006; Jenkins et al. 2006; Stewart et al. 2008; Quesnel et al. 2009). However, the patient's self-perceived cognitive dysfunction is integrally linked to increased psychological distress (Wefel et al. 2004a). Boykoff et al. (2009) published compelling qualitative evidence of the negative effects of "chemobrain" on the economic, emotional, and interpersonal aspects of breast cancer survivors' lives. Furthermore, a recent prospective study of 101 patients with breast cancer noted that self-perceived cognitive dysfunction was significantly related to negative affectivity ($p = .015$) and depression ($p < .001$; Hermelink et al. 2010). Thus, even in the setting of cancer "cure" following chemotherapy, breast cancer survivors continue to face the critical barrier of worsened cognition and its downstream emotional distress in their daily lives.

Ovarian Failure

The risk of chemotherapy-related ovarian failure is related to the dose and type of chemotherapy and the age at diagnosis (Goodwin et al. 1999). Specifically, risk of ovarian failure is markedly increased when the chemotherapy regimen includes cyclophosphamide or anthracycline and is administered to women older than 35 years. Patients with breast cancer may experience hot flashes, vaginal dryness, and mood changes. Early evaluation and symptomatic treatment is essential to facilitate improved quality of life. Furthermore, early ovarian failure increases the risk of osteopenia or osteoporosis, for which close monitoring should occur. Treatment with calcium, vitamin D, and bisphosphonates may be necessary to maintain adequate bone health in this setting (Hillner et al. 2003; see algorithm for breast cancer survivorship bone health, presented at the end of this chapter).

Second Malignancies

Research from our institution has demonstrated a small increased risk of acute myeloid leukemia after adjuvant chemotherapy (1.8% vs 1.2%) in women older than 65 years (Patt et al. 2007). Use of more intense regimens that included two or more cycles containing 2,400 mg/m^2 cyclophosphamide with granulocyte colony-stimulating factor support resulted in a cumulative incidence of acute myeloid leukemia of 1.01% (95% confidence interval, 0.63–1.62%), compared with 0.21% (95% confidence interval, 0.11–0.41%) for patients treated with standard AC (doxorubicin and cyclophosphamide) regimens (Smith et al. 2003). Although the benefit from adjuvant chemotherapy exceeds the risk of developing acute myeloid leukemia, appropriate understanding of this risk is necessary for long-term follow-up.

Radiation Therapy

Cardiovascular Toxicity

Historically, postmastectomy radiation was found to increase the risk of cardiovascular toxicity. A large retrospective study of breast cancer survivors demonstrated a significant increase in overall mortality rates in patients who had received postmastectomy radiation; this effect was attributed to deaths from cardiovascular disease (Jones and Ribeiro 1989). However, with advances in radiation therapy and development of adaptive techniques to reduce cardiac exposure to radiation, recent randomized trials evaluating patients who received postmastectomy radiation therapy have shown no increase in cardiovascular morbidity (Hojris et al. 1999). But even with modern radiation therapy techniques, careful monitoring for symptoms of cardiac toxicity remains essential during follow-up visits.

Second Malignancies

Although they are rare, secondary malignancies are a potential late effect of radiation for the treatment of breast cancer. A retrospective study of the Surveillance, Epidemiology, and End Results (SEER) Cancer Incidence Database demonstrated that, at 15 years after diagnosis of breast cancer, the cumulative incidence of angiosarcoma was 0.9 per 1,000 patients who had received radiation therapy, compared with 0.1 per 1,000 patients who had not received radiation therapy (Yap et al. 2002). In patients who have received radiation therapy, an angiosarcoma presents in the irradiated field as a purple macule or papule; clinical suspicion of malignancy should lead to immediate core biopsy for further assessment. In addition to risk of solid tumor malignancies such as angiosarcoma, risk of hematologic malignancies such as acute myeloid leukemia and myelodysplastic syndrome is also slightly increased following radiation therapy (Kaplan et al. 2011).

Furthermore, data from the SEER database have demonstrated that, at 10 years after the breast cancer diagnosis, patients who had received radiation therapy had a relative risk of 2.0 for developing lung cancer, compared with patients who had not received radiation therapy (Neugut et al. 1993). This risk affected all three major subtypes of breast cancer: small cell, squamous cell, and adenocarcinoma. Similar risks for esophageal cancer were observed with older radiation techniques; these risks have declined with the implementation of new radiation techniques that enable greater exclusion of the esophagus from the irradiated field (Levi et al. 2005).

The risk of developing contralateral breast cancer is also slightly increased with older radiation therapy techniques; the Early Breast Cancer Trialists' Collaborative Group found a significantly increased incidence of contralateral breast cancer (rate ratio, 1.18) in patients who had received radiation therapy (Clarke et al. 2005). A more recent study found that patients younger than 45 years, particularly those with strong family histories, appeared to have an increased risk of developing contralateral breast cancer following postmastectomy radiation therapy (Hooning et al. 2008).

Hormonal Therapy

Tamoxifen

Although tamoxifen has been shown to reduce the risk of recurrence of early-stage breast cancer, it acts as a selective estrogen receptor modulator and may increase the risk of endometrial carcinoma and uterine sarcomas. Careful monitoring of each patient with an intact uterus who has taken or is taking tamoxifen is therefore essential. Tamoxifen also increases the risk of deep venous thrombosis, and patients should be educated regarding the signs and symptoms of deep venous thrombosis. Furthermore, because tamoxifen is associated with ocular toxicity (although rarely), patients should be counseled to maintain close follow-up with their ophthalmologist.

Aromatase Inhibitors

The ATAC (anastrozole, tamoxifen, alone or in combination) trial demonstrated that anastrozole, compared with tamoxifen, reduced the risk of recurrence of early-stage breast cancer (Cuzick et al. 2010). As a result, aromatase inhibitors have become the standard of care for the treatment of hormone receptor-positive breast cancer in postmenopausal woman. However, although aromatase inhibitors have a favorable side effect profile compared with tamoxifen, they have a negative effect on bone health through estrogen deprivation (Eastell et al. 2011). As a result, patients should undergo regular monitoring with bone density studies and receive counseling regarding bone health to reduce their risk of developing worsening osteopenia or osteoporosis.

Psychosocial Functioning

An important aspect of follow-up with breast cancer survivors is the true acknowledgment of the grief and sadness that is associated with the loss of all or part of the female breast. Furthermore, following treatment, many patients enter into to a period of increased anxiety, depression, and stress (Khan et al. 2012). Many patients may benefit from participation in breast cancer support groups, particularly those that are geared toward their specific demographic. For example, young breast cancer survivors often gravitate to the Young Survival Coalition, which focuses on meeting the needs of young women who have been diagnosed with breast cancer. The Sisters Network provides strength and support to young and old African-American women who are breast cancer survivors. In addition, many breast cancer survivors find benefit in individual counseling sessions, which may focus on mindfulness and meditation to reduce fears of recurrence (Tacon 2011).

Key Practice Points

- Current guidelines support surveillance of breast cancer survivors with a physical examination and a mammogram; use of more intensive monitoring is not recommended.
- Mammography remains the primary imaging technique for breast cancer because it is the only imaging method that has consistently been found to reduce breast cancer–related mortality.
- Risk of anthracycline-related cardiomyopathy increases with age, combination with trastuzumab, and combination with mediastinal radiation therapy.
- Risk of ovarian failure is increased when the chemotherapy regimen includes cyclophosphamide or anthracycline and is administered to women older than 35 years.
- Tamoxifen may increase the risk of endometrial carcinoma, uterine sarcoma, deep venous thrombosis, and ocular toxicity.
- Patients who are treated with aromatase inhibitors should undergo regular monitoring with bone density studies and receive counseling regarding bone health to reduce their risk of developing worsening osteopenia or osteoporosis.

Suggested Readings

Beaulac SM, McNair LA, Scott TE, et al. Lymphedema and quality of life in survivors of early-stage breast cancer. *Arch Surg* 2002;137:1253–1257.
Bender CM, Sereika SM, Berga SL, et al. Cognitive impairment associated with adjuvant therapy in breast cancer. *Psychooncology* 2006;15:422–430.

Berry DA, Cronin KA, Plevritis SK, et al. Effect of screening and adjuvant therapy on mortality from breast cancer. *N Engl J Med* 2005;353:1784–1792.

Boykoff N, Moieni M, Subramanian SK. Confronting chemobrain: an in-depth look at survivors' reports of impact on work, social networks, and health care response. *J Cancer Surviv* 2009;3: 223–232.

Bristow MR, Mason JW, Billingham M, et al. Dose-effect and structure-function relationships in doxorubicin cardiomyopathy. *Am Heart J* 1981;102:709–718.

Chaudary MA, Millis RR, Hoskins EO, et al. Bilateral primary breast cancer: a prospective study of disease incidence. *Br J Surg* 1984;71:711–714.

Clarke M, Collins R, Darby S, et al. Effects of radiotherapy and of differences in the extent of surgery for early breast cancer on local recurrence and 15-year survival: an overview of the randomised trials. *Lancet* 2005;366:2087–2106.

Correa DD, Ahles TA. Neurocognitive changes in cancer survivors. *Cancer J* 2008;14:396–400.

Cozen W, Bernstein L, Wang F, et al. The risk of angiosarcoma following primary breast cancer. *Br J Cancer* 1999;81:532–536.

Cuzick J, Sestak I, Baum M, et al. Effect of anastrozole and tamoxifen as adjuvant treatment for early-stage breast cancer: 10-year analysis of the ATAC trial. *Lancet Oncol* 2010;11:1135–1141.

Early Breast Cancer Trialists' Collaborative Group. Comparisons between different polychemo-therapy regimens for early breast cancer: meta-analyses of long-term outcome among 100,000 women in 123 randomised trials. *Lancet* 2012;379:432–444.

Eastell R, Adams J, Clack G, et al. Long-term effects of anastrozole on bone mineral density: 7-year results from the ATAC trial. *Ann Oncol* 2011;22:857–862.

Fajardo LL, Roberts CC, Hunt KR. Mammographic surveillance of breast cancer patients: should the mastectomy site be imaged? *Am J Roentgenol* 1993;161:953–955.

GIVIO Investigators. Impact of follow-up testing on survival and health-related quality of life in breast cancer patients. A multicenter randomized controlled trial. *JAMA* 1994;271: 1587–1592.

Goodwin PJ, Ennis M, Pritchard KI, et al. Risk of menopause during the first year after breast cancer diagnosis. *J Clin Oncol* 1999;17:2365–2370.

Hermelink K, Kuchenhoff H, Untch M, et al. Two different sides of "chemobrain": determinants and nondeterminants of self-perceived cognitive dysfunction in a prospective, randomized, multicenter study. *Psychooncology* 2010;19:1321–1328.

Hillner BE, Ingle JN, Chlebowski RT, et al. American Society of Clinical Oncology 2003 update on the role of bisphosphonates and bone health issues in women with breast cancer. *J Clin Oncol* 2003;21:4042–4057.

Hojris I, Overgaard M, Christensen JJ, et al. Morbidity and mortality of ischaemic heart disease in high-risk breast-cancer patients after adjuvant postmastectomy systemic treatment with or without radiotherapy: analysis of DBCG 82b and 82c randomised trials. Radiotherapy Committee of the Danish Breast Cancer Cooperative Group. *Lancet* 1999;354:1425–1430.

Hooning MJ, Aleman BM, Hauptmann M, et al. Roles of radiotherapy and chemotherapy in the development of contralateral breast cancer. *J Clin Oncol* 2008;26:5561–5568.

Hurria A, Rosen C, Hudis C, et al. Cognitive function of older patients receiving adjuvant chemo-therapy for breast cancer: a pilot prospective longitudinal study. *J Am Geriatr Soc* 2006;54: 925–931.

Jenkins V, Shilling V, Deutsch G, et al. A 3-year prospective study of the effects of adjuvant treat-ments on cognition in women with early stage breast cancer. *Br J Cancer* 2006;94:828–834.

Jones JM, Ribeiro GG. Mortality patterns over 34 years of breast cancer patients in a clinical trial of post-operative radiotherapy. *Clin Radiol* 1989;40:204–208.

Kaplan HG, Malmgren JA, Atwood MK. Increased incidence of myelodysplastic syndrome and acute myeloid leukemia following breast cancer treatment with radiation alone or combined with chemotherapy: a registry cohort analysis 1990–2005. *BMC Cancer* 2011;11:260.

Keefe DL. Trastuzumab-associated cardiotoxicity. *Cancer* 2002;95:1592–1600.

Khan F, Amatya B, Pallant JF, et al. Factors associated with long-term functional outcomes and psychological sequelae in women after breast cancer. *Breast* 2012;21:314–320.

Khatcheressian JL, Wolff AC, Smith TJ, et al. American Society of Clinical Oncology 2006 update of the breast cancer follow-up and management guidelines in the adjuvant setting. *J Clin Oncol* 2006;24:5091–2097.

Kuhl CK, Schrading S, Leutner CC, et al. Mammography, breast ultrasound, and magnetic resonance imaging for surveillance of women at high familial risk for breast cancer. *J Clin Oncol* 2005;23:8469–8476.

Levi F, Randimbison L, Te VC, et al. Increased risk of esophageal cancer after breast cancer. *Ann Oncol* 2005;16:1829–1831.

Lu W, de Bock GH, Schaapveld M, et al. The value of routine physical examination in the follow up of women with a history of early breast cancer. *Eur J Cancer* 2011;47:676–682.

Neugut AI, Robinson E, Lee WC, et al. Lung cancer after radiation therapy for breast cancer. *Cancer* 1993;71:3054–3057.

Patt DA, Duan Z, Fang S, et al. Acute myeloid leukemia after adjuvant breast cancer therapy in older women: understanding risk. *J Clin Oncol* 2007;25:3871–3876.

Pinder MC, Duan Z, Goodwin JS, et al. Congestive heart failure in older women treated with adjuvant anthracycline chemotherapy for breast cancer. *J Clin Oncol* 2007;25:3808–3815.

Quesnel C, Savard J, Ivers H. Cognitive impairments associated with breast cancer treatments: results from a longitudinal study. *Breast Cancer Res Treat* 2009;116:113–123.

Shilling V, Jenkins V, Morris R, et al. The effects of adjuvant chemotherapy on cognition in women with breast cancer—preliminary results of an observational longitudinal study. *Breast* 2005; 14:142–150.

Smith RE, Bryant J, DeCillis A, et al. Acute myeloid leukemia and myelodysplastic syndrome after doxorubicin-cyclophosphamide adjuvant therapy for operable breast cancer: the National Surgical Adjuvant Breast and Bowel Project experience. *J Clin Oncol* 2003;21: 1195–1204.

Stewart A, Collins B, Mackenzie J, et al. The cognitive effects of adjuvant chemotherapy in early stage breast cancer: a prospective study. *Psychooncology* 2008;17:122–130.

Tabar L, Vitak B, Chen HH, et al. Beyond randomized controlled trials: organized mammographic screening substantially reduces breast carcinoma mortality. *Cancer* 2001;91:1724–1731.

Tacon AM. Mindfulness: existential, loss, and grief factors in women with breast cancer. *J Psychosoc Oncol* 2011;29:643–656.

Wefel JS, Lenzi R, Theriault R, et al. "Chemobrain" in breast carcinoma?: a prologue. *Cancer* 2004a;101:466–475.

Wefel JS, Lenzi R, Theriault RL, et al. The cognitive sequelae of standard-dose adjuvant chemotherapy in women with breast carcinoma: results of a prospective, randomized, longitudinal trial. *Cancer* 2004b;100:2292–2299.

Yap J, Chuba PJ, Thomas R, et al. Sarcoma as a second malignancy after treatment for breast cancer. *Int J Radiat Oncol Biol Phys* 2002;52:1231–1237.

Survivorship Algorithms

These cancer survivorship algorithms have been specifically developed for MD Anderson using a multidisciplinary approach and taking into consideration circumstances particular to MD Anderson, including the following: MD Anderson's specific patient population, MD Anderson's services and structure, and MD Anderson's clinical information. These algorithms are provided for informational purposes only and are not intended to replace the independent medical or professional judgment of physicians or other health care providers. Moreover, these algorithms should not be used to treat pregnant women.

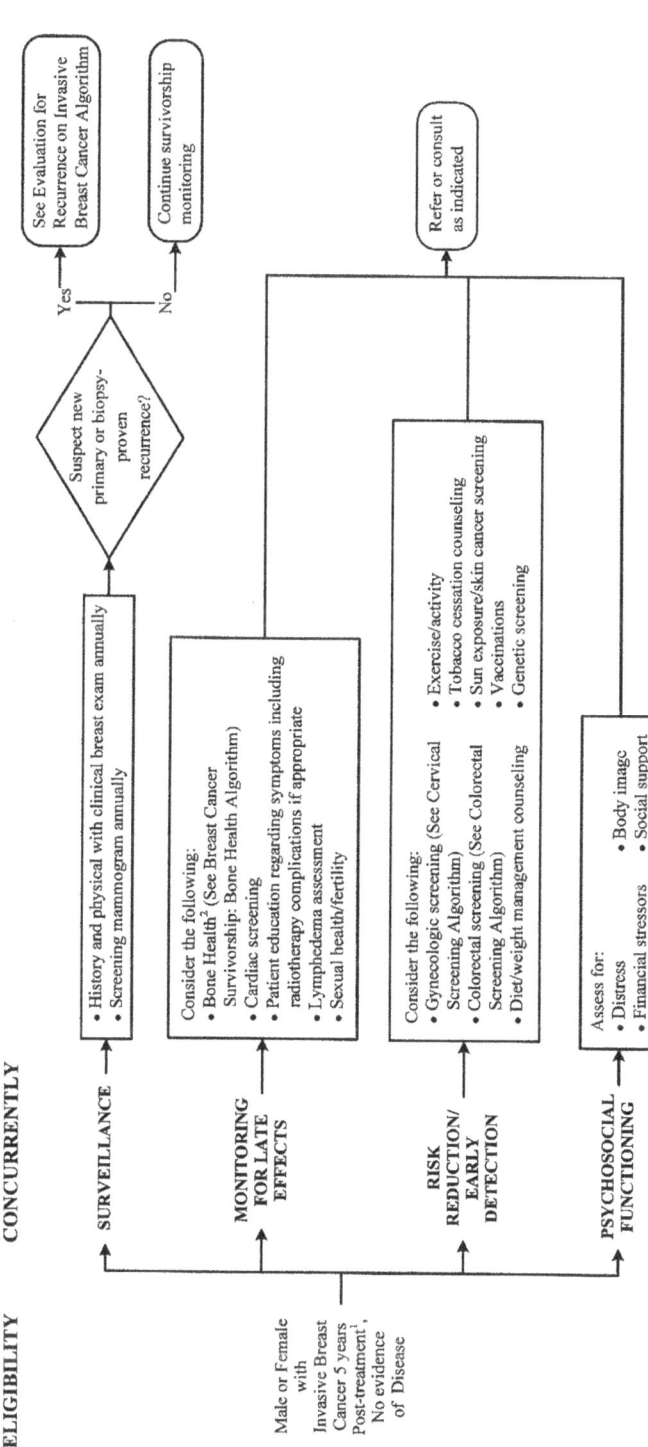

Algorithm 5.1 Survivorship—invasive breast cancer

68   P.K. Morrow

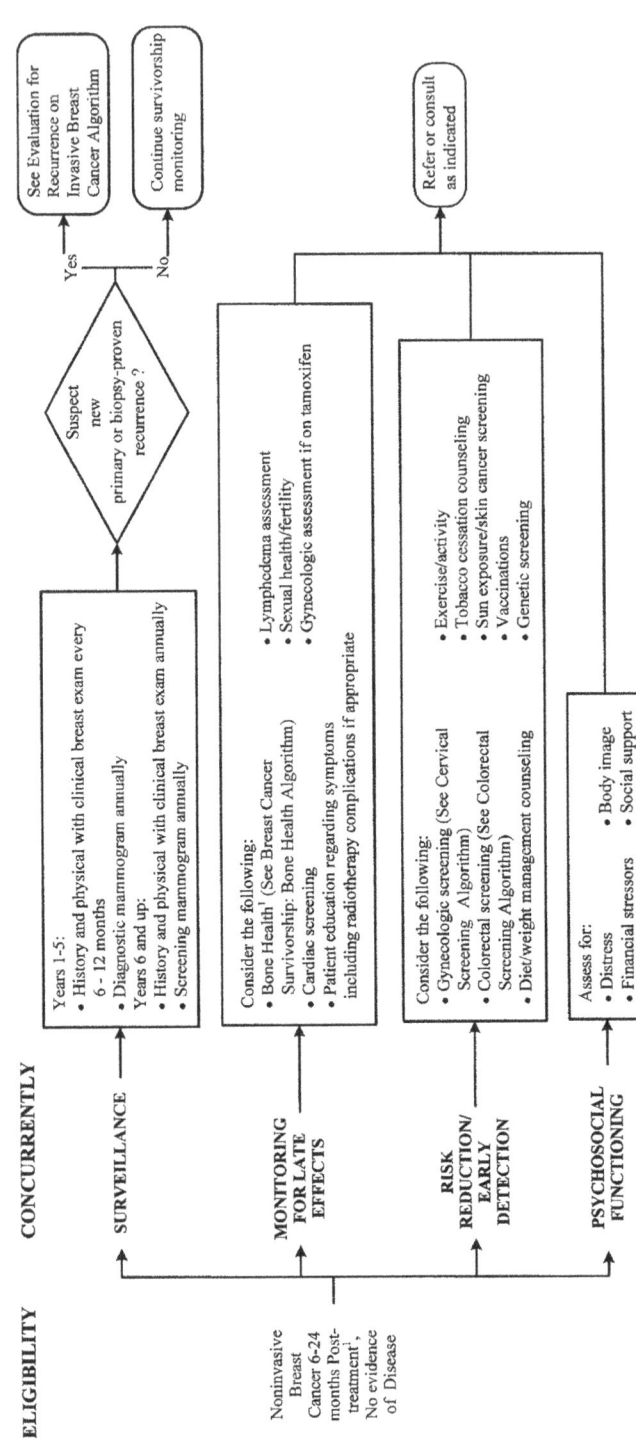

Algorithm 5.2 Survivorship—noninvasive breast cancer

[1] Completion of all treatment with the exception of hormonal agents
[2] Premenopausal women on tamoxifen or hormonal therapy

Department of Clinical Effectiveness V4
Approved by the Executive Committee of the Medical Staff 10/30/2012

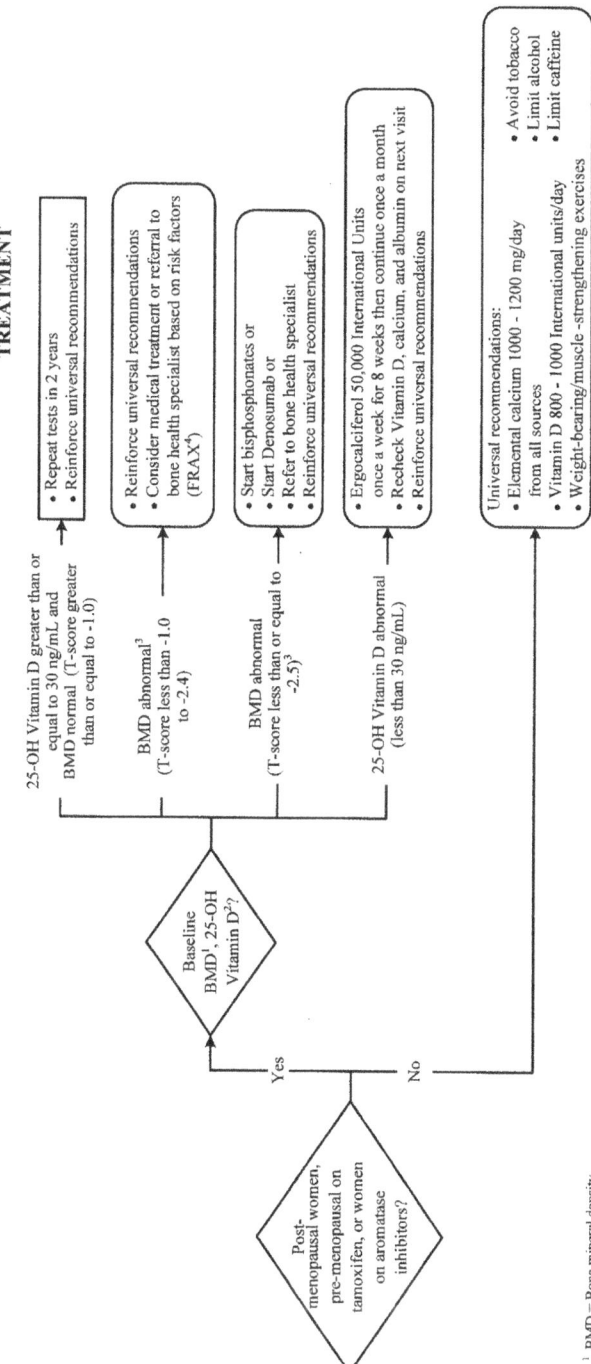

TREATMENT

Baseline BMD[1], 25-OH Vitamin D[2]?

Post-menopausal women, pre-menopausal on tamoxifen, or women on aromatase inhibitors?

Yes

No

25-OH Vitamin D greater than or equal to 30 ng/mL and BMD normal (T-score greater than or equal to -1.0)
- Repeat tests in 2 years
- Reinforce universal recommendations

BMD abnormal[3] (T-score less than -1.0 to -2.4)
- Reinforce universal recommendations
- Consider medical treatment or referral to bone health specialist based on risk factors (FRAX[4])

BMD abnormal (T-score less than or equal to -2.5)[3]
- Start bisphosphonates or
- Start Denosumab or
- Refer to bone health specialist
- Reinforce universal recommendations

25-OH Vitamin D abnormal (less than 30 ng/mL)
- Ergocalciferol 50,000 International Units once a week for 8 weeks then continue once a month
- Recheck Vitamin D, calcium, and albumin on next visit
- Reinforce universal recommendations

Universal recommendations:
- Elemental calcium 1000 - 1200 mg/day from all sources
- Vitamin D 800 - 1000 International units/day
- Weight-bearing/muscle -strengthening exercises
- Avoid tobacco
- Limit alcohol
- Limit caffeine

Department of Clinical Effectiveness V3
Approved by the Executive Committee of the Medical Staff 10/30/2012

[1] BMD = Bone mineral density
[2] 25-hydroxyvitamin D, also know as 25-hydroxycholecalciferol, calcidiol or abbreviated as 25-OH Vitamin D, the main vitamin D metabolite circulating in plasma
[3] Abnormal BMD: Osteopenia, T-score between -1.0 and -2.4; Osteoporosis, T-score less than or equal to -2.5
[4] FRAX WHO Fracture Risk Assessment Tool at www.shef.ac.uk/frax

Copyright 2012 The University of Texas M.D. Anderson Cancer Center

Algorithm 5.3 Breast cancer survivorship: bone health

Chapter 6
Colorectal Cancer Survivorship Management

Shahab U. Ahmed and Cathy Eng

Contents

L.E. Foxhall, M.A. Rodriguez (eds.), *Advances in Cancer Survivorship Management*,   71
MD Anderson Cancer Care Series, DOI 10.1007/978-1-4939-0986-5_6,
© The University of Texas M.D. Anderson Cancer Center 2015

Chapter Overview An estimated 96,830 new cases of colon cancer and 40,000 new cases of rectal cancer occurred in 2014, according to the most recent estimates from the American Cancer Society. The Centers for Disease Control and Prevention found that the number of survivors of all types of cancer increased from 9.8 million in 2001 to 11.7 million in 2007, and about 10% of these were survivors of colorectal cancer (CRC). By the year 2030, the number of patients with CRC is estimated to increase by as much as 30%. Given these overwhelming demographic changes, it is extremely important to improve our understanding of the essential health care needs and management issues of long-term CRC survivors. The term "cancer survivor" is now commonly used to describe a person from the time of cancer diagnosis through the remaining years of life. This chapter addresses CRC survivorship care and management issues, including risk evaluation, proper staging, available treatment options, surveillance recommendations, quality of life concerns, and prevention of recurrence.

Components of Survivorship Care

Four components are essential to comprehensive survivorship care: proper treatment and prevention, surveillance, intervention, and coordination of care. Prevention means using efficacious methods to prevent recurrence of the original cancer and occurrence of new cancers or late effects. Surveillance indicates monitoring for cancer spread, recurrence, or second cancers, as well as for medical and psychosocial late effects. Intervention means using sensible methods to address the consequences of cancer and its treatment. Coordination of care includes the arrangement and integration of necessary follow-up care between specialists and primary care providers to ensure that the survivor's health needs are met.

Noninterventional Risk Evaluation

Researchers have found that the following noninterventional risk factors may increase a person's chance of developing colorectal polyps or CRC:

- Age: about 90% of people diagnosed with CRC are older than 50 years
- Ethnicity: in the United States, African Americans have the highest incidence of CRC and CRC-related mortality (American Cancer Society 2011)
- Personal history of colorectal polyps or CRC
- Personal history of inflammatory bowel disease (ulcerative colitis or Crohn disease)

Table 6.1 Relative risk of developing colorectal cancer (CRC) with a family history of the disease

Family history	Relative risk (95% confidence interval)
No family history	1
1 first-degree relative with CRC	2.3 (2.0–2.5)
>1 first-degree relative with CRC	4.3 (3.0–6.1)
1 first-degree relative diagnosed with CRC before age 45 years	3.9 (2.4–6.2)
1 first-degree relative with colorectal adenoma	2.0 (1.6–2.6)

Source: Johns and Houlston (2001)

- Family history of CRC: Table 6.1 shows the relationship between family history and relative risk of developing CRC
- Inherited syndromes: the two most common inherited syndromes linked with CRC are familial adenomatous polyposis and hereditary non-polyposis CRC (Lynch syndrome)

Patient Reactions to a Colorectal Cancer Diagnosis

A CRC diagnosis can be very challenging for the patient. Some patients with CRC have found the following actions helpful for managing the difficult feelings they experienced after hearing of their diagnosis:

- Finding a physician that the patient feels comfortable with
- Working with the physician to establish a treatment plan, which helps the patient feel more settled and regain a sense of control over their life
- Trying to do as many usual activities as possible
- Joining CRC support group(s) though organizations such as www. CCAlliance.org, www.acor.org, www.cancercare.org, www.cancer.org, or www.fightcolorectalcancer.org

Survival Rates and Staging

According to the American Cancer Society (2011), only 39% of patients diagnosed with CRC between 1999 and 2006 had localized disease, for which the 5-year relative survival rate was 90%; 5-year relative survival rates for patients diagnosed with regional and distant CRC were 70% and 12%, respectively. The 5-year relative survival rate for CRC in general has increased from 51% for patients diagnosed in the mid-1970s to 67% for patients diagnosed between 1999 and 2006 (National Cancer Institute 2011). The following are 5-year relative survival rates according to the location of the cancer (Gatta et al. 2003):

- Rectum: 59%
- Right colon: 59%
- Transverse colon: 59%
- Rectosigmoid junction: 62%
- Ascending colon: 63%
- Left colon: 65%
- Descending colon: 66%

Stages are often labeled using Roman numerals I through IV. According to the American Joint Committee on Cancer (2009), CRC is staged as follows:

- Stage 0: very early cancer on the innermost layer of the intestine
- Stage I (T1-2, N0, M0): cancer is in the inner layers of the colon
- Stage II (T3-4b, N0, M0): cancer has spread through the muscle wall of the colon
- Stage III (any T, N1-N2a-b, M0): cancer has spread to the lymph nodes
- Stage IV (M1a-b with any T or N): cancer has spread to other organs

Treatment Modalities

Surgery

Surgery is the only definitive treatment modality for cure of nonmetastatic disease (stage I-III). For patients undergoing curative surgical resection of CRC, overall survival with surgery alone mimics that of the general population.

For surgically resectable metastatic lesions (limited in number, satisfactory organ preservation possible), a course of stage IV neoadjuvant chemotherapy or chemoradiation (for rectal cancer) is usually considered. Surgery can be performed safely 4 weeks after the last cycle of chemotherapy, assuming no anti–vascular endothelial growth factor (VEGF) agents were used (Van Cutsem et al. 2010).

Chemotherapy

Adjuvant chemotherapy for 6 months is indicated for stage III CRC but not for stage II CRC. However, chemotherapy may be considered for high-risk stage II CRC that includes any of the following: T4 primary tumor, histologic findings of poor differentiation, lymphovascular invasion, perineal invasion, bowel obstruction or perforation, fewer than 12 regional lymph nodes in the surgical specimen, positive margin(s), or microsatellite instability (Wolpin et al. 2007). Chemotherapy is also used to improve symptoms and prolong survival in patients with stage IV colon cancer.

Several chemotherapeutic agents are available for the treatment of metastatic CRC. Conventional agents include fluoropyrimidine, capecitabine (Xeloda), oxaliplatin, and irinotecan. Targeted agents include bevacizumab (anti-VEGF), cetuximab (HER monoclonal antibody), and panitumumab (HER monoclonal antibody).

Radiation

Radiation alone has a limited role in the treatment of CRC; it is usually combined with chemotherapy for patients with locally advanced rectal cancer. However, radiation may be used for palliation of metastases in certain locations, such as the sacrum or brain.

Chemoradiation

Patients with clinical stage II or stage III rectal cancer who underwent radiation therapy (45–50 Gy in 25–28 fractions of 1.8 Gy over a period of 5.5 weeks) and chemotherapy (fluorouracil or capecitabine) before surgery were found to have fewer problems after treatment was completed and a lower risk of cancer recurrence in the rectum than patients who underwent radiation and chemotherapy after surgery (Bosset et al. 2006). The patients who underwent neoadjuvant chemoradiation also underwent more sphincter-sparing procedures, experienced fewer toxic effects during therapy, and adhered better to the chemotherapy than patients in the other group.

Other

For patients with stage IV disease that has spread to the liver, various treatments other than surgery that are directed specifically at the liver can be used. These may include radiofrequency ablation. For additional details, see http://www.mdanderson.org/education-and-research/resources-for-professionals/clinical-tools-and-resources/practice-algorithms/ca-treatment-colon-web-algorithm.pdf.

Surveillance

The proportion of CRC patients undergoing resection with curative intent increased from 6.7% during the 1976–1984 period to 23.7% during the 1994–2003 period (P<0.001) for those with distant metastases and from 15.9% to 58.1% (P<0.001) for those with local recurrence (Guyot et al. 2005). According to another study, patients with hepatic CRC metastases detected at follow-up were significantly more likely to have a potentially curative operation than patients with hepatic CRC metastases who did not receive regular follow-up (Child et al. 2005).

In 2000, the American Society of Clinical Oncology (ASCO) introduced clinical practice guidelines for follow-up care and recurrence prevention for patients with stage II and III CRC (Benson et al. 2004). These guidelines were updated in 2005 (Desch et al. 2005). The ASCO Colon Cancer Survivorship Care Plan is a 1-page document that outlines the components of follow-up care (physician visit, carcinoembryonic antigen test, computed tomographic scan, and colonoscopy). Surveillance recommendations for colon (Table 6.2) and rectal (Table 6.3) cancer were developed at MD Anderson using the ASCO guidelines.

Genetic Tests Predicting Recurrence

Nonmetastatic Disease

Currently, about 75–85% of patients with stage II CRC can be cured with surgery alone (Donna 2007), but there is no way to identify these patients. Moreover, the absolute survival benefit of chemotherapy is relatively small, about 3–6%, whereas the risk of serious side effects is about 25% (Laino 2009). According to reports from the 45th annual ASCO meeting in 2009, new molecular tools can help physicians identify patients who might benefit most from chemotherapy. To date, 3 gene expression tests for CRC have been or are being studied: Oncotype DX (Genomic Health, Redwood City, CA), Coloprint (Agendia, Irvine, CA), and OncoDefender-CRC (Everist Genomics, Ann Arbor, MI). Oncotype DX is currently the only gene expression test out of the 3 that is approved by the US Food and Drug Administration (FDA).

Oncotype DX

The Oncotype DX colon cancer recurrence score for stage II cancer is calculated from the quantitated expression of seven recurrence genes and five reference genes in the tumor tissue and is expressed as an individual recurrence score ranging from 0 to 100 (Oncotype DX 2011). A linear relationship was demonstrated between the recurrence score and colon cancer recurrence risk in the QUASAR validation study (Kerr et al. 2009). The recurrence score also provides information about treatment outcome for patients with stage II and III CRC. In the NSABP C-07 study, it was suggested that the addition of oxaliplatin showed greater benefit in patients with high recurrence scores (i.e., >40%) than in patients with low recurrence scores (i.e., <30%).

Coloprint

Coloprint analyzes 18 genes, compared with 12 genes in Oncotype DX, and identifies patients as either high risk or low risk. In the first validation study, Coloprint was superior to the ASCO criteria in assessing the risk of cancer recurrence without prescreening for microsatellite instability (Salazar 2011).

Table 6.2 Colon cancer observation/surveillance recommendations used at MD Anderson

Surveillance technique	Stage I, stage II (low risk)	Stage II (high risk), stage III	Stage IV/no evidence of disease
Physical examination	Every 3–6 months for the first 2 years, then every 6 months for 3 years	Every 3 months for 3 years, then every 6 months for 2 years	Every 3–4 months for 2 years, then every 6 months for 3 years
Carcinoembryonic antigen test	Every 3–6 months for 1–2 years, then every 6 months for 3 years	Every 3 months for 3 years, then every 6 months for 2 years	Every 3–4 months for 3 years, then every 6 months for 3 years
Contrast-enhanced computed tomographic scan of the chest and contrast-enhanced computed tomographic scan or magnetic resonance imaging of the abdomen/pelvis	Every 12 months for 5 years	Every 12 months for 5 years	Every 3 months as needed to monitor therapy; upon reaching no evidence of disease, every 3–6 months for 2–3 years, then yearly as dictated by primary site, response, and site of metastasis if clinically appropriate
Colonoscopy	After 1 year, then (if normal) after 3 years, then every 5 years	After 1 year, then (if normal) after 3 years, then every 5 years	For patients with unresected, intact primary tumors, endoscopic surveillance is recommended every 3–6 months to ensure luminal patency

Table 6.3 Rectal cancer observation/surveillance recommendations used at MD Anderson

Surveillance technique	Stage I	Stage II (low risk)	Stage II (high risk), stage III	Stage IV/no evidence of disease
Physical examination	Every 3–6 months for 3 years, then every 6 months for 2 years	Every 3–6 months for 3 years, then every 6 months for 2 years	Every 3 months for 3 years, then every 6 months for 2 years	Every 3–4 months for 2 years, then every 6 months for 3 years
Carcinoembryonic antigen test	Every 3–6 months for 3 years, then every 6–12 months for 2 years	Every 3 months for 3 years, then every 6 months for 2 years	Every 3 months for 3 years, then every 6 months for 2 years	Every 3–4 months for 3 years, then every 6 months for 3 years
Contrast-enhanced computed tomographic scan of the chest and contrast-enhanced computed tomographic scan or magnetic resonance imaging of the abdomen/pelvis	Every 12 months for at least 3 years	Every 12 months for at least 5 years	Every 12 months for at least 5 years	Every 3 months; upon reaching no evidence of disease, every 6 months, then yearly as dictated by primary site, response, and site of metastasis if clinically appropriate
Proctoscopy	Every 6 months for 3 years, then every 6–12 months for 2 years	Every 6 months for 3 years, then every 6–12 months for 2 years	Every 6 months for 3 years, then every 6–12 months for 2 years	
Colonoscopy	After 1 year, then (if normal) after 3 years, then every 5 years	After 1 year, then (if normal) after 3 years, then every 5 years	After 1 year, then (if normal) after 3 years, then every 5 years	

OncoDefender-CRC

OncoDefender evaluates the expression levels of five specific genes (identified by Everist Genomics as predictors of recurrence). It is the only molecular prognostic test that can predict the risk of recurrence in patients with previously surgically treated stage I/II colon cancer and stage I rectal cancer (for stage I colon cancer: sensitivity 69%, specificity 88%, accuracy 79%; for stage II colon cancer: sensitivity 70%, specificity 55%, accuracy 61%).

Metastatic Disease

The *K-RAS* gene, a human homolog of the Kirsten rat sarcoma-2 virus oncogene, is linked with cellular signaling pathways, including those involving the epidermal growth factor receptor. A *K-RAS* mutation on codon 12 has been found to predict unresponsiveness to epidermal growth factor receptor–targeted monoclonal antibodies (cetuximab or panitumumab) in previously treated patients or in patients undergoing first-line therapy for metastatic CRC (Chang et al. 2009).

Quality of Life Management

Quality of life is generally measured by structured questionnaires that can be scored and quantified. For evaluating quality of life after surgery, the Functional Assessment of Cancer Therapy-Colorectal (FACT-C) questionnaire system is reliable and has been validated in patients with CRC. The European Organization for Research and Treatment questionnaire template (QLC-C30) is a more reliable and valid assessment of quality of life for patients with advanced disease than the FACT-C (Silpakit et al. 2006).

Surgery-Related Issues

Care of Stomata

For patients requiring a stoma, enterostomal therapists or surgical oncology staff nurses provide preoperative support, postoperative education, and state-of-the-art supplies (DeCosse and Cennerazzo 1997).

Most patients with left-sided or sigmoid colostomy learn to perform habitual stomal irrigation. Small security pads or pouches are available for use between irrigations (DeCosse and Cennerazzo 1997). Stomal irrigation is not advised if the patient is substantially obese, has poor vision, or has another disabling factor that limits or precludes personal stomal management (DeCosse and Cennerazzo 1997). Thin-walled translucent or opaque pouches adhere well and are secure, comfortable, odor-proof, non-irritating, and inconspicuous (DeCosse and Cennerazzo 1997). To ensure proper sealing on the cicatricial skin, strategic application of skin barrier paste and powder (Stomahesive) is useful (DeCosse and Cennerazzo 1997). Avoiding foods such as fish, onions, garlic, broccoli, asparagus, and cabbage and eating yogurt or drinking buttermilk may help reduce odor production. It is important that patients manage the stoma with reasonable efficiency because Medicare reimbursement is restricted and provision of stomal supplies is limited (DeCosse and Cennerazzo 1997).

Patients should call the doctor if one or more of the following symptoms occur (www.upmc.com):

- Purple, black, or white stoma
- Severe cramps lasting more than 6 hours
- Severe watery discharge from the stoma lasting more than 6 hours
- No output from the colostomy for 3 days
- Excessive bleeding from the stoma

Effects of Rectal Surgery

Unsurprisingly, all patients who undergo abdominoperineal resection tend to have a permanent stoma, and patients who undergo low anterior resection are more likely to have a stoma than patients who undergo high anterior resection (Engel et al. 2003). Patients who undergo low anterior resection also are usually less depressed and have better sexual function and social adaptation than patients who undergo high anterior resection (Engel et al. 2003). For patients who undergo a low rectal anastomosis, irregular bowel movements are common for weeks or even months after the surgery (DeCosse and Cennerazzo 1997).

Pelvic radiation therapy and temporary fecal diversion may contribute to a narrowed anastomosis that may require dilatation (DeCosse and Cennerazzo 1997). Bulk in the diet, with added fiber or with a psyllium hydrophilic mucilloid (Metamucil), helps keep bowel movements stable.

The current rate of urinary dysfunction after surgery for rectal cancer is between 30% and 70% (Calpista 2007). Several factors, aside from preservation of nerve fibers, are involved in the pathophysiology of mild urinary incontinence. Loss of sympathetic innervations owing to damage of the hypogastric nerve or parasympathetic innervations owing to damage of the sacral splanchnic plexus may be responsible for urgency or stress incontinence and sexual dysfunction. Sexual dysfunction is more difficult to assess in women. Following rectal surgery, many women experience dyspareunia and fear of stool leakage, both of which limit sexual activity. A nerve-sparing surgical approach to the rectum could minimize damage to the pelvic nerves, but this technique is difficult owing the complex anatomy of the various neural branches.

Table 6.4 Drugs used to treat symptoms commonly associated with chemotherapeutic agents (DeCosse and Cennerazzo 1997; Saif and Reardon 2005; Surjushe et al 2009; Laura 2010; Ocvirk and Cencelj 2010)

Symptom	Drug	Route
Mild nausea	Trimethobenzamide	Oral, rectal
	Prochlorparazine	Oral, rectal
	Lorazepam	Oral
Severe nausea	Granisetron	Intravenous
	Ondansetron	Oral, intravenous
Gastric stasis	Metoclopromide	Oral
	Cisapride	Oral
Diarrhea (fluorouracil, capecitabine, irinotecan)	Loperamide	Oral
	Attapulgite	Oral
	Diphenoxylate hydrochloride with sulfate	Oral
	Sandostatin	Intravenous
Peripheral neuropathy (oxaliplatin)	Glutathione	Intravenous
	Ca^{++}/Mg^{++}	Intravenous
	Carbamazepine	Oral
	Gabapentin	Oral
Mucositis (fluorouracil, capecitabine)	Magic brand mouth wash, analgesics, topical steroids	Topical, oral
Hand and foot syndrome (palmar-plantar erythrodysesthesia; capecitabine, fluorouracil)	Emollient, vitamin B_6	Topical
Acne-like rash (cetuximab)	Emollient, antibiotic	Topical

Chemotherapy-Related Issues

Anticancer agents may cause anemia, neutropenia, diarrhea, nausea, vomiting, hypertension, neuropathy, and anorexia; however, these toxic effects are often treatable.

Table 6.4 lists drugs that help control common problems associated with chemotherapeutics used to treat CRC. Uridine triacetate (Vistonuridine) has been used to treat fluorouracil and capecitabine overdose in cancer patients (Bamat 2011) under an FDA emergency-use Investigational New Drug waiver. Patients treated with uridine triacetate have fully recovered from the fluorouracil overdose even in cases in which a lethal outcome otherwise would have been expected.

According to the *Journal of Allergy and Clinical Immunology*, rapid desensitization has been safely and effectively used to treat oxaliplatin-induced allergic reactions.

Hematologic side effects, such as severe anemia and neutropenia, can hinder a patient's immune response and result in severe infection and can even be fatal. Such side effects can necessitate cessation of ongoing therapy. Erythropoietin, a glycoprotein that stimulates red blood cell production, can be used to treat anemia, and filgastrim, a granulocyte colony-stimulating factor, can be used to treat neutropenia. However, erythropoietin has been linked to an increased risk of thrombosis, and care should be taken when treating patients at risk for developing venous thromboembolism (Barbera and Thomas 2010).

The most common and significant side effect of bevacizumab is hypertension, which is caused by decreased production of nitric oxide, a potent vasodilator, through inhibition of VEGF. The decision to start standard antihypertensive medication(s) should be made on an individual basis, taking into consideration the presence of other risk factors for cardiovascular disease and the persistence of blood pressure readings above 150/100 mmHg (Arriaga and Becerra 2006). Angiotensin-converting enzyme inhibitors (e.g., enalapril, lisinopril) are recommended for the initial management of bevacizumab-induced hypertension.

Other side effects of bevacizumab include epistaxis, thrombosis, and gastrointestinal bleeding. Prophylactic anticoagulation is not recommended, and clinicians should consider the risk-benefit ratio when prescribing bevacizumab to patients at high risk for thrombotic events (age >65 years with a history of arterial thromboembolism; Arriaga and Becerra 2006). Patients taking bevacizumab should also talk to a health care provider before taking acetaminophen, aspirin, ibuprofen, ketoprofen, or naproxen (Stenerson 2009).

The following drugs may interact with capecitabine (Stenerson 2009): antacids with aluminum or magnesium, folic acid, leucovorin, medicines to increase blood counts, phenytoin, vaccines, and warfarin.

Radiation-Related Issues

Short-Term Effects

Potential side effects of pelvic radiation therapy include tenesmus, proctitis, diarrhea, intestinal obstruction, stricture, fistula, and dysuria during the course of the therapy. The addition of chemotherapy may increase the toxic effects (DeCosse and Cennerazzo 1997). About 3–5% of patients receiving therapeutic levels of pelvic radiation may require operative management (DeCosse and Cennerazzo 1997). Eating a nutritious diet is a very important way to manage these side effects.

Radiation-induced perianal dermatitis can be bothersome to the patient. Skin care after radiation therapy is advised as follows (DeCosse and Cennerazzo 1997):

- Use hydrophilic lubricants (e.g., Eucerin, Aquaphor, Lubriderm) two or three times per day on the irradiated areas
- Use ointments combined with vitamins A and D or zinc oxide to protect anal area if diarrhea is present
- Cleanse the perianal area with tepid water and pat dry after each bowel movement
- Wear cotton undergarments to reduce moisture build-up by allowing adequate air exchange

Long-Term Effects

Pelvic irradiation increases the risk of hip fractures in women aged 65 years or older (Baxter et al. 2005). Combined-modality therapies (i.e., chemoradiation) may exacerbate the toxic effects of radiation on bone density; medications and lack of estrogen may further contribute to the risk of osteoporosis. Therefore, bone density of CRC survivors should be monitored regularly and evaluated carefully when symptoms develop that suggest fractures.

Palliation

Palliation is defined by quality rather than by quantity of remaining life. Patients with incurable distal rectal cancer often have persistent bleeding, and the risks and morbidity of a palliative abdominoperineal resection may outweigh any benefits (DeCosse and Cennerazzo 1997). In the setting of pelvic recurrence, quality of life could be improved by pelvic exenteration in 88% of selected patients (Yeung et al. 1994).

Pain Management

Pain control is by far one of the most important quality-of-life issues for patients with recurrent CRC. Radiation therapy is considered the primary treatment for symptomatic pelvic and bone metastases of CRC.

The need for analgesics should be obvious. Anticholinergics are the preferable treatment for gastrointestinal spasm, and corticosteroids are useful for treating nerve pain. Policies for the control of chronic malignant pain are different from those for the control of acute pain. The following are important things to keep in mind when treating chronic malignant pain (DeCosse and Cennerazzo 1997):

- Morphine should be administered on a scheduled regimen with regular use of stool softeners
- Analgesics should be given sufficiently, despite risk of potential addiction
- Oral administration is preferable
- Nonsteroidal anti-inflammatory drugs, antidepressants, and corticosteroids should be used as additional support
- Titration of incremental doses should be considered until pain relief is achieved
- Transdermal patches are useful for maintenance but should not be used as initial therapy because their stickiness is limited by the amount of body hair and perspiration

Pregnancy

In general, pregnant patients with CRC present with more advanced disease than other patients, and the majority of pregnant patients die within 1 year of diagnosis; the estimated median survival duration is less than 5 months (Chan et al. 1999).

Clinicians should perform the diagnostic and prognostic tests outlined in Table 6.5. Surgery could be performed safely before 20 weeks of gestation when

Table 6.5 Special considerations for diagnostic and prognostic tools for colorectal cancer in pregnant patients (Minter et al 2005; Saif 2005)

Tool	Notes
Carcinoembryonic antigen test	Level not affected by pregnancy
Abdominal computed tomographic scan	Contraindicated in pregnancy, consider ultrasound
Magnetic resonance imaging	Avoids maternal and fetal exposure to ionizing radiation and is useful for assessment of maternal disease of the abdomen during pregnancy
Colonoscopy	Considered a relative contraindication in pregnancy; partial colonoscopy is often considered instead

appropriate (Cohen-Kerem et al. 2005). After 20 weeks of gestation, surgery should be delayed to allow reasonable maturation of the fetus (Yaghoobi et al. 2009). It has also been proposed that colon surgery can be performed immediately after an uncomplicated cesarean section.

Adjuvant chemotherapy is not indicated in the first trimester because of the potential teratogenic effects of fluorouracil (irinotecan may also harm a fetus), but it can be administered during the second and third trimesters (Cappell 1998). Oxaliplatin has been found to be useful for treating CRC in pregnant patients, but only during the second and third trimesters (Gensheimer et al. 2009). However, oxaliplatin can be considered during the first trimester in patients with meta-static disease and for high-risk groups. No adjuvant or neoadjuvant radiation is recommended during pregnancy until after delivery or elective abortion (Cappell 1998).

Following the surgery, the placenta should be thoroughly examined for metastasis. Breast feeding is contraindicated during anticancer chemotherapy.

Prevention of Recurrence

Current dietary and lifestyle recommendations for the prevention of CRC can be summarized as follows (American Cancer Society 2011): get screened regularly, maintain a healthy weight throughout life, adopt a physically active lifestyle, and consume a healthy diet with an emphasis on plant sources.

Diet

The following foods are recommended:

- High-fiber foods
- 5–8 servings of fruits and vegetables daily

- 100% whole-grain breads and pastas
- Dairy foods and vitamin D: assessment of a cohort from the National Cancer Institute–sponsored Polyp Prevention Trial (the Third National Health and Nutrition Examination Survey; Hartman et al. 2005; Freedman et al. 2007) showed that patients who had previously had one or more adenomas removed during a qualifying colonoscopy who had high vitamin D blood levels ($\geq$80 nmol/L) had a 72% lower risk of CRC-related death than those with low vitamin D blood levels (<50 nmol/L)
- Calcium: orally ingested calcium has been conjectured to lower the risk of colon cancer by binding bile acids and fatty acids, thereby reducing exposure to toxic intraluminal compounds
- Nuts and seeds
- Fish oil: 1–2 capsules or 1–3 tablespoons daily of omega-3 fatty acids is beneficial for patients with CRC (Daniel et al. 2009)

These foods should be avoided:

- High amounts of red meat and processed meat
- Meat from farms that use antibiotics, hormones, and large amounts of corn and soy feed
- Refined and processed grains and sugar
- Fried foods

Activity

Research supports a connection between exercise and cancer prevention. A study released in February 2009 showed that active individuals were 24% less likely to develop colon cancer than sedentary individuals. For patients with stage III CRC who survive and are recurrence-free approximately 6 months after completion of adjuvant chemotherapy, physical activity appears to reduce the risk of cancer recurrence and mortality (Meyerhardt et al. 2006). Recommended exercise can include walking, dancing, rollerblading, swimming, cycling, or team sports, after setting goals.

Alcohol and Tobacco

In a meta-analysis of eight cohort studies, the relative risk of developing CRC among those who consumed 45 g of alcohol per day (i.e., about 3 standard drinks per day) compared with nondrinkers was 1.41 (95% confidence interval, 1.16–1.72; Cho et al. 2004).

Cigarette smoking has been shown to be associated with an increased risk of colorectal adenoma and CRC (Pande et al. 2010). In the Cancer Prevention Study II, multivariate-adjusted CRC-related mortality rates were highest among current smokers, intermediate among former smokers, and lowest in nonsmokers, with an increased risk observed after 20 or more years of smoking in both men and women (Chao et al. 2000).

Aspirin

According to a 2011 analysis conducted by the National Cancer Institute, the 20-year hazard ratio for CRC-related mortality among patients in clinical trials who took aspirin for at least 5 years was 0.60 (95% confidence interval, 0.45–0.81; Rothwell et al. 2011).

Hormone Replacement Therapy

Various study results have suggested a decreased risk of colon cancer among users of postmenopausal female hormone supplements. However, most studies assessing risk of rectal cancer have shown no benefit or a slightly elevated risk of rectal cancer associated with hormone replacement therapy.

Physician Support

Physician support has been shown to be associated with low levels of patient distress and helplessness/hopelessness and a high level of "fighting spirit." However, physicians must be mindful of the problems they face when communicating bad news to their patients, including lack of sufficient time, difficulty being honest without causing distress, and challenges in dealing with patients' families, responding to patients' emotions, and discussing life expectancy.

Key Practice Points

- Active individuals are 24% less likely to develop colon cancer than sedentary individuals.
- For rectal cancer, preoperative magnetic resonance imaging or an endoscopic ultrasound is required to determine whether the patient clinically has high-risk stage II or stage III disease, in which case neoadjuvant chemoradiation is indicated.

- Prior colon resection does not preclude resection of hepatic or pulmonary metastatic CRC lesions.
- Stage II disease does not always require adjuvant chemotherapy or chemoradiation.
- *K-RAS* mutations on codon 12 indicate resistance to cetuximab and panitumumab.
- Sexual dysfunction is more difficult to assess in women.
- Pregnancy does not alter the carcinoembryonic antigen level.
- Aspirin may decrease CRC-related mortality.
- Orally ingested calcium lowers the risk of colon cancer by binding bile acids and fatty acids.
- Maintain optimal pain medication.

Acknowledgment We thank Jonathan Phillips, Department of Medical Oncology, for assisting us with editing this chapter.

Suggested Readings

Abdalla EK, Vauthey JN, Ellis L, et al. Recurrence and outcomes following hepatic resection, radiofrequency ablation, and combined resection/ablation for colorectal liver metastases. *Ann Surg* 2004;239(6):818–825.

Adam R, Avisar E, Ariche A, et al. Five-year survival following hepatic resection after neoadjuvant therapy for nonresectable colorectal cancer. *Ann Surg Oncol* 2001;8(4):347–353.

Alberts SR, Horvath WL, Sternfeld WC, et al. Oxaliplatin, fluorouracil, and leucovorin for patients with unresectable liver-only metastases from colorectal cancer: a North Central Cancer Treatment Group phase II study. *J Clin Oncol* 2005;23(36):9243–9249.

American Cancer Society. Colorectal cancer facts and figures 2011–2013. Atlanta: American Cancer Society; 2011.

American Joint Committee on Cancer. *Cancer Staging Manual*. 7th ed. Chicago: AJCC; 2009.

Arriaga Y, Becerra, CR. Adverse effects of bevacizumab and their management in solid tumors. *Support Cancer Ther* 2006;3(4):247–250.

American Society of Clinical Oncology. 2005 update of ASCO practice guideline recommendations for colorectal cancer surveillance: guideline summary. *JOP* 2005;1(4):137–139.

Baddi L, Benson A III. Adjuvant therapy in stage II colon cancer: current approaches. *The Oncologist* 2005;10(5):325–331.

Bamat M. Uridine triacetate: an orally administered, life-saving antidote for 5-FU overdose. *J Clin Oncol* 2011;28:15s.

Barbera L, Thomas G. Erythropoiesis stimulating agents, thrombosis and cancer. *Radiother Oncol* 2010;95(3):269–276.

Baxter NN, Habermann EB, Tepper JE, Durham SB, Virnig BA. Risk of pelvic fractures in older women following pelvic irradiation. *JAMA* 2005;294(20):2587–2593.

Benson AB III, Schrag D, Somerfield MR, et al. American Society of Clinical Oncology recommendations on adjuvant chemotherapy for stage II colon cancer. *J Clin Oncol* 2004;22(16):3408–3419.

Bosset JF, Collette L, Calais G, et al. Chemotherapy with preoperative radiotherapy in rectal cancer. *N Engl J Med* 2006;355(11):1114–1123.

Calder K, Pollitz K. What cancer survivors need to know about health insurance. http://www.
canceradvocacy.org/assets/documents/health-insurance-publication-2012.pdf.   Accessed
November 12, 2012.

Calpista A. Functional urological complications after colo-rectal cancer. *Pelviperineology*
2007;26:38–40.

Cappell MS. Colon cancer during pregnancy. The gastroenterologist's perspective. *Gastroenterol
Clin North Am* 1998;27(1):225–256.

Chan YM, Ngai SW, Lao TT. Colon cancer in pregnancy. A case report. *J Reprod Med*
1999;44(8):733–736.

Chang DZ, Kumar V, Ma Y, Li K, Kopetz S. Individualized therapies in colorectal cancer: KRAS
as a marker for response to EGFR-targeted therapy. *J Hematol Oncol* 2009;2:18.

Chao A, Thun MJ, Jacobs EJ, Henley SJ, Rodriguez C, Calle EE. Cigarette smoking and colorectal
cancer mortality in the cancer prevention study II. *J Natl Cancer Inst* 2000;92(23):1888–1896.

Child, PW, Yan TD, Perera DS, Morris DL. Surveillance-detected hepatic metastases from colorectal
cancer had a survival advantage in seven-year follow-up. *Dis Colon Rectum* 2005;48(4):744–748.

Cho E, Smith-Warner SA, Ritz J, et al. Alcohol intake and colorectal cancer: a pooled analysis of
8 cohort studies. *Ann Intern Med* 2004;140(8):603–613.

Cohen-Kerem R, Railton C, Oren D, Lishner M, Koren G. Pregnancy outcome following non-
obstetric surgical intervention. *Am J Surg* 2005;190(3):467–473.

Colon Cancer Alliance. Quality of life issues. http://www.ccalliance.org/issues/quality_ostomy.
html. Published 2012. Accessed November 12, 2012.

Daniel CR, McCullough ML, Patel RC, et al. Dietary intake of omega-6 and omega-3 fatty acids
and risk of colorectal cancer in a prospective cohort of U.S. men and women. *Cancer Epidemiol
Biomarkers Prev* 2009;18(2):516–525.

DeCosse JJ, Cennerazzo WJ. Quality-of-life management of patients with colorectal cancer.
CA Cancer J Clin 1997;47(4):198–206.

Denlinger CS, Barsevick AM. The challenges of colorectal cancer survivorship. *J Natl Compr
Canc Netw* 2009;7(8):883–893.

Desch CE, Benson AB III, Somerfield MR, et al. Colorectal cancer surveillance: 2005 update of an
American Society of Clinical Oncology practice guideline. *J Clin Oncol* 2005;23(33):8512–8519.

Donna M (2007). Colorectal cancer fast facts. http://coloncancer.about.com/od/fastfacts/a/FF_
CRC_Survival.htm. Published 2007. Accessed November 12, 2012.

Engel J, Kerr J, Schlesinger-Raab A, Eckel R, Sauer H, Holzel D. Quality of life in rectal cancer
patients: a four-year prospective study. *Ann Surg* 2003;238(2):203–213.

Freedman DM, Looker AC, Chang SC, Graubard BI. Prospective study of serum vitamin D and
cancer mortality in the United States. *J Natl Cancer Inst* 2007;99(21):1594–1602.

Gatta G, Ciccolallo L, Capocaccia R, et al. Differences in colorectal cancer survival between
European and US populations: the importance of sub-site and morphology. *Eur J Cancer*
2003;39(15):2214–2222.

Gensheimer M, Jones CA, Graves CR, Merchant NB, Lockhart AC. Administration of oxaliplatin
to a pregnant woman with rectal cancer. *Cancer Chemother Pharmacol* 2009;63(2):371–373.

Guyot F, Faivre J, Manfredi S, Meny B, Bonithon-Kopp C, Bouvier AM. Time trends in the treatment and survival of recurrences from colorectal cancer. *Ann Oncol* 2005;16(5):756–761.

Hartman TJ, Albert PS, Snyder K, et al. The association of calcium and vitamin D with risk of
colorectal adenomas. *J Nutr* 2005;135(2):252–259.

Johns LE, Houlston RS. A systemic review and meta-analysis of familial colorectal cancer.
Am J Gastroenterol 2001;96(10):1992–3003.

Kerr D, Gray R, Quirke P, et al. A quantitative multigene RT-PCR assay for prediction of recurrence in stage II colon cancer: selection of the genes in four large studies and results of the
independent, prospectively designed QUASAR validation study. *J Clin Oncol* 2009;27:15s
(suppl; abstract 4000).

Laino C. Gene test predicts colon cancer recurrence risk. *Oncology Times* 2009;6(7):14.

Laura D. Knocking out the side effects of colorectal cancer treatment. http://www.ccalliance.org/
treatment/side_effects_knockingout.html. Published 2010. Accessed November 12, 2012.

Meyerhardt JA, Heseltine D, Niedzwiecki D, et al. Impact of physical activity on cancer recurrence
and survival in patients with stage III colon cancer: findings from CALGB 89803. *J Clin Oncol*
2006;24(22):3535–3541.

Minter A, Malik R, Ledbetter L, Winokur TS, Hawn MT, Saif MW. Colon cancer in pregnancy. *Cancer Control* 2005;12(3):196–202.

National Cancer Institute. Surveillance Epidemiology and End Results (SEER) fact sheets: colon and rectum. http://seer.cancer.gov/statfacts/html/colorect.html. Published 2011. Accessed November 12, 2012.

National Coalition for Cancer Survivorship. Self advocacy: a cancer survivor's handbook. http://www.canceradvocacy.org/assets/documents/self-advocacy-publication.pdf. Published July 15, 2011. Accessed November 12, 2012.

Ocvirk J, Cencelj S. Management of cutaneous side-effects of cetuximab therapy in patients with metastatic colorectal cancer. *J Eur Acad Dermatol Venereol* 2010;24(4):453–459.

Pande M, Amos CI, Eng C, Frazier ML. Interactions between cigarette smoking and selected polymorphisms in xenobiotic metabolizing enzymes in risk for colorectal cancer: a case-only analysis. *Mol Carcinog* 2010;49(11):974–980.

Oncotype DX. Validated clinical benefits of the Onco*type* DX® colon cancer assay. http://www.oncotypedx.com/en-US/Colon/HealthcareProfessionals/ColonCancerAssay/ClinicalSummary. Published November 2011. Accessed November 2012.

Popat S, Hubner R, Houlston RS. Systematic review of microsatellite instability and colorectal cancer prognosis. *J Clin Oncol* 2005;23(3):609–618.

Rothwell PM, Fowkes FG, Belch JF, Ogawa H, Warlow CP, Meade TW. Effect of daily aspirin on long-term risk of death due to cancer: analysis of individual patient data from randomised trials. *Lancet* 2011;377(9759):31–41.

Saif MW. Management of colorectal cancer in pregnancy: a multimodality approach. *Clin Colorectal Cancer* 2005;5(4):247–256.

Saif MW, Reardon J. Management of oxaliplatin-induced peripheral neuropathy. *Ther Clin Risk Manag* 2005;1(4):249–258.

Salazar R. Gene expression signature to improve prognosis prediction of stage II and III colorectal cancer. *J Clin Oncol* 2011;29(1):17–24.

Silpakit C, Sirilerttrakul S, Jirajarus M, Sirisinha T, Sirachainan E, Ratanatharathorn V. The European Organization for Research and Treatment of Cancer Quality of Life Questionnaire (EORTC QLQ-C30): validation study of the Thai version. *Qual Life Res* 2006;15(1):167–172.

Stenerson M. Chemotherapy drugs list for colon cancer. http://www.coloncancerresource.com/chemotherapy-drugs-list.html. Published 2009. Accessed November 12, 2012.

Surjushe A, Vasani R, Medhekar S, Thakre M, Saple DG. Hand-foot syndrome due to capecitabine. *Indian J Dermat* 2009;54(3):301–302.

The University of Texas MD Anderson Cancer Center. Cancer survivorship. http://www.mdanderson.org/topics/survivorship. Published 2012. Accessed November 12, 2012.

Van Cutsem E, Nordlinger B, Cervantes A. Advanced colorectal cancer: ESMO Clinical Practice Guidelines for treatment. *Ann Oncol* 2010;21(Suppl 5):93–97.

Wolpin BM, Meyerhardt JA, Mamon HJ, Mayer RJ. Adjuvant treatment of colorectal cancer. *CA Cancer J Clin* 2007;57(3):168–185.

Yaghoobi M, Koren G, Nulman I. Challenges to diagnosing colorectal cancer during pregnancy. *Can Fam Physician* 2009;55(9):881–885.

Yeung RS, Moffat FL, Falk RE. Pelvic exenteration for recurrent colorectal carcinoma: a review. *Cancer Invest* 1994;12(2):176–188.

Survivorship Algorithms

These cancer survivorship algorithms have been specifically developed for MD Anderson using a multidisciplinary approach and taking into consideration circumstances particular to MD Anderson, including the following: MD Anderson's specific patient population, MD Anderson's services and structure, and MD Anderson's clinical information. These algorithms are provided for informational purposes only and are not intended to replace the independent medical or professional judgment of physicians or other health care providers. Moreover, these algorithms should not be used to treat pregnant women.

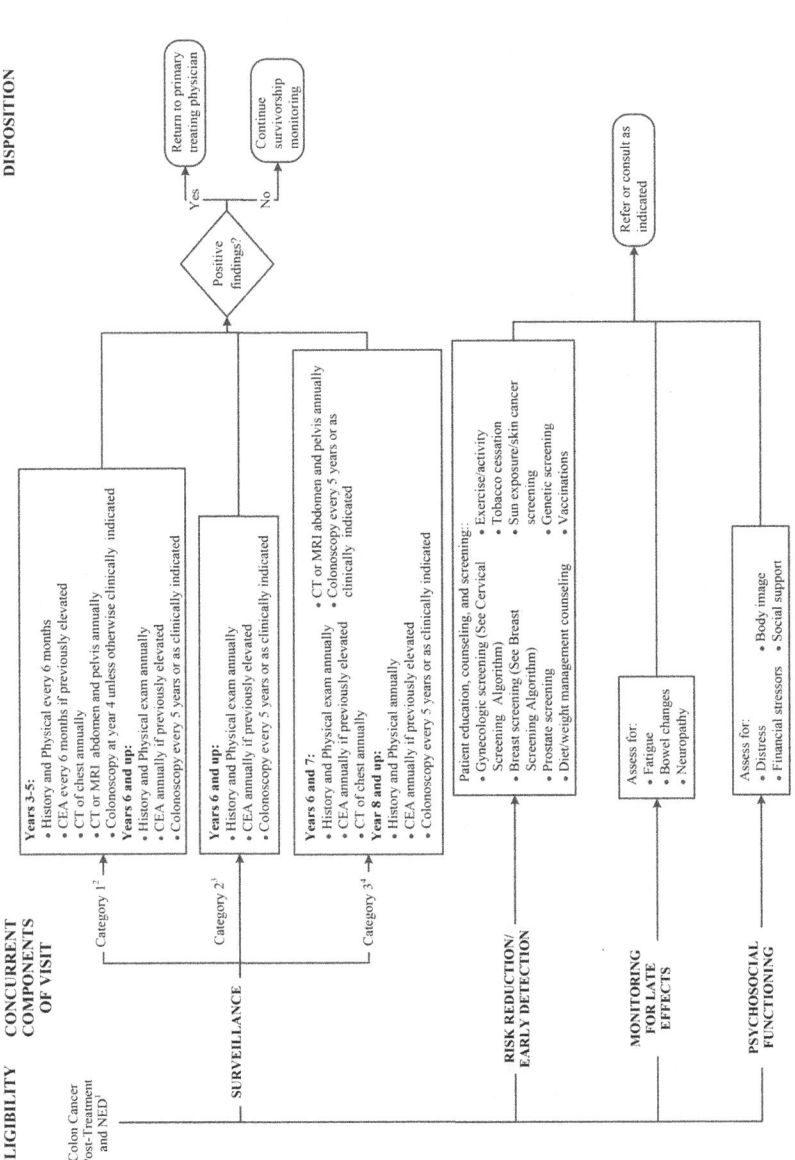

Algorithm 6.1a Survivorship—colon cancer (page 1)

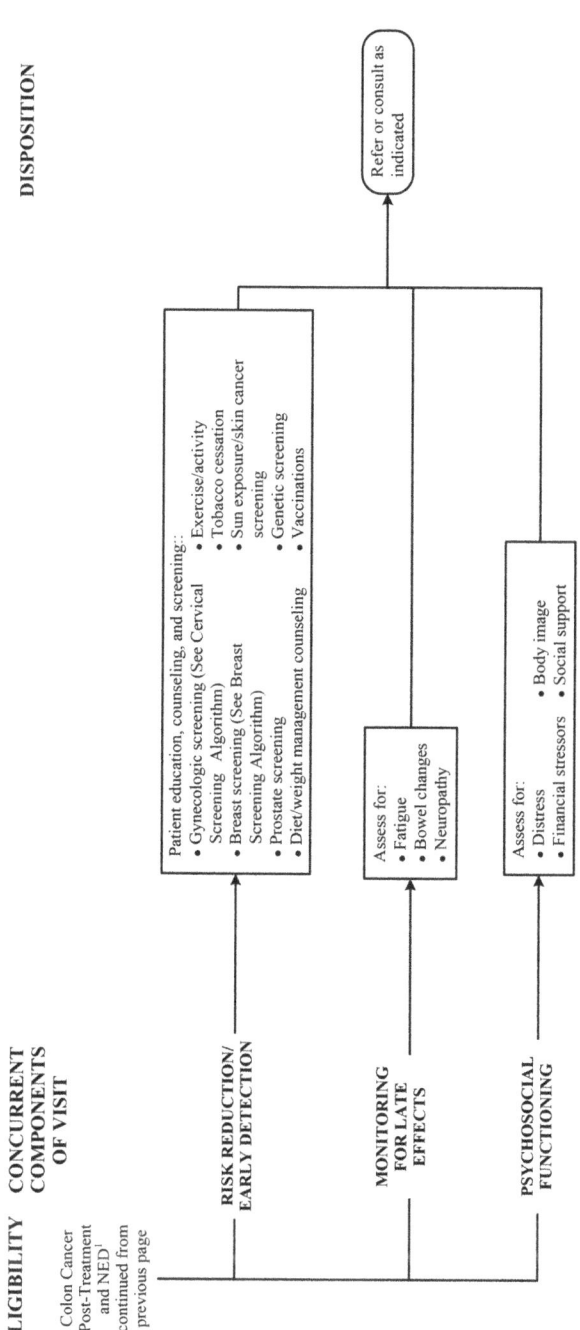

DISPOSITION

Refer or consult as indicated

ELIGIBILITY

Colon Cancer Post-Treatment and NED[1] continued from previous page

CONCURRENT COMPONENTS OF VISIT

RISK REDUCTION/ EARLY DETECTION

Patient education, counseling, and screening::
- Gynecologic screening (See Cervical Screening Algorithm)
- Breast screening (See Breast Screening Algorithm)
- Prostate screening
- Diet/weight management counseling
- Exercise/activity
- Tobacco cessation
- Sun exposure/skin cancer screening
- Genetic screening
- Vaccinations

MONITORING FOR LATE EFFECTS

Assess for:
- Fatigue
- Bowel changes
- Neuropathy

PSYCHOSOCIAL FUNCTIONING

Assess for:
- Distress
- Financial stressors
- Body image
- Social support

[1]NED = No Evidence of Disease

Department of Clinical Effectiveness V1
Approved by The Executive Committee of the Medical Staff 11/29/2011

Algorithm 6.1b Survivorship—colon cancer (page 2)

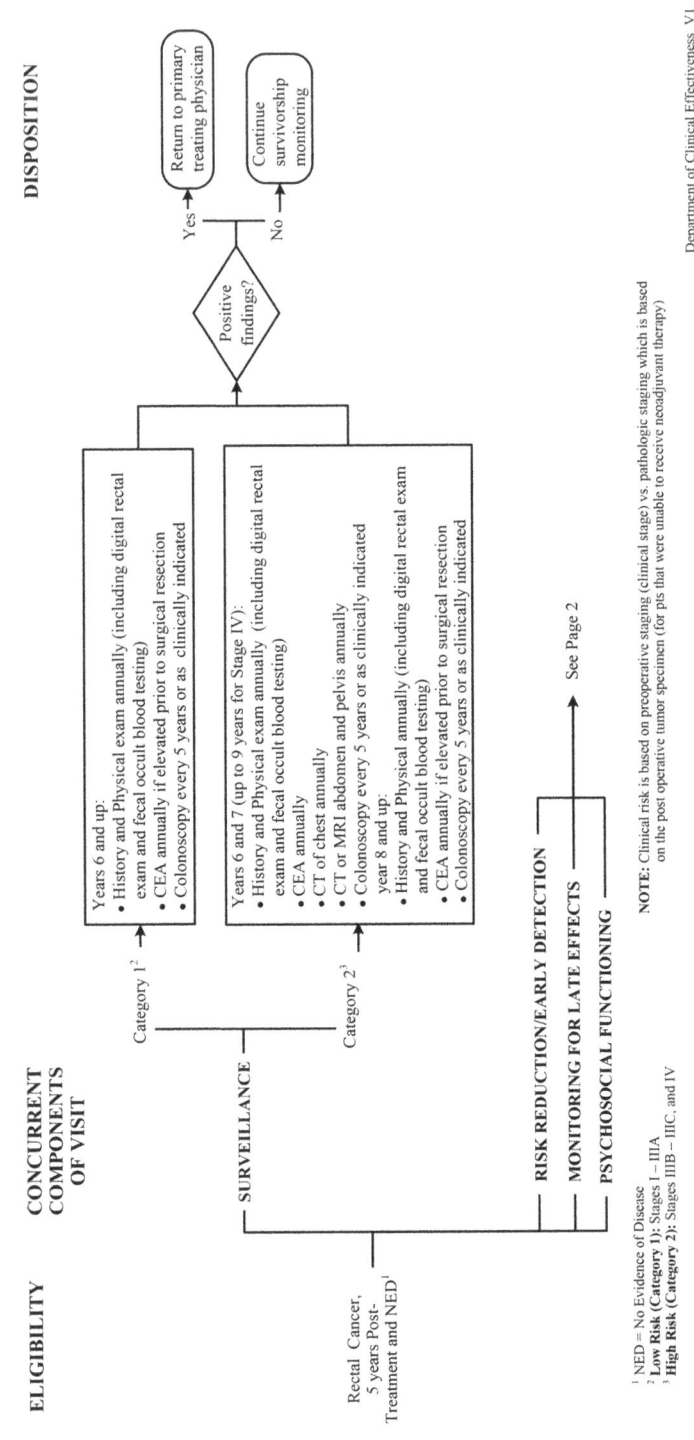

ELIGIBILITY

CONCURRENT COMPONENTS OF VISIT

DISPOSITION

Rectal Cancer, 5 years Post-Treatment and NED[1]

SURVEILLANCE

Category 1[2]

Years 6 and up:
- History and Physical exam annually (including digital rectal exam and fecal occult blood testing)
- CEA annually if elevated prior to surgical resection
- Colonoscopy every 5 years or as clinically indicated

Category 2[3]

Years 6 and 7 (up to 9 years for Stage IV):
- History and Physical exam annually (including digital rectal exam and fecal occult blood testing)
- CEA annually
- CT of chest annually
- CT or MRI abdomen and pelvis annually
- Colonoscopy every 5 years or as clinically indicated

year 8 and up:
- History and Physical annually (including digital rectal exam and fecal occult blood testing)
- CEA annually if elevated prior to surgical resection
- Colonoscopy every 5 years or as clinically indicated

RISK REDUCTION/EARLY DETECTION

MONITORING FOR LATE EFFECTS

PSYCHOSOCIAL FUNCTIONING

See Page 2

Positive findings?

Yes → Return to primary treating physician

No → Continue survivorship monitoring

NOTE: Clinical risk is based on preoperative staging (clinical stage) vs. pathologic staging which is based on the post operative tumor specimen (for pts that were unable to receive neoadjuvant therapy)

[1] NED = No Evidence of Disease
[2] **Low Risk (Category 1):** Stages I – IIIA
[3] **High Risk (Category 2):** Stages IIIB – IIIC, and IV

Department of Clinical Effectiveness V1
Approved by The Executive Committee of the Medical Staff 11/29/2011

Algorithm 6.2a Survivorship—rectal cancer (page 1)

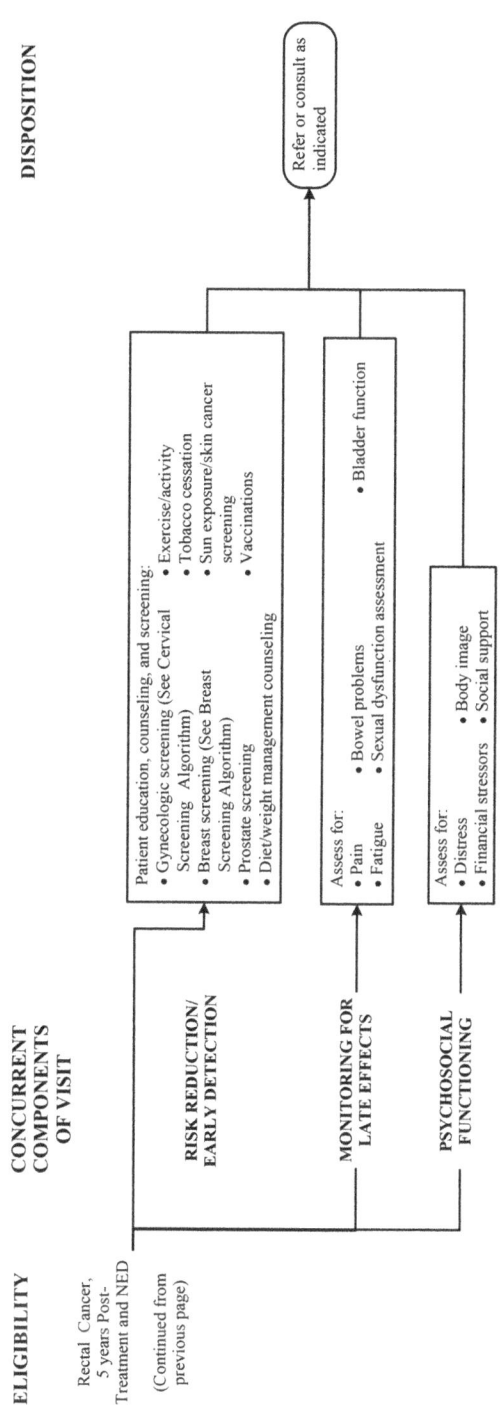

DISPOSITION

Refer or consult as indicated

CONCURRENT COMPONENTS OF VISIT

ELIGIBILITY

Rectal Cancer, 5 years Post-Treatment and NED

(Continued from previous page)

RISK REDUCTION/ EARLY DETECTION

Patient education, counseling, and screening:
- Gynecologic screening (See Cervical Screening Algorithm)
- Breast screening (See Breast Screening Algorithm)
- Prostate screening
- Diet/weight management counseling
- Exercise/activity
- Tobacco cessation
- Sun exposure/skin cancer screening
- Vaccinations

MONITORING FOR LATE EFFECTS

Assess for:
- Pain
- Fatigue
- Bowel problems
- Sexual dysfunction assessment
- Bladder function

PSYCHOSOCIAL FUNCTIONING

Assess for:
- Distress
- Financial stressors
- Body image
- Social support

[1]NED = No Evidence of Disease

Copyright 2011 The University of Texas MD Anderson Cancer Center

Department of Clinical Effectiveness V1
Approved by The Executive Committee of the Medical Staff 11/29/2011

Algorithm 6.2b Survivorship—rectal cancer (page 2)

Chapter 7
Genitourinary Cancer Survivorship Management

Marcia L. Patterson, John W. Davis, Jeri Kim, Karen E. Hoffman, William E. Osai, and Deborah A. Kuban

Contents

L.E. Foxhall, M.A. Rodriguez (eds.), *Advances in Cancer Survivorship Management*,
MD Anderson Cancer Care Series, DOI 10.1007/978-1-4939-0986-5_7,
© The University of Texas M.D. Anderson Cancer Center 2015

Chapter Overview Genitourinary (GU) cancer encompasses several cancers, occurring in both the young and the old, and affecting predominantly men. Survivors of GU cancers constitute more than 50% of male cancer survivors, and primary care clinicians and specialists will likely see an increasing number of GU cancer survivors in their practice. Long-term cancer survivors have ongoing needs, and evidence-based guidelines can assist busy clinicians in understanding and confidently managing these needs. This chapter summarizes the needs of long-term GU cancer survivors, using evidence-based cancer-specific algorithms. The algorithms were developed for the purpose of addressing the many needs of long-term survivors, on the basis of the Institute of Medicine's survivorship model of care.

Introduction

Genitourinary (GU) cancer is a diverse group of diseases that includes prostate, testicular, bladder, kidney, and penile cancer. The population affected is heterogeneous in terms of age at diagnosis, risk factors, treatment, and prognosis, although the most common characteristic is male sex. According to the Institute of Medicine (Hewitt et al. 2005), more than 50% of male cancer survivors are survivors of GU cancer. The high rate of GU cancer survivorship is a testament to the success of treatment modalities, but long-term monitoring of these patients presents a challenge for two main reasons: (1) a broad knowledge base is needed because of the heterogeneity of GU cancers, and (2) recommendations for surveillance beyond 3 years are inconsistent or lacking and fail to address quality-of-life issues and management of late effects specific to each type of cancer (Hewitt et al. 2005).

    The GU survivorship clinical practice algorithms included with this chapter provide an evidence-based standard of care for long-term survivors of GU cancer who have completed treatment at least 2–5 years previously and show no evidence of recurrent disease. The algorithms were developed by translating existing evidence into recommendations under four concurrent components of the survivorship visit. A more detailed description of the models of care can be found in Chap. 2. A discussion of each disease-specific algorithm will be the focus of the remainder of this chapter.

Kidney Cancer (Renal Cell Carcinoma)

Renal cell carcinoma (RCC) accounts for up to 90% of kidney cancer. Several histologic types of RCC exist, but 85% are classified as clear cell carcinoma (DeVita et al. 2008). Other histologic types include papillary, chromophobe, and collecting duct; sarcomatoid differentiation is associated with poor outcome (National Comprehensive Cancer Network 2011). RCC incidence has steadily increased since 1975, and the increase is attributed mostly to early-stage disease found incidentally (National Cancer Institute 2011). Environmental risk factors include tobacco use, obesity, and hypertension. Hereditary conditions such as Von Hippel-Lindau disease account for only a small percentage of RCC diagnoses (American Cancer Society 2012).

Surgical resection of the primary tumor remains the standard of care for localized tumors, and this treatment results in cure for most low-grade, early-stage tumors. Radical nephrectomy, used to treat locally advanced tumors, involves removal of the kidney, adrenal gland, perirenal fat, and Gerota fascia. Nephron-sparing partial nephrectomy is performed in select cases. Lymphadenectomy may also be performed (National Cancer Institute 2011). Newer, less invasive surgical approaches such as radiofrequency ablation and cryotherapy are offered to some patients, especially those for whom a traditional surgical approach is too risky.

Prognosis with RCC is inversely correlated with both stage and grade at diagnosis. Five-year overall survival rates with RCC range from 5% to 94%, depending on stage, histologic findings, and source of the malignancy (Chin et al. 2006). The Fuhrman nuclear grading system is used to grade clear cell tumor morphology. Grades range from 1 to 4, and grade is inversely correlated with prognosis independent of stage (Chin et al. 2006). The University of California Los Angeles Integrated Staging System is a validated system that places patients into low-, intermediate-, and high-risk categories on the basis of tumor stage and grade.

Surveillance and Eligibility for Care at the MD Anderson Survivorship Clinic

Most patients who are eligible for care in our survivorship clinic have been treated definitively with partial or radical nephrectomy. However, a few patients have been treated with systemic therapy such as interferon, interleukin-2, or, more recently, molecular targeted therapies. Patients with hereditary RCC (Von Hippel-Lindau disease) are not eligible because of the high recurrence rate associated with this disease. Patients whose primary treatment modality was an ablative therapy are also not eligible because of the lack of reported 5-year survival and recurrence rates associated with this treatment. Although cases of late metastases from RCC are documented, 93% of recurrences occur within 5 years of nephrectomy. The most common metastatic sites are lungs, bones, liver, and renal fossa (Shuch et al. 2012). Lung lesions and local recurrence can be detected by imaging of the chest and abdomen. Liver metastases can be diagnosed by findings on computed tomographic (CT) imaging and elevated transaminases or bilirubin levels. Bone metastases most often occur within the first 3 years after completion of treatment and generally manifest as pain and elevated alkaline phosphatase levels. Therefore, routine surveillance of bones is not recommended for long-term survivors of RCC (Chin et al. 2006; Shuch et al. 2012).

The role of CT imaging during the long-term phase of survivorship is not as clear as it is in the first 2–3 years after therapy, when the risk of recurrence is much higher. The risks of CT imaging must be balanced by its contribution to the management of recurrences and complications because the cumulative dose of radiation from frequent CTs can be significant, especially in young patients. Additionally, the nephrotoxic effect of contrast dye in a patient with a solitary kidney must be considered, as well as the unnecessary expense and anxiety created from false positive findings. The type and frequency of diagnostic studies recommended in the algorithm are therefore based on risk of recurrence and metastatic patterns of RCC, as well as potential late effects of treatment.

Annual visits are recommended between years 5 and 15 after treatment is completed, and during each visit a thorough history and physical examination is essential. Although occult metastases can occur in the absence of symptoms, many patients with recurrence have constitutional or organ-specific symptoms. A CT scan is omitted in patients with low-grade, low-risk T1 tumors. After year 10, imaging is performed only as clinically indicated.

Late Effects: Monitoring and Management

Renal insufficiency is the main adverse effect of treatment because most patients undergo nephrectomy as the primary therapy. Even when creatinine levels are normal, a patient with a solitary kidney is at risk for renal compromise if exposed to certain conditions. The patient must be educated regarding his or her role in the prevention and management of this lifelong treatment effect. Nephrotoxic medications are particularly dangerous, and patients must be instructed to minimize or avoid use of nonsteroidal anti-inflammatory drugs. Depending on the glomerular filtration rate, medications for the treatment of intercurrent illnesses and chronic conditions may require dose reduction.

Blood pressure control is imperative. Hypertension can be prevented through lifestyle modification but may require pharmacotherapy. Weight management protects renal function, not only directly through reduction in body mass, but also by reducing the risk of diseases such as diabetes and hypertension that are associated with kidney disease. Adequate hydration is also important, especially if the patient must undergo diagnostic studies that use nephrotoxic contrast media. Renal function is easily monitored by annual laboratory testing of blood urea nitrogen and creatinine. Many patients with kidney cancer have a significant comorbidity that already predisposes them to renal dysfunction, and after nephrectomy, they often meet the criteria for stage II–III chronic kidney disease (Chapman et al. 2010). These patients need more frequent creatinine monitoring and may require referral to a nephrologist. Systemic therapy such as interferon, interleukin-2, and, more recently, molecular targeted therapies are generally reserved for patients with advanced RCC. In the rare case that a patient is disease-free 5 years after chemotherapy, he or she will likely require surveillance that exceeds the recommendations of the current kidney cancer survivorship algorithm.

Urothelial Cancer: Bladder/Ureter/Renal Pelvis

Urothelial cell carcinoma of the bladder (transitional cell carcinoma) is associated with a wide variety of clinical behaviors and responses to treatment. In simple terms, the disease is categorized into a low-grade/low-stage "superficial" form and a high-grade/progressive-stage form. The superficial form is more of a nuisance cancer in that cystoscopic resection is generally successful, but recurrent tumors are common, requiring surveillance with periodic cystoscopy.

For patients with invasive disease who undergo extirpation of the bladder, recurrence and progression are significant problems, occurring in approximately 50% of patients by 2 years after surgery. Recurrence beyond 2 years is increasingly uncommon. Patients undergoing cystectomy also undergo a pelvic lymph node dissection and a urinary diversion. Urinary diversions can be categorized in three common categories: conduit (incontinent), continent catheterizable reservoir, and continent neobladder.

Surveillance and Eligibility for Care at the MD Anderson Survivorship Clinic

Patients with superficial bladder cancer are not eligible for the survivorship care outlined in bladder/ureter/renal pelvis cancer survivorship algorithm (presented at the end of the chapter) owing to the nature of recurrences and need for frequent endoscopic surveillance. Most patients entering the survivorship clinic have been treated definitively with cystectomy and urinary diversion. A small percentage of patients have received systemic chemotherapy in the adjuvant or neoadjuvant setting. Annual surveillance recommendations take into account the probability and locations of disease recurrence, with the goal of optimizing quality of life and managing possible deterioration of renal function or metabolic abnormalities from the urinary diversion.

Metastatic recurrence is very rare at 5 or more years after completion of treatment, and follow-up should emphasize functional status (Jaske et al. 2006). New primary urothelial tumors may occur in the upper tract or retained urethra; however, vigorous imaging-based screening is of unclear benefit as opposed to standard evaluation for bleeding or other clinical presentations (Sanderson and Roupret 2007). In a review by Studer et al. (2006), urethral recurrence after orthotopic substitution occurred in 25 (5%) of 482 cases, with a median time to recurrence of 14 months (range 3–158 months). Upper tract recurrence was diagnosed in 15 (3%) of 482 cases at a median of 31 months (range 12–72 months). Intravenous pyelogram is recommended every other year between years 5 and 10 after completion of treatment for monitoring and management of functional issues and new upper tract lesions, with the addition of a CT urogram if clinically indicated. The diagnostic yield of urine cytology is controversial, but urine cytology remains the standard of care in most guidelines (National Comprehensive Cancer Network 2011).

It is also noteworthy that the most common risk factor for bladder cancer is smoking, and therefore survivors of this disease may experience additional smoking-related health concerns and cessation needs.

Late Effects: Monitoring and Management

Although cancer recurrence is not anticipated after 5 years, declining functional status, stoma issues, and bowel complications may occur. The simplest form of urinary diversion is the ileal conduit, in which the ureters are attached to a 15–20-cm isolated segment of the distal ileum and the distal end is exteriorized as an incontinent diversion to an external appliance. Madersbacher et al. (2003) reported that the overall conduit-related complication rate was 66%. The 5-year complication rate was 45%, but this increased to 50% at 10 years, 54% at 15 years, and 94% at more than 15 years after surgery. The main causes of complications were upper tract changes (hydronephrosis) and urolithiasis. For stoma-related problems (e.g., hernia), the median time to development of the complication was 54 months (range 4–274 months); most occurred within the first 5 years. However, stomal stenosis occurred in 6% of patients in this series. Bowel-related complications also occurred mostly within the first 5 years.

Shimko et al. (2011) analyzed another large single-institution cohort of 1,057 patients who underwent either ileal or colonic conduit urinary diversion. The cumulative rate of complications was 60.8% (643 patients), and 1,453 complications were attributable to the conduit. Incidence rates for complications were as follows: bowel, 20.3%; renal, 20.2%; infectious, 16.5%; stomal, 15.4%; urolithiasis, 15.3%; metabolic, 12.8%; and hydronephrosis, 11.5%. In terms of follow-up length, of 276 patients surviving for more than 5 years after surgery without complications, 116 (42%) eventually experienced a complication. Renal replacement therapy was necessary in 26 patients (2.5%) at a median of 8.4 years (range 0.9–23.5 years), and another 22 patients (2.1%) experienced loss of a functional renal unit at a median of 2.4 years (range 0.2–23.5 years).

Patients selected for orthotopic neobladder urinary diversion are generally younger and more fit than those who undergo ileal conduit urinary diversion. However, stage of disease and predicted survival are not necessarily the driving selection factors; younger patients are less likely to suffer adverse effects from complications of the procedure. Therefore, non–disease-related mortality rates may be decreased in the short term by selecting younger patients. Both populations (i.e., those who undergo neobladder urinary diversion and those who undergo ileal conduit urinary diversion) also undergo a significant primary surgery to remove the bladder and stage the lymph nodes, and in both populations, the bowel is reconstructed and subject to leakage, fistula, and obstruction at any time in the future. The key difference is that approximately 40 additional centimeters of ileum are harvested for a neobladder urinary diversion.

Long-term and short-term metabolic changes occur after a urinary diversion procedure. The extent of these changes depends on the type of procedure and length of bowel used for the diversion. In Studer et al. (2006), a common postoperative management decision for patients who underwent an ileal neobladder urinary diversion was administration of 2–6 g of oral sodium bicarbonate daily to prevent acidosis. Rehospitalization occurred in 30 (6.2%) of 482 patients. Of the patients surviving beyond 10 years after surgery, none had to continue the bicarbonate therapy. Patients surviving 15–20 years after surgery had bone densities matching those of age-matched controls. Vitamin B12 levels were subnormal in 37 (12%) of 314 patients, and 15 (5%) received vitamin B12 replacement therapy. Comparing two series from the same surgeon (Madersbacher et al. 2003; Studer et al. 2006), one could conclude that the upper tract preservation and metabolic acid disturbance rates were not significantly different between the two urinary diversion techniques. Choice of the neobladder construction technique or ileal conduit diversion is a matter of surgeon preference and training, in addition to patient preference. Regardless of the surgical technique used, clinicians should monitor patients for bone demineralization, electrolyte imbalance, and bowel symptoms if clinically indicated.

In general, urinary continence is satisfactory after neobladder urinary diversion, but never as good as prior to surgery. In the Studer series (Studer et al. 2006), overall daytime continence was 92%, achieving a plateau at 12 months and remaining stable for 7 years. Nighttime continence rates were lower—79%—and many used an alarm clock to ensure at least one nighttime void. Hypercontinence is possible, especially in woman undergoing a neobladder urinary diversion. In the Studer series, 7% of patients used intermittent self-catheterization or an indwelling catheter.

Erectile function rates are difficult to capture in patients with urothelial cancer owing to multiple comorbidities and age. In the Studer series, 99 (22.4%) of 442 evaluable men reported at least one successful erection without medical assistance and 68 (15.4%) reported at least one with medical assistance. In clinical practice, many patients with aggressive disease are not selected for a nerve-sparing procedure, and therefore support for erectile dysfunction needs should be anticipated (see Chap. 25 on sexuality).

Some patients receive chemotherapy, generally platinum-based. These patients may experience long-term effects such as prolonged bone marrow suppression, peripheral neuropathy, or renal insufficiency, and symptoms should be managed accordingly. The algorithm recommends annual blood urea nitrogen and creatinine testing; an annual complete blood count is also reasonable for monitoring purposes.

Urothelial Cancer: Upper Tract

Patients surviving upper tract urothelial cancer show a heterogeneous range of outcomes. Their follow-up issues reported more than 5 years after completion of treatment are not significantly different from those of patients with RCC who undergo nephrectomy, and most issues involve management of the remaining renal unit. Before the 5-year mark, patients undergo frequent cystoscopic evaluations of the bladder because bladder recurrence may be as high as 50%. For patients with high-grade tumors, management is similar but is more likely to involve definitive resection if the patient has a normal contralateral kidney. Many of these procedures are performed using laparoscopic techniques, and the time-honored tradition is to resect the entire ureter and a cuff of bladder where the ureter enters. Muntener et al. (2007) reviewed a contemporary series of upper tract disease managed with laparoscopic techniques and found that the overall results were similar to those in patients undergoing open surgery.

Appropriate surveillance and care for survivors of transitional cell carcinoma of the upper tract is covered by the bladder/ureter/renal pelvis cancer survivorship algorithm. Surveillance tests for transitional cell carcinoma of the upper tract from years 5 through 20 after completion of treatment parallel surveillance tests for bladder cancer, with the addition of annual monitoring of electrolyte levels. The late effects of treatment are similar to those noted in the kidney cancer survivorship algorithm.

Prostate Cancer

Prostate cancer is the second-most common cancer diagnosed in men worldwide and is the most common cancer diagnosed in men in developed countries (Jemal et al. 2011). In 2013, an estimated 238,590 men will be diagnosed with prostate cancer in the United States and 39,720 men will die from the disease (American Cancer Society 2012). Since the introduction of prostate specific antigen (PSA) screening in the early 1990s, most men with prostate cancer are diagnosed with disease that has not spread beyond the prostate and immediately surrounding tissue. Men with clinically localized disease are categorized into low-, intermediate-, and high-risk groups on the basis of tumor (T) stage, Gleason score, and PSA level. Treatment decisions are guided by extent of disease, other medical conditions, and patient preference. Common treatments for prostate cancer include active surveillance, surgical resection, brachytherapy, external beam radiation therapy, and androgen deprivation therapy. Some men receive treatment that combines two or more of these treatment modalities.

Survival after treatment is typically long-term. For all stages, the 5-year survival rate is 99%, the 10-year survival rate is 95%, and the 15-year survival rate is 82%

(American Cancer Society 2012). Because of the long-term survival, men often live with the medical and psychosocial effects of treatment for multiple decades. The likelihood and character of medical late effects of treatment vary with the treatment received; late effects may include urinary incontinence, rectal bleeding, and impotence.

Surveillance and Eligibility for Care at the MD Anderson Survivorship Clinic

The prostate cancer survivorship algorithm (presented at the end of the chapter) addresses care of men who have completed treatment for prostate cancer at least 2 years previously and show no evidence of disease. To be eligible for care at the survivorship clinic, men who underwent prostatectomy must have a PSA level of less than 0.1 ng/ml and men who received radiation therapy must have a PSA level of less than 1.0 ng/ml that is not rising.

Prostate cancer survivors are evaluated annually for disease recurrence, late effects of treatment, and psychosocial distress. Although most men treated for localized prostate cancer do not develop recurrent disease, recurrence can arise many years after treatment. Men with high-risk features at initial diagnosis are at increased risk for disease recurrence, but all men should be followed for possible recurrence because early detection and treatment of recurrence may improve outcomes.

At the annual evaluation, clinicians should perform a general physical examination and digital rectal examination and determine PSA levels to evaluate for disease recurrence. Testosterone levels are determined for select men if clinically indicated, including men whose testosterone level did not return to normal after androgen deprivation therapy. A rise in PSA levels or an abnormal digital rectal examination may trigger further diagnostic workup. If the patient is found to have recurrent disease, he should be referred back to his primary treating oncologist.

Late Effects: Monitoring and Management

Because the survival duration after prostate cancer is typically long, men can live with the late effects of treatment for multiple decades. Medical late effects of treatment include sexual, urinary, and bowel dysfunction. The likelihood and character of late effects depend on the treatment. Men who underwent prostatectomy are more likely to have urinary incontinence, whereas men who received radiation therapy are more likely to have rectal symptoms (Sanda et al. 2008). In addition to undergoing assessment of potential sexual, urinary, and bowel late effects of treatment, men who received androgen deprivation therapy should be evaluated for possible bone and endocrine effects of therapy.

Erectile Dysfunction

Sexual dysfunction, both erectile and orgasmic, is common after both prostatectomy and radiation therapy (Penson et al. 2003). Please see Chap. 25 on sexuality for more information about the treatment of erectile and orgasmic dysfunction. Therapy for erectile dysfunction includes phosphodiesterase-5 inhibitors, penile self-injection programs with vasoactive drugs, vacuum erection devices, and penile prosthesis.

Postsurgical Incontinence

Reported post-prostatectomy incontinence rates vary. Generally, less than 10% of men experience significant urinary incontinence, but a larger proportion of men have stress urinary incontinence or require pads for protection (Wilson and Gilling 2011). Additional improvement in urinary control is unlikely more than 2 years after surgery. Men with bothersome incontinence may be eligible for surgical interventions, including an artificial urinary sphincter or a bulbourethral sling.

Lower Urinary Tract Symptoms

Men who received radiation therapy may exhibit lower urinary tract symptoms, either urinary obstruction (because they still have a prostate in place) or overactive bladder. Men who underwent prostatectomy may also experience lower urinary tract symptoms from an overactive bladder. If symptoms are from bladder outlet obstruction, patients may be treated with alpha blockers or 5-alpha reductase inhibitors, keeping in mind the impact of 5-alpha reductase inhibitors on the interpretation of PSA values. Similarly, anticholinergic agents can be considered for men with an overactive bladder, keeping in mind the side effect profile of anticholinergic medications in elderly individuals.

Although uncommon, urinary stricture can develop after radiation therapy or after prostatectomy. Symptoms include decreased strength of urinary stream that can progress to urinary obstruction or urinary retention. Survivors with urinary stricture should be referred to a urologist for evaluation and treatment. Another rare late side effect of radiation therapy is radiation cystitis, which often presents as hematuria.

Rectal Symptoms

Chronic radiation proctitis can develop any time after radiation therapy, resulting in rectal irritation or urgency and the presence of mucous or blood in the stool. With modern radiation techniques and dose constraints, less than 10% of men are expected to develop significant rectal bleeding (Pederson et al. 2012). Initial treatment for proctitis symptoms is often steroid suppositories. If symptoms persist or recur, colonoscopy and consideration of additional therapies such as argon plasma coagulation is necessary.

Late Effects of Hormonal Therapy

Men who received androgen deprivation therapy as a component of their treatment need to be monitored for the potential long-term effects of testosterone suppression. Gonadotropin-releasing hormone agonists can decrease bone mineral density, thereby predisposing survivors to osteoporosis and bone fractures (Saad et al. 2008). Survivors should be counseled to optimize bone health by taking calcium and vitamin D nutritional supplements, decreasing caffeine intake, refraining from smoking, and participating in weight-bearing and resistance exercise. Depending on the length of hormonal therapy and the baseline bone density measurement, periodic reassessment of bone mineral density may be appropriate. If osteopenia is present, bisphosphonate therapy should be considered (please see the Chap. 21 on endocrinologic issues for additional information on bone health). Testosterone suppression can decrease lean body mass, increase body fat, decrease muscle strength, reduce insulin sensitivity, and increase low-density lipoprotein cholesterol and triglyceride levels (Smith et al. 2002). Men treated with testosterone suppression may have lingering body composition and metabolic changes as ongoing treatment effects. Survivors should be counseled to exercise and maintain a healthy weight. They should also undergo regular screening for elevated cholesterol and diabetes.

Penile Cancer

Penile cancer, like RCC and urothelial cancer, typically has a short interval between treatment and any eventual recurrence. Cure is best obtained with adequate local control from surgery or radiation to the primary tumor. In addition, limited lymph node metastasis to the inguinal chain can be cured with surgical removal, whereas more extensive metastasis through the inguinal chain and into the pelvic chain is associated with high rates of relapse and cancer-related mortality. Chemotherapy may be used as a component of multimodal upfront therapy for tumors that present at an advanced stage, as well as for relapse, but it is not curative in most circumstances.

Efforts to achieve a cure with local and regional therapy are often successful but may be associated with long-term side effects such as sexual dysfunction (i.e., partial to complete amputation of the penis) and lymphedema from an inguinal lymph node dissection. Larger lesions with high-grade features according to biopsy findings or advanced clinical staging may require partial or complete amputation. In general, urinary control is maintained because the sphincter muscles are rarely involved. Sexual dysfunction may occur depending on penile length-sparing efforts and other features of surgical intervention (Pizzocaro et al. 2010). Low-grade distal lesions may be eligible for organ-sparing treatments such as circumcision, local excision, Mohs microsurgery, laser ablation, brachytherapy, or external beam radiation.

Thuret et al. (2011) gathered a large cohort from the SEER database to assess the odds of survival during follow-up. The overall survival rate was 84.3% for all patients just after treatment, and this increased to 95% at 2 years and 97.8% at 5 years of disease-free follow-up. The authors concluded that penile cancer–related mortality at 5 or more years after completion of treatment is very rare.

Surveillance and Eligibility for Care at the MD Anderson Survivorship Clinic

As shown in the penile cancer survivorship algorithm (presented at the end of the chapter), patients diagnosed with early-stage disease (pT1 and pT2 tumors with no lymph node involvement) are eligible for care in the survivorship clinic 3 or more years after completion of treatment if they have remained disease-free since treatment. Patients with localized or metastatic disease (any pT3, pT4, or any lymph node involvement) are eligible if they have remained disease-free for at least 5 years since completing treatment. The risk of recurrence after 3–5 years is rare, yet new primary penile lesions are possible, depending on the patient's risk factors. The cornerstone for diagnosing recurrent disease is physical assessment: careful examination of the penis and thorough palpation of the inguinal lymph nodes is essential. Surveillance imaging is reserved for patients in whom obesity precludes a thorough examination or in those whose examination revealed suspicious lesions. Long-term self-examination and prompt follow-up is necessary, and patients should be instructed accordingly.

Late Effects: Monitoring and Management

The major potential late effects requiring follow-up are incontinence, lymphedema, sexual dysfunction, and emotional distress. Depending on their age, patients may also require further cancer screening such as colorectal and prostate cancer screening. Although incontinence is not expected after surgical resection of the primary cancer, urinary strictures and fistulae are potential late effects of radiation and brachytherapy techniques. Incidence of necrosis and stenosis varies by case series in the literature; necrosis occurs in 3–23% of patients, and stenosis occurs in 10–44% of patients (Pettaway et al. 2007). These complications may require additional dilation or reconstructive procedures. In addition, penile necrosis, pain, and edema requiring a secondary penectomy are possible.

Compared with the extended pelvic lymph node dissection performed for prostate and bladder cancer, the inguinal lymph node dissection performed with penile cancer is associated with a much higher rate of lymphoceles and lymphedema. Spiess et al. (2009) reviewed the published literature and found lymphocele incidence rates of 9–87% and lymphedema incidence rates of 17–50%. Standard extremity lymphedema management with physical therapy experts is warranted; management techniques include compressive garments and lymphatic massage. New-onset edema requires a de novo workup to exclude deep vein thrombosis, phlebitis, or medical sources of edema (e.g., cardiopulmonary dysfunction, renal insufficiency).

Testicular Cancer

Germ cell tumors (GCTs) occur in germinal cells. GCTs occurring in the testicle are called testicular GCTs and those occurring outside the testicle are called extragonadal GCTs. Testicular GCTs are the most common malignancy in men aged 18–34 years; an estimated 7,920 new cases and 370 deaths will occur in 2013 (America Cancer Society 2012). Histologically, GCTs are classified as seminoma or nonseminoma, each comprising approximately 50% of cases. A nonseminoma is further classified as an embryonal tumor, yolk sac tumor, choriocarcinoma, or teratoma (mature and immature); tumors often occur with a mixture of these components and may additionally include seminoma. Risk factors for GCTs include cryptorchidism, family history, white race, and a history of testicular cancer (Holzik et al. 2004).

The 5-year progression-free survival rate is 80–95% for all stages. The American Joint Committee on Cancer staging system and the International Germ Cell Cancer Collaborative Group staging and prognostic methods are the predominant classification systems. Further information about staging and management of testicular cancer can be found elsewhere (International Germ Cell Cancer Collaborative Group 1997; Albers et al. 2011). All patients with a testicular GCT undergo orchiectomy. Some patients with stage I disease may be offered surveillance and others may receive additional treatment, including platinum-based chemotherapy, paraaortic lymph node radiation, or retroperitoneal lymph node dissection, either alone or in the appropriate combination. Salvage therapy is administered for refractory or recurrent disease.

Surveillance and Eligibility for Care at the MD Anderson Survivorship Clinic

Testicular cancer survivorship algorithms, including eligibility criteria, are presented at the end of the chapter. Testicular cancer survivors must have survived at least 2 years after completion of primary treatment and show no evidence of disease, regardless of histologic findings and stage at the time of diagnosis, to be eligible for care in the survivorship clinic. Advances in chemotherapy and radiation therapy have improved the cure rates for testicular cancer, resulting in a 72–86% 5-year overall survival rate for patients with seminoma and a 48–92% 5-year overall survival rate for patients with nonseminoma (Albers et al. 2011). At 5 or more years after completion of treatment, the risk of recurrence is low—cumulative incidence rates of 1.1% at 5 years and 4% at 10 years have been reported (Gerl et al. 1997). However, curative treatments have been associated with second malignancies, bone marrow suppression, cardiovascular disease, infertility, hypogonadism, neurotoxicity, and renal insufficiency. These effects occur during or shortly after completion of treatment (early effects) or several years or decades after completion of treatment (late effects). Because survivors have a relatively long life expectancy, it is essential that the oncologist and the primary care physician collaborate in managing morbidities associated with treatment for testicular cancer.

The testicular cancer survivorship algorithms specify certain activities for long-term monitoring of survivors, including annual physical examinations, diagnostic studies, and weight and body mass index monitoring. Imaging at 5 or more years after completion of treatment is minimized because of the potential risk for secondary cancers from cumulative radiation doses and kidney damage from CT contrast dye. Each potential long-term effect is discussed below.

Late Effects: Monitoring and Management

Hypogonadism

Impaired levels of follicle-stimulating hormone, luteinizing hormone, and testosterone have been observed in patients with testicular cancer, before and after treatment (Pont and Albrecht 1997). When hypogonadism occurs after chemotherapy or radiation therapy, hormone levels generally return to pretreatment levels following treatment (Peterson et al. 1999). Absolute serum testosterone levels may not capture subclinical hypogonadism; therefore, annual tracking of hormone levels is recommended. In patients who display symptoms but have normal serum testosterone levels, checking the luteinizing hormone, follicle-stimulating hormone, and sex hormone-binding globulin levels may be helpful in detecting subclinical or compensated hypogonadism.

Infertility

Infertility in survivors may be the result of impaired spermatogenesis due to treatment-related or non–treatment-related effects (Carroll et al. 1987). Impaired spermatogenesis develops in 5% of men treated with orchiectomy only, 11% of men treated with orchiectomy plus radiation therapy, and 20% of men treated with orchiectomy plus cisplatin chemotherapy (Gerl et al. 2001). Treatment-induced impaired spermatogenesis generally resolves 2 years after completion of treatment in 94–97% of patients (Gandini et al. 2006). Sperm banking before primary treatment is the preferred choice for preserving fertility. For patients who did not bank sperm and remain oligospermic or azoospermic at 2 or more years after completion of treatment, testicular sperm extraction, donor sperm, and adoption are viable options.

Metabolic Syndrome and Cardiovascular Disease

Risk of developing metabolic syndrome or cardiovascular disease as defined by the National Cholesterol Education Program adult treatment panel III (Lorenzo et al. 2007) occurs disproportionately in testicular cancer survivors compared with unaffected cohorts, depending on the primary treatment modality following orchiectomy. Chemotherapy and radiation therapy administered alone or in combination increase the risk for metabolic syndrome (Huddart et al. 2003). Survivors are at risk for metabolic syndrome and should be monitored for cardiovascular risk factors with annual serum creatinine analysis, lipid panel, and weight and diet counseling. Statin therapy should be initiated if therapeutic lifestyle changes fail.

Renal Insufficiency

Cisplatin and radiation therapy both decrease the glomerular filtration rate and increase blood urea nitrogen levels in a dose-dependent fashion (Fossa et al. 2002). Reduced renal function occurs as early as 3 months after chemotherapy or 3–5 years after radiation therapy. Monitoring of creatinine levels, glomerular filtration rate, and blood urea nitrogen levels at least annually is essential in these patients. The National Kidney Foundation recommends close monitoring of glomerular filtration rate, reduced salt intake, and optimum blood pressure control in patients with chronic kidney disease regardless of etiology. A >4 ml/minutes per annum decline in glomerular filtration rate is prognostic for eventual renal failure (National Kidney Foundation 2004). Other measures to preserve kidney function include avoiding nephrotoxic agents such as nonsteroidal anti-inflammatory drugs.

Neurotoxicity

Peripheral neuropathy and hearing loss are common in testicular cancer survivors who have undergone chemotherapy or radiation therapy (Tuxen and Hansen 1994). Symptoms of peripheral neuropathy include numbness and tingling of the extremities, diminished deep tendon reflexes, and loss of proprioception that may affect the ability to walk (Roelofs et al. 1984). Ototoxicity attributed to hair loss in the organ of Corti results in hearing loss, usually in the high-frequency range, in 21–33% of patients (Strumberg et al. 2002). Audiology examinations determine the characteristics of the hearing loss and the appropriate treatment, but rarely do patients need hearing aids.

Marrow Failure/Secondary Malignancies

Bone marrow toxicity in testicular cancer survivors occurs as a result of the toxic effects of chemotherapy and radiation therapy. Although rapidly dividing cancerous cells are targeted for destruction, normal rapidly dividing cells of the bone marrow, intestine, and skin are not spared. Normal cells recover after treatment; however, misrepair of DNA double-strand breaks can lead to genomic instability and development of second cancers in survivors (Allan and Travis 2005). Solid and hematologic tumors occur more often in testicular cancer survivors than in the general population, and the risk increases with time after completion of treatment (Travis et al. 1997).

Current treatment strategies minimize chemotherapy and radiation therapy doses without reducing the cure rate. Nonetheless, some patients with disseminated disease still require high cumulative doses of chemotherapy and radiation as primary or salvage therapy. In addition to obtaining age-appropriate screening for colorectal and prostate cancers, testicular cancer survivors should maintain monitoring throughout life for second tumors, depending on the treatment received.

Extragonadal Germ Cell Tumors

Extragonadal GCTs in men are malignancies that develop from germinal cells located outside the testicles. Extragonadal GCTs occur in the pineal gland, retroperitoneum, and mediastinum. Although extragonadal GCTs share similar histology (seminoma and nonseminoma) and are treated similarly to their testicular counterparts, prognoses are dissimilar (International Germ Cell Cancer Collaborative Group 1997; Albers et al. 2011). Rodney et al. (2012) reported a 54% progression-free survival rate at a median of 33.3 months after chemotherapy and surgery for patients with extragonadal GCTs. Patients who survive therapy for extragonadal GCTs have similar post-therapy complications to those observed in patients with testicular GCTs, and management is similar to that used for testicular GCTs, as discussed earlier. The testicular cancer survivorship algorithm for stages II-IIIC (presented at the end of the chapter) can be used to guide care of extragonadal GCT survivors; however, the frequency and type of imaging studies may vary according to the tumor site and extent of previous tumor involvement.

In conclusion, survivors of testicular and extragonadal GCTs are at risk for multiple treatment-related morbidities such as renal insufficiency, hearing loss, neuropathy, cardiovascular disease, second malignancies, and infertility. Survivorship care at 3 or more years after completion of treatment should focus on anticipating these potential medical issues and monitoring accordingly. The algorithms provided in this chapter can guide the cancer specialist and primary care physician in managing survivorship care.

Table 7.1 Unmet needs reported by genitourinary cancer survivors	Number of unmet needs	Percentage reporting
	0	32%
	1	22%
	2	11%
	3	6%
	4	6%
	>4	23%

Risk Reduction and Early Detection

Like survivors of other types of cancer, GU cancer survivors can reduce modifiable risk factors associated with cancer and undergo cancer screening appropriate for their age. More detailed information about risk reduction activities for primary and secondary cancers is provided in section III on cancer prevention and screening.

Psychosocial Functioning

Psychosocial support is essential as the survivor begins to fully experience the impact of permanent late effects on his or her quality of life. The late effect may be physical, but it can carry a psychological, social, or economic burden. For example, a testicular cancer survivor may have chemotherapy-related neuropathy that prevents him from working full time, or may be unable to secure health insurance because of his cancer history. A prostate cancer survivor may have erectile dysfunction or urinary dribbling that leads to social withdrawal and depression. Bladder cancer survivors with external urinary diversions can experience body image changes. Although these late effects are physical, they can each result in altered psychosocial functioning and reduced quality of life.

Several factors influence a cancer survivor's perception of needs, perhaps most notably the type of cancer and treatment. Additional factors include sex, age, education, life experience, cultural and socioeconomic factors, and personality. Understanding the impact of late effects on long-term survivors is essential to the continually evolving standard of care in oncology. Research will play an invaluable role in understanding unmet needs of cancer survivors and is necessary for the creation of appropriate resources. Most research on psychosocial needs has been done with breast cancer survivors. The authors of this chapter conducted a multi-item survey of GU cancer survivors to evaluate unmet needs in several domains. Patients surveyed were predominantly prostate cancer survivors, but also included kidney, testicular, bladder, and penile cancer survivors, all of whom met the eligibility criteria in the algorithms. Table 7.1 summarizes the percentage of patients reporting unmet needs in the survey. Almost one-fourth of the patients (23%) reported more than four unmet needs, and 68% reported at least one unmet need. The most commonly reported unmet needs were sexual problems, concerns with cancer recurrence, and coordination of care among the patient's other health care providers.

As recommended under the psychosocial functioning component of the GU survivorship algorithms, the patient should be assessed for stressors during each visit, and referrals should be made to a counselor, mental health practitioner, social worker, or social service agency as indicated. More detailed information about psychosocial functioning can be found in Chap. 27 on sexuality.

Conclusion

In summary, cancer survivors face a complex array of health issues that range from physiologic to psychological to social. Guidelines serve as a roadmap for clinicians involved in the care of cancer survivors. Health care providers feel confident that they are providing comprehensive and appropriate care, and patients feel comforted in knowing that their follow-up is based on a plan of care that is derived from the current literature. Outcomes can be tracked and measured, and management strategies can be improved. Guidelines and algorithms will play a central role as the field of cancer survivorship evolves.

Key Practice Points

- GU cancer survivors represent a growing population with a wide range of needs, and clinicians are likely to encounter such patients in their practice.
- Data-driven algorithms are needed to guide decision-making regarding various aspects of long-term cancer survivorship care, from surveillance to psychosocial care. The algorithms presented at the end of this chapter are intended to assist clinicians in this effort.
- Visits after 10 years focus primarily on management of late effects and risk reduction through primary and secondary prevention.
- The applicable body of research for long-term cancer survivors is limited, and further research is needed as the standard of care evolves.
- When applied to large populations, guidelines can serve as a vehicle for research through consistency of care, collection of data, and measurement of outcomes that will ultimately be translated back into clinical care and future guidelines.

Suggested Readings

Albers P, Albrecht W, Algaba F, et al. EAU guidelines on testicular cancer: 2011 update. *Eur Urol* 2011;60:304–319.

Allan JM, Travis LB. Mechanisms of therapy-related carcinogenesis. *Nat Rev Cancer* 2005;5:943–955.

American Cancer Society. Cancer facts & figures 2012. http://www.cancer.org/research/cancerfactsstatistics/cancerfactsfigures2012/index. Published 2012. Accessed July 20, 2013.

Carroll PR, Whitmore WF Jr, Herr HW, et al. Endocrine and exocrine profiles of men with testicular tumors before orchiectomy. *J Urol* 1987;137:420–423.

Chapman D, Moore R, Klarenbach S, et al. Residual renal function after partial or radical nephrectomy for renal cell carcinoma. *Can Urol Assoc J* 2010;4:337–243.

Chin AI, Lam JS, Figlin RA, et al. Surveillance strategies for renal cell carcinoma patients following nephrectomy. *Rev Urol* 2006;8:1–7.

DeVita VT Jr, Chu E. A history of cancer chemotherapy. *Cancer Res* 2008;68:8643–8653.

DeVita VT, Lawrence TS, Rosenberg SA, et al. *Cancer Principles and Practice of Oncology.* 8th ed. Philadelphia: Lippincott Williams & Wilkins; 2008.

Fossa SD, Aass N, Winderen M, et al. Long-term renal function after treatment for malignant germ-cell tumours. *Ann Oncol* 2002;13:222–228.

Gandini L, Sgro P, Lombardo F, et al. Effect of chemo- or radiotherapy on sperm parameters of testicular cancer patients. *Hum Reprod* 2006;21:2882–2889.

Gerl A, Clemm C, Schmeller N, et al. Late relapse of germ cell tumors after cisplatin-based chemotherapy. *Ann Oncol* 1997;8:41–47.

Gerl A, Muhlbayer D, Hansmann G, et al. The impact of chemotherapy on Leydig cell function in long term survivors of germ cell tumors. *Cancer* 2001;91:1297–1303.

Hewitt M, Greenfield S, Stovall E, eds. From Cancer Patient to Cancer Survivor: Lost in Transition. Washington, DC: The National Academies Press; 2005.

Holzik MFL, Rapley EA, Hoekstra HJ, et al. Genetic predisposition to testicular germ-cell tumours. *Lancet Oncology* 2004;5:363–371.

Huddart RA, Norman A, Shahidi M, et al. Cardiovascular disease as a long-term complication of treatment for testicular cancer. *J Clin Oncol* 2003;21:1513–1523.

International Germ Cell Cancer Collaborative Group. International Germ Cell Consensus Classification: a prognostic factor-based staging system for metastatic germ cell cancers. *J Clin Oncol* 1997;15:594–603.

Jaske G, Algaba F, Fossa S, et al. Guidelines on bladder cancer: muscle-invasive and metastatic. http://www.uroweb.org/guidelines/online-guidelines/. Published 2006. Accessed June 11, 2011.

Jemal A, Bray F, Center MM, et al. Global cancer statistics. *CA: Cancer J Clin* 2011;61:69–90.

Kidney Disease Outcomes Quality Initiative. K/DOQI clinical practice guidelines on hypertension and antihypertensive agents in chronic kidney disease. *Am J Kidney Dis* 2004;43:S1-290.

Lorenzo C, Williams K, Hunt KJ, et al. The National Cholesterol Education Program—Adult Treatment Panel III, International Diabetes Federation, and World Health Organization definitions of the metabolic syndrome as predictors of incident cardiovascular disease and diabetes. *Diabetes Care* 2007;30:8–13.

Madersbacher S, Schmidt J, Eberle JM, et al. Long-term outcome of ileal conduit diversion. *J Urol* 2003;169:985–990.

Muntener M, Nielsen ME, Romero FR, et al. Long-term oncologic outcome after laparoscopic radical nephroureterectomy for upper tract transitional cell carcinoma. *Eur Urol* 2007;51: 1639–1644.

National Cancer Institute. Renal cell cancer treatment PDQ 2011. http://www.cancer.gov/cancertopics/pdq/treatment/renalcell/HealthProfessional. Published 2011. Accessed July 29, 2013.

National Comprehensive Cancer Network. NCCN clinical practice guidelines in oncology: bladder cancer and kidney cancer (version 2.2011). http://www.nccn.org/professionals/physician_gls/f_guidelines.asp. Accessed June 6, 2011.

National Kidney Foundation. K/DOQI clinical practice guidelines on hypertension and antihypertensive agents in chronic kidney disease. *Am J Kidney Dis* 2004;43(suppl 1):S1-S290.

Oosterlinck W, Lobel B, Jakse G, et al. Guidelines on bladder cancer. *Eur Urol* 2002;41:105–112.

Pederson AW, Fricano J, Correa D, et al. Late toxicity after intensity-modulated radiation therapy for localized prostate cancer: an exploration of dose-volume histogram parameters to limit genitourinary and gastrointestinal toxicity. *Int J Radiat Oncol Biol Phys* 2012;82:235–241.

Penson DF, Litwin MS, Aaronson NK. Health related quality of life in men with prostate cancer. *J Urol* 2003;169:1653–1661.

Petersen PM, Skakkebaek NE, Rorth M, et al. Semen quality and reproductive hormones before and after orchiectomy in men with testicular cancer. *J Urol* 1999;161:822–826.

Pettaway CA, Lynch DF, Davis JW. Tumors of the penis. In: Wein AJ, ed. *Campbell-Walsh Urology*. 9th ed. Philadelphia: Saunders Elsevier; 2007.

Pizzocaro G, Algaba F, Horenblas S, et al. EAU Penile Cancer Guidelines 2009. *Eur Urol* 2010;57: 1002–1012.

Pont J, Albrecht W. Fertility after chemotherapy for testicular germ cell cancer. *Fertil Steril* 1997;68:1–5.

Rodney AJ, Tannir NM, Siefker-Radtke AO, et al. Survival outcomes for men with mediastinal germ-cell tumors: The University of Texas M. D. Anderson Cancer Center experience. *Urol Oncol* 2012;30:879–885.

Roelofs RI, Hrushesky W, Rogin J, et al. Peripheral sensory neuropathy and cisplatin chemotherapy. *Neurology* 1984;34:934–938.

Saad F, Adachi JD, Brown JP, et al. Cancer treatment-induced bone loss in breast and prostate cancer. *J Clin Oncol* 2008;26:5465–5476.

Sanda MG, Dunn RL, Michalski J, et al. Quality of life and satisfaction with outcome among prostate-cancer survivors. *N Engl J Med* 2008;358:1250–1261.

Sanderson KM, Roupret M. Upper urinary tract tumour after radical cystectomy for transitional cell carcinoma of the bladder: an update on the risk factors, surveillance regimens and treatments. *BJU Int* 2007;100:11–16.

Shimko MS, Tollefson MK, Umbreit EC, et al. Long-term complications of conduit urinary diversion. *J Urol* 2011;185:562–567.

Shuch B, Pantuck AJ, Klatte T. Surveillance for metastatic disease after nephrectomy for renal cell carcinoma. http://www.uptodate.com/contents/surveillance-for-metastatic-disease-after-nephrectomy-for-renal-cell-carcinoma. Published 2012. Accessed July 29, 2013.

Silberstein JL, Parsons JK. Evidence-based principles of bladder cancer and diet. *Urology* 2010;75:340–346.

Smith MR, Finkelstein JS, McGovern FJ, et al. Changes in body composition during androgen deprivation therapy for prostate cancer. *J Clin Endocrinol Metab* 2002;87:599–603.

Spiess PE, Hernandez MS, Pettaway CA. Contemporary inguinal lymph node dissection: minimizing complications. *World J Urol* 2009;27:205–212.

Stephenson AJ, Chetner MP, Rourke K, et al. Guidelines for the surveillance of localized renal cell carcinoma based on the patterns of relapse after nephrectomy. *J Urol* 2004;172:58–62.

Strumberg D, Brugge S, Korn MW, et al. Evaluation of long-term toxicity in patients after cisplatin-based chemotherapy for non-seminomatous testicular cancer. *Ann Oncol* 2002;13:229–236.

Studer UE, Burkhard FC, Schumacher M, et al. Twenty years experience with an ileal orthotopic low pressure bladder substitute—lessons to be learned. *J Urol* 2006;176:161–166.

Thuret R, Sun M, Abdollah F, et al. Conditional survival predictions after surgery for patients with penile carcinoma. *Cancer* 2011;117:3723–3730.

Travis LB, Curtis RE, Storm H, et al. Risk of second malignant neoplasms among long-term survivors of testicular cancer. *J Natl Cancer Inst* 1997;89:1429–1439.

Tuxen MK, Hansen SW. Neurotoxicity secondary to antineoplastic drugs. *Cancer Treat Rev* 1994;20:191–214.

Wilson LC, Gilling PJ. Post-prostatectomy urinary incontinence: a review of surgical treatment options. *BJU Int* 2011;107(Suppl 3):7–10.

Survivorship Algorithms

These cancer survivorship algorithms have been specifically developed for MD Anderson using a multidisciplinary approach and taking into consideration circumstances particular to MD Anderson, including the following: MD Anderson's specific patient population, MD Anderson's services and structure, and MD Anderson's clinical information. These algorithms are provided for informational purposes only and are not intended to replace the independent medical or professional judgment of physicians or other health care providers. Moreover, these algorithms should not be used to treat pregnant women.

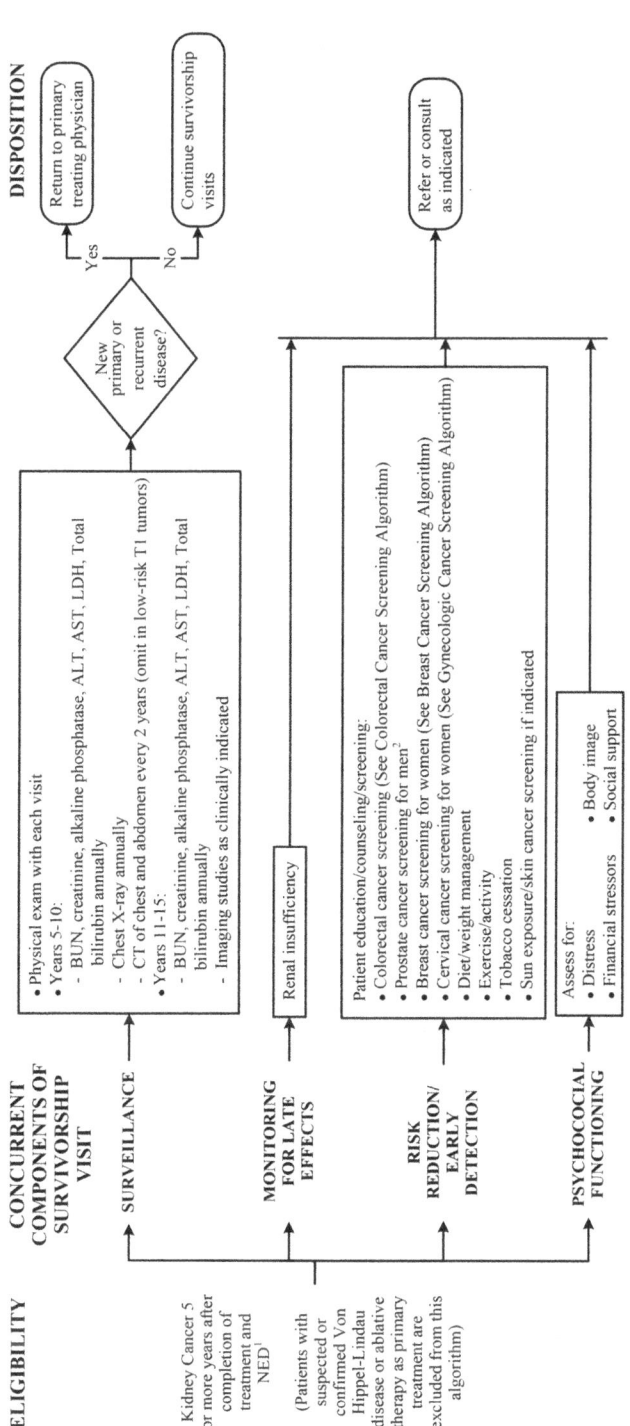

ELIGIBILITY

Kidney Cancer 5 or more years after completion of treatment and NED[1]

(Patients with suspected or confirmed Von Hippel-Lindau disease or ablative therapy as primary treatment are excluded from this algorithm)

CONCURRENT COMPONENTS OF SURVIVORSHIP VISIT

SURVEILLANCE

- Physical exam with each visit
- Years 5–10:
  - BUN, creatinine, alkaline phosphatase, ALT, AST, LDH, Total bilirubin annually
  - Chest X-ray annually
  - CT of chest and abdomen every 2 years (omit in low-risk T1 tumors)
- Years 11–15:
  - BUN, creatinine, alkaline phosphatase, ALT, AST, LDH, Total bilirubin annually
  - Imaging studies as clinically indicated

MONITORING FOR LATE EFFECTS

Renal insufficiency

RISK REDUCTION/ EARLY DETECTION

Patient education/counseling/screening:
- Colorectal cancer screening (See Colorectal Cancer Screening Algorithm)
- Prostate cancer screening for men[2]
- Breast cancer screening for women (See Breast Cancer Screening Algorithm)
- Cervical cancer screening for women (See Gynecologic Cancer Screening Algorithm)
- Diet/weight management
- Exercise/activity
- Tobacco cessation
- Sun exposure/skin cancer screening if indicated

PSYCHOCOCIAL FUNCTIONING

Assess for:
- Distress
- Financial stressors
- Body image
- Social support

DISPOSITION

New primary or recurrent disease?

Yes → Return to primary treating physician

No → Continue survivorship visits

Refer or consult as indicated

[1] NED = No Evidence of Disease
[2] Beginning at age 50 (45 for family history and/or African American) until age 75.

Copyright 2013 The University of Texas MD Anderson Cancer Center

Department of Clinical Effectiveness V3
Approved by the Executive Committee of the Medical Staff 11/27/2012

Algorithm 7.1 Survivorship—kidney cancer

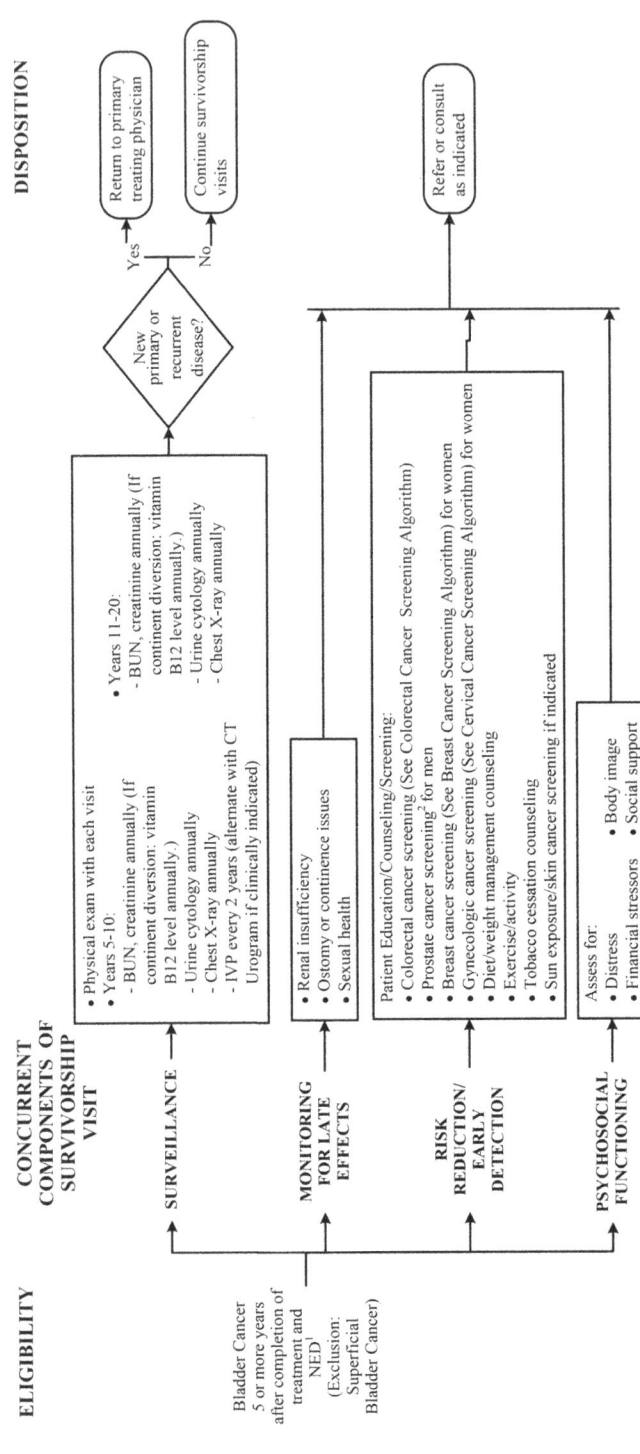

[1] NED = No evidence of Disease

[2] Beginning at age 50 (45 for family history and/or African American) until age 75.

Algorithm 7.2 Survivorship—bladder/ureter/renal pelvis cancer

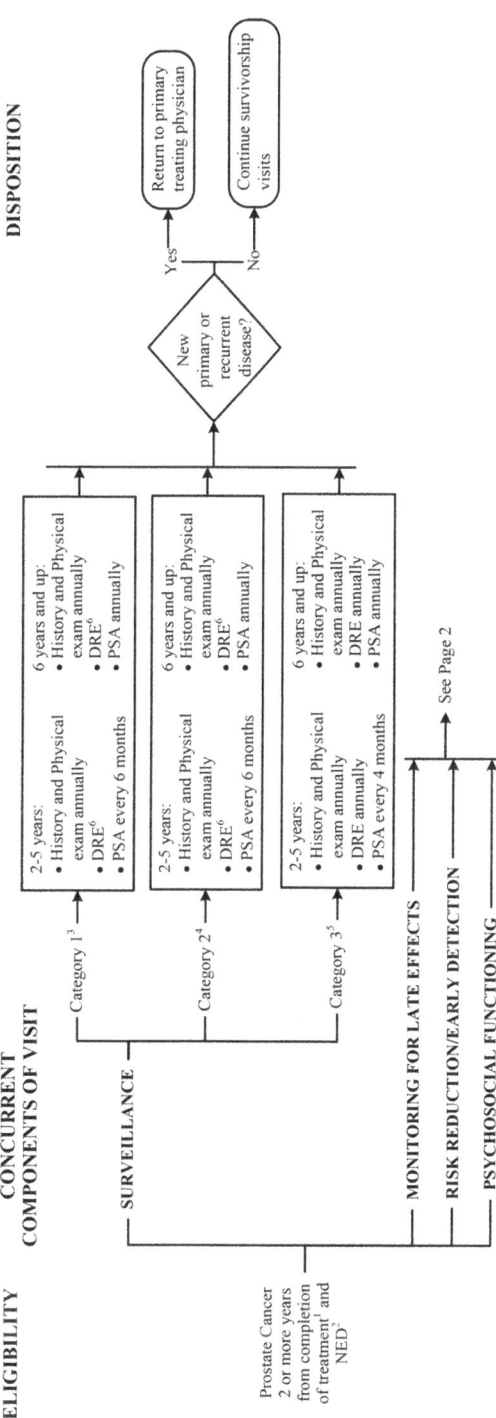

ELIGIBILITY

Prostate Cancer 2 or more years from completion of treatment[1] and NED[2]

CONCURRENT COMPONENTS OF VISIT

SURVEILLANCE

Category 1[3]

2-5 years:
- History and Physical exam annually
- DRE[6]
- PSA every 6 months

6 years and up:
- History and Physical exam annually
- DRE[6]
- PSA annually

Category 2[4]

2-5 years:
- History and Physical exam annually
- DRE[6]
- PSA every 6 months

6 years and up:
- History and Physical exam annually
- DRE[6]
- PSA annually

Category 3[5]

2-5 years:
- History and Physical exam annually
- DRE annually
- PSA every 4 months

6 years and up:
- History and Physical exam annually
- DRE annually
- PSA annually

MONITORING FOR LATE EFFECTS — See Page 2

RISK REDUCTION/EARLY DETECTION

PSYCHOSOCIAL FUNCTIONING

DISPOSITION

New primary or recurrent disease?

Yes → Return to primary treating physician

No → Continue survivorship visits

[1] PSA less than 0.1 for status post prostatectomy and less than 1.0 for status post radiation therapy.
[2] NED = No Evidence of Disease
[3] Category 1: status-post radical prostatectomy or radiation therapy: Pathologic stage: pT2, N0, M0, negative margins, or Clinical stage cT2, N0, M0, Gleason less than or equal to 7 and PSA less than 0.1 ng/mL or less than 1 ng/mL if treated with radiation therapy.
[4] Category 2: status-post prostatectomy or status-post prostatectomy plus radiation therapy. Pathologic stage: pT2, N0, M0, positive margins, Gleason less than or equal to 7, PSA less than 0.1 ng/mL
[5] Category 3: status-post prostatectomy or status-post prostatectomy plus radiation therapy or status-post radiation therapy. Pathologic staging: pT3, N0, M0; Clinical stage, cT3, N0, M0; Gleason 8-10, and PSA less than 0.1 ng/mL or less than 1 ng/mL if treated with radiation therapy only.
[6] DRE: Digital rectal examination annually for patients treated with radiation therapy or every 2 years for patients treated with radical prostatectomy and PSA is undetectable.

Department of Clinical Effectiveness V3
Approved by The Executive Committee of the Medical Staff 11/27/2012

Algorithm 7.3a Survivorship—prostate cancer (page 1)

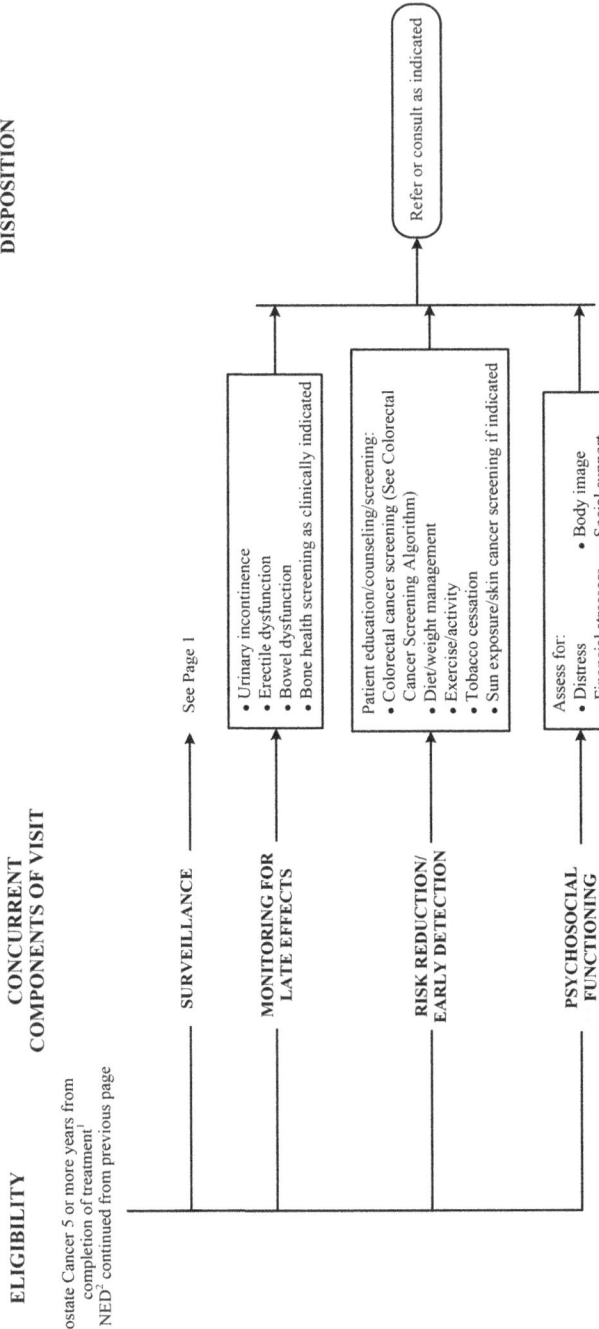

DISPOSITION

Refer or consult as indicated

ELIGIBILITY

Prostate Cancer 5 or more years from
completion of treatment[1]
and NED[2] continued from previous page

CONCURRENT COMPONENTS OF VISIT

SURVEILLANCE → See Page 1

MONITORING FOR LATE EFFECTS
- Urinary incontinence
- Erectile dysfunction
- Bowel dysfunction
- Bone health screening as clinically indicated

RISK REDUCTION/ EARLY DETECTION
Patient education/counseling/screening:
- Colorectal cancer screening (See Colorectal Cancer Screening Algorithm)
- Diet/weight management
- Exercise/activity
- Tobacco cessation
- Sun exposure/skin cancer screening if indicated

PSYCHOSOCIAL FUNCTIONING
Assess for:
- Distress
- Financial stressors
- Body image
- Social support

[1] PSA less than 0.1 for status post prostatectomy and less than 1.0 for status post radiation therapy.
[2] NED = No Evidence of Disease

Copyright 2013 The University of Texas MD Anderson Cancer Center

Department of Clinical Effectiveness V3
Approved by The Executive Committee of the Medical Staff 11/27/2012

Algorithm 7.3b Survivorship—prostate cancer (page 2)

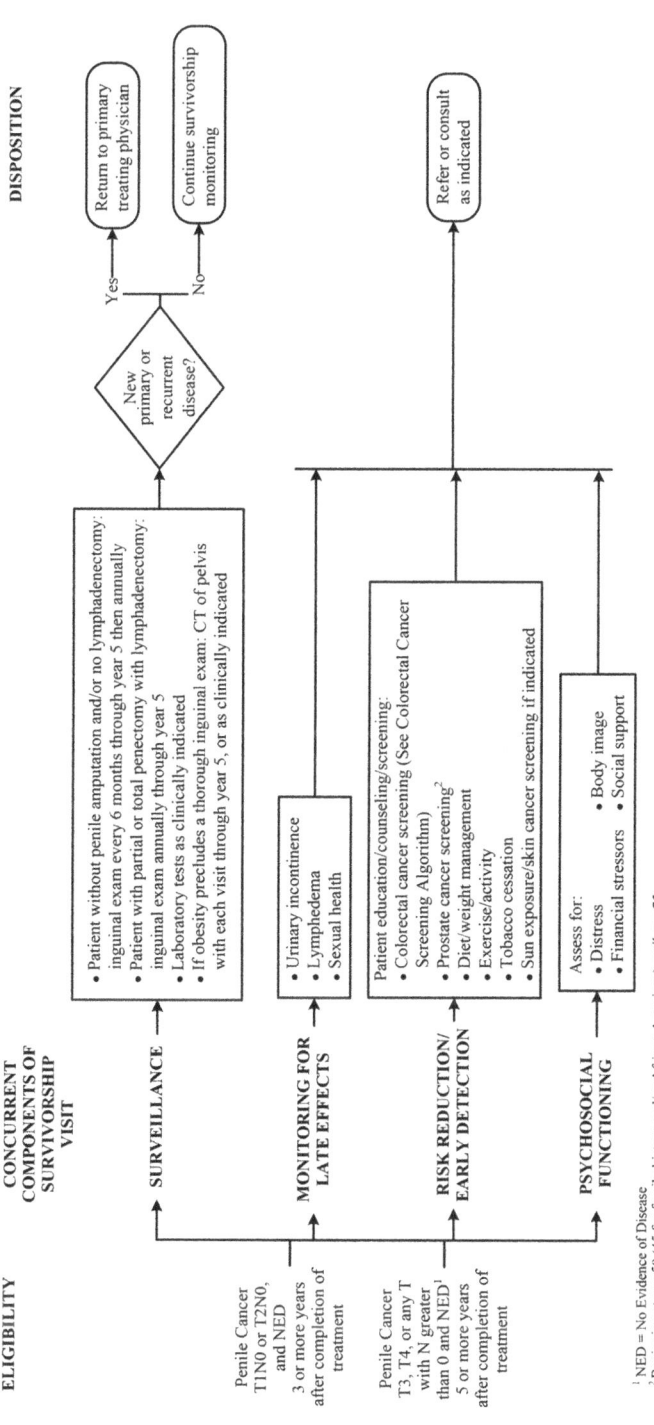

Algorithm 7.4 Survivorship—penile cancer

DISPOSITION

Return to primary treating physician

Continue survivorship monitoring

Refer or consult as indicated

Yes

No

New primary or recurrent disease?

CONCURRENT COMPONENTS OF SURVIVORSHIP VISIT

SURVEILLANCE

- Patient without penile amputation and/or no lymphadenectomy: inguinal exam every 6 months through year 5 then annually
- Patient with partial or total penectomy with lymphadenectomy: inguinal exam annually through year 5
- Laboratory tests as clinically indicated
- If obesity precludes a thorough inguinal exam: CT of pelvis with each visit through year 5, or as clinically indicated

MONITORING FOR LATE EFFECTS

- Urinary incontinence
- Lymphedema
- Sexual health

RISK REDUCTION/ EARLY DETECTION

Patient education/counseling/screening:
- Colorectal cancer screening (See Colorectal Cancer Screening Algorithm)
- Prostate cancer screening[2]
- Diet/weight management
- Exercise/activity
- Tobacco cessation
- Sun exposure/skin cancer screening if indicated

PSYCHOSOCIAL FUNCTIONING

Assess for:
- Distress
- Financial stressors
- Body image
- Social support

ELIGIBILITY

Penile Cancer T1N0 or T2N0, and NED
3 or more years after completion of treatment

Penile Cancer T3, T4, or any T with N greater than 0 and NED[1]
5 or more years after completion of treatment

[1] NED = No Evidence of Disease
[2] Beginning at age 50 (45 for family history and/or African American) until age 75.

Copyright 2013 The University of Texas MD Anderson Cancer Center

Department of Clinical Effectiveness V3
Approved by the Executive Committee of the Medical Staff 11/27/2012

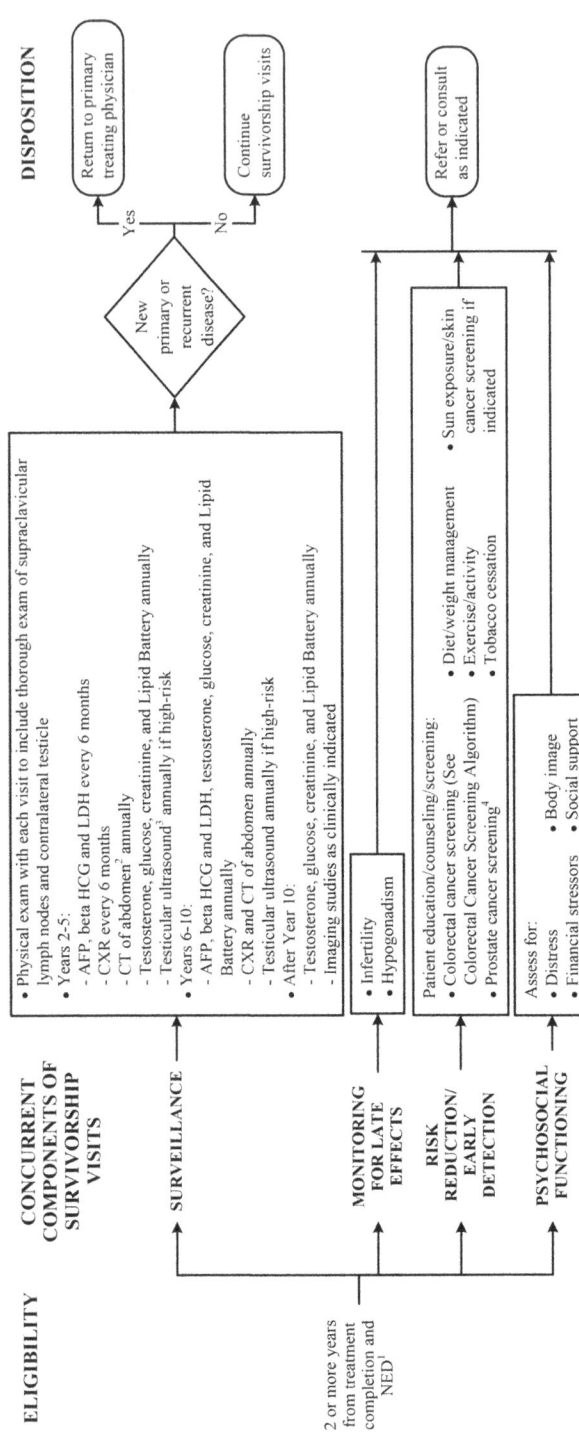

[1] NED = no evidence of disease
[2] Also obtain CT of pelvis if previous scrotal interference or pelvic surgery
[3] Annual ultrasound of contralateral testicle if one of the following present: Diagnosis of seminoma and less than 30 years old when diagnosed or testicular maldescent or infertility.
[4] Beginning at age 50, men should discuss risks and benefits of prostate testing with their doctor.

Department of Clinical Effectiveness V3
Approved by the Executive Committee of the Medical Staff 11/27/2012

Algorithm 7.5 Survivorship—testicular cancer, germ cell: stage I seminoma surveillance

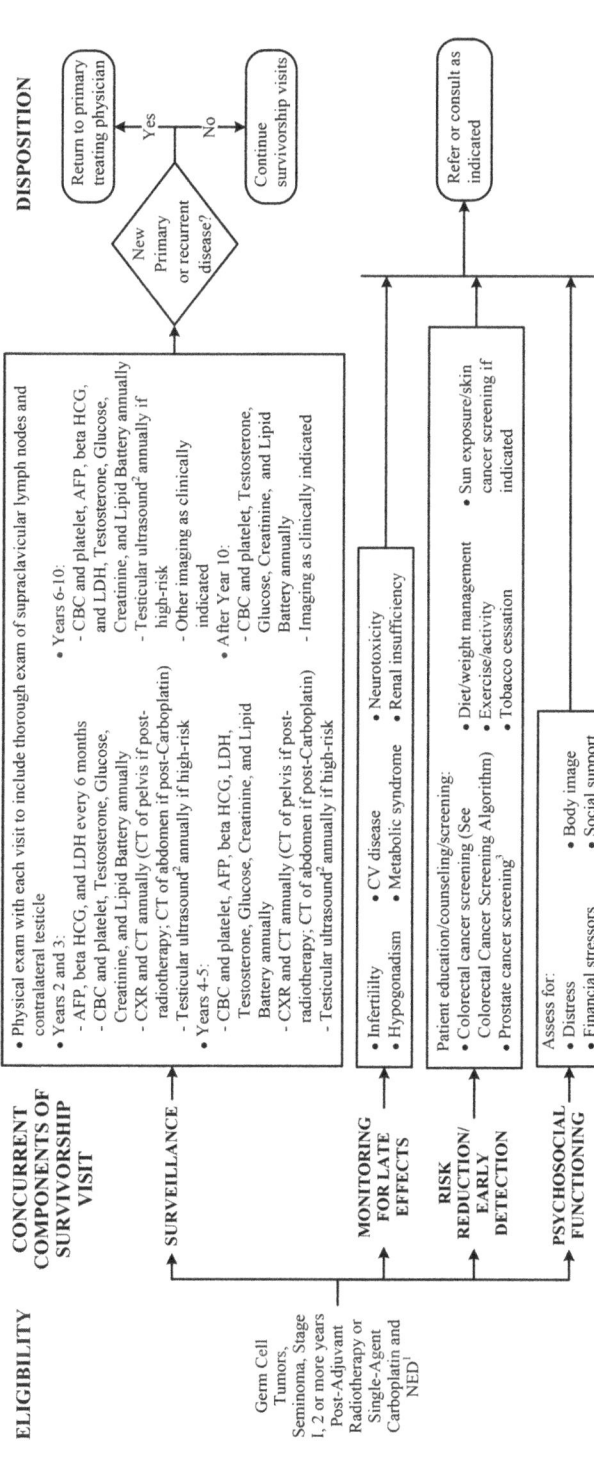

ELIGIBILITY

Germ Cell Tumors, Seminoma, Stage I, 2 or more years Post-Adjuvant Radiotherapy or Single-Agent Carboplatin and NED[1]

CONCURRENT COMPONENTS OF SURVIVORSHIP VISIT

SURVEILLANCE

- Physical exam with each visit to include thorough exam of supraclavicular lymph nodes and contralateral testicle
- Years 2 and 3:
  - AFP, beta HCG, and LDH every 6 months
  - CBC and platelet, Testosterone, Glucose, Creatinine, and Lipid Battery annually
  - CXR and CT annually (CT of pelvis if post-radiotherapy; CT of abdomen if post-Carboplatin)
  - Testicular ultrasound[2] annually if high-risk
- Years 4-5:
  - CBC and platelet, AFP, beta HCG, LDH, Testosterone, Glucose, Creatinine, and Lipid Battery annually
  - CXR and CT annually (CT of pelvis if post-radiotherapy; CT of abdomen if post-Carboplatin)
  - Testicular ultrasound[2] annually if high-risk
- Years 6-10:
  - CBC and platelet, AFP, beta HCG, and LDH, Testosterone, Glucose, Creatinine, and Lipid Battery annually
  - Testicular ultrasound[2] annually if high-risk
  - Other imaging as clinically indicated
- After Year 10:
  - CBC and platelet, Testosterone, Glucose, Creatinine, and Lipid Battery annually
  - Imaging as clinically indicated

MONITORING FOR LATE EFFECTS

- Infertility
- Hypogonadism
- CV disease
- Metabolic syndrome
- Neurotoxicity
- Renal insufficiency

RISK REDUCTION/ EARLY DETECTION

Patient education/counseling/screening:
- Colorectal Cancer screening (See Colorectal Cancer Screening Algorithm)
- Prostate cancer screening[3]
- Diet/weight management
- Exercise/activity
- Tobacco cessation
- Sun exposure/skin cancer screening if indicated

PSYCHOSOCIAL FUNCTIONING

Assess for:
- Distress
- Financial stressors
- Body image
- Social support

DISPOSITION

New Primary or recurrent disease?

Yes → Return to primary treating physician

No → Continue survivorship visits

Refer or consult as indicated

[1] NED = No Evidence of Disease

[2] Annual ultrasound of contralateral testicle if one of the following is present: diagnosis of seminoma and less than 30 years old when diagnosed or testicular maldescent, or infertility.

[3] Beginning at age 50, men should discuss risks and benefits of prostate testing with their doctor.

Department of Clinical Effectiveness V3
Approved by the Executive Committee of the Medical Staff 11/27/2012

Algorithm 7.6 Survivorship—testicular cancer, germ cell: seminoma, stage I, after adjuvant radiotherapy or single-agent carboplatin

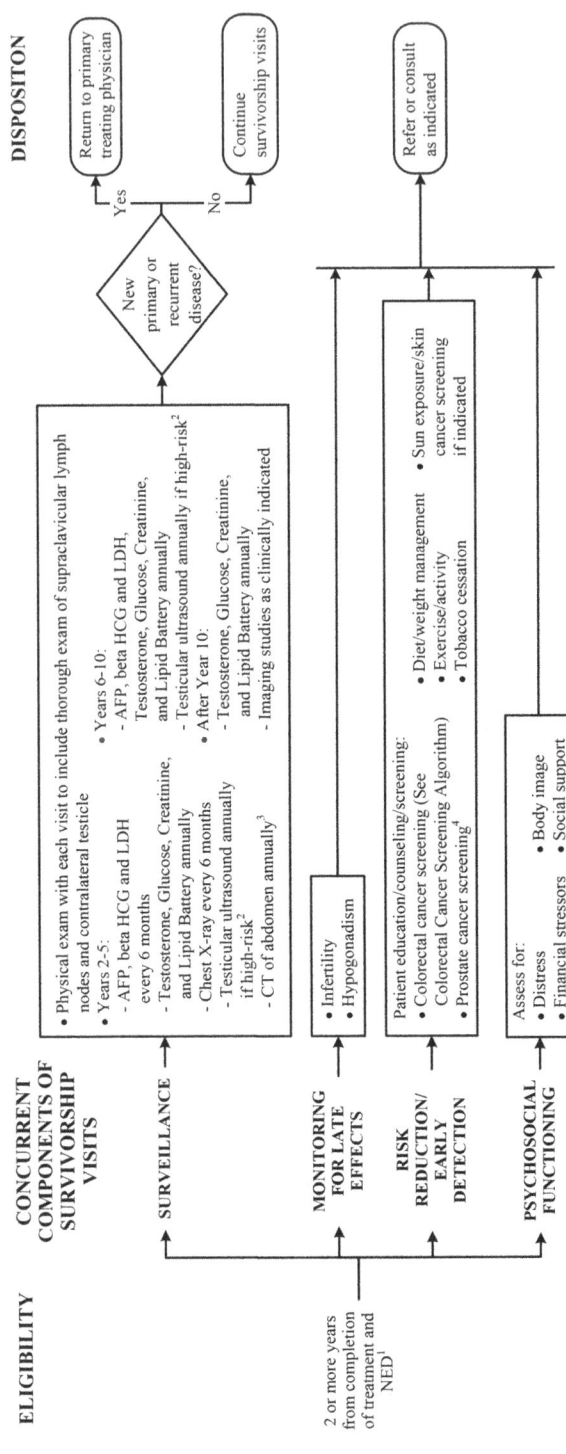

Algorithm 7.7 Survivorship—testicular cancer, germ cell: stage I nonseminoma surveillance

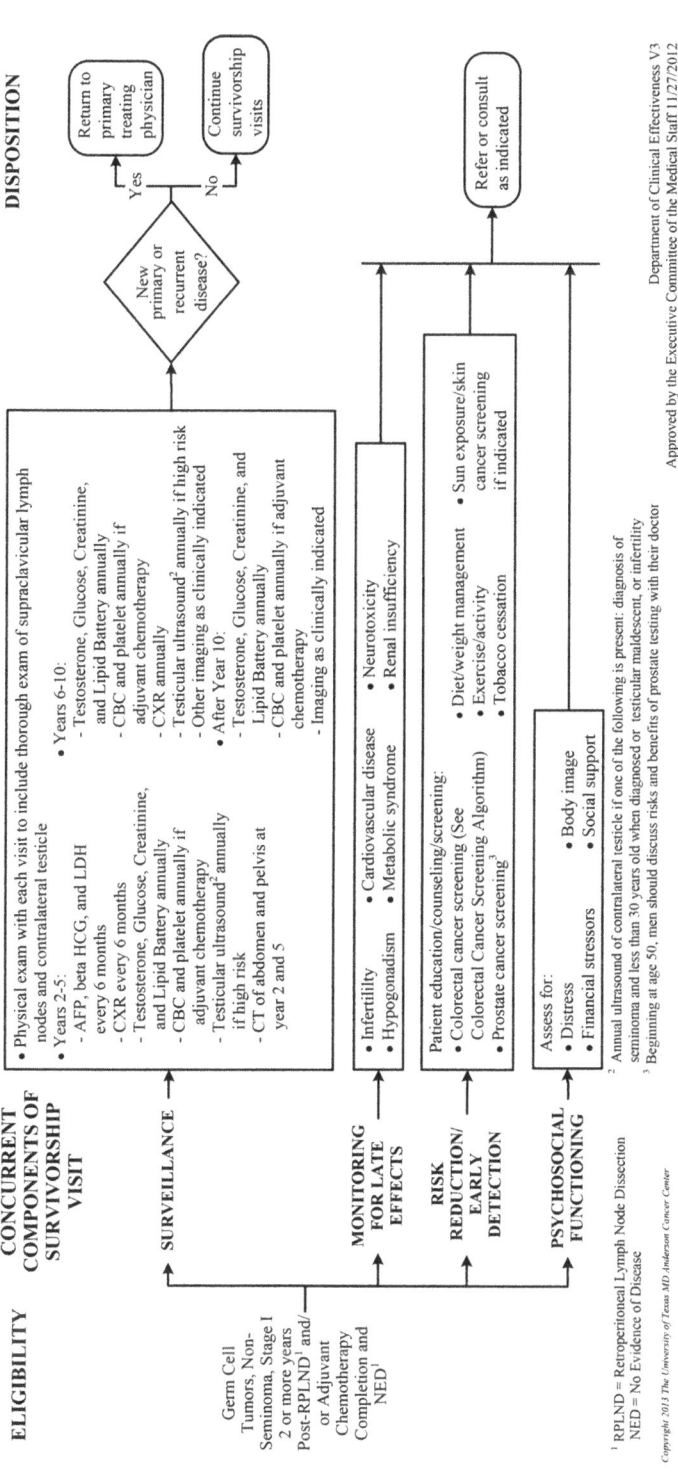

Algorithm 7.8 Survivorship—testicular cancer; germ cell: nonseminoma, stage I, after retroperitoneal lymph node dissection or adjuvant chemotherapy

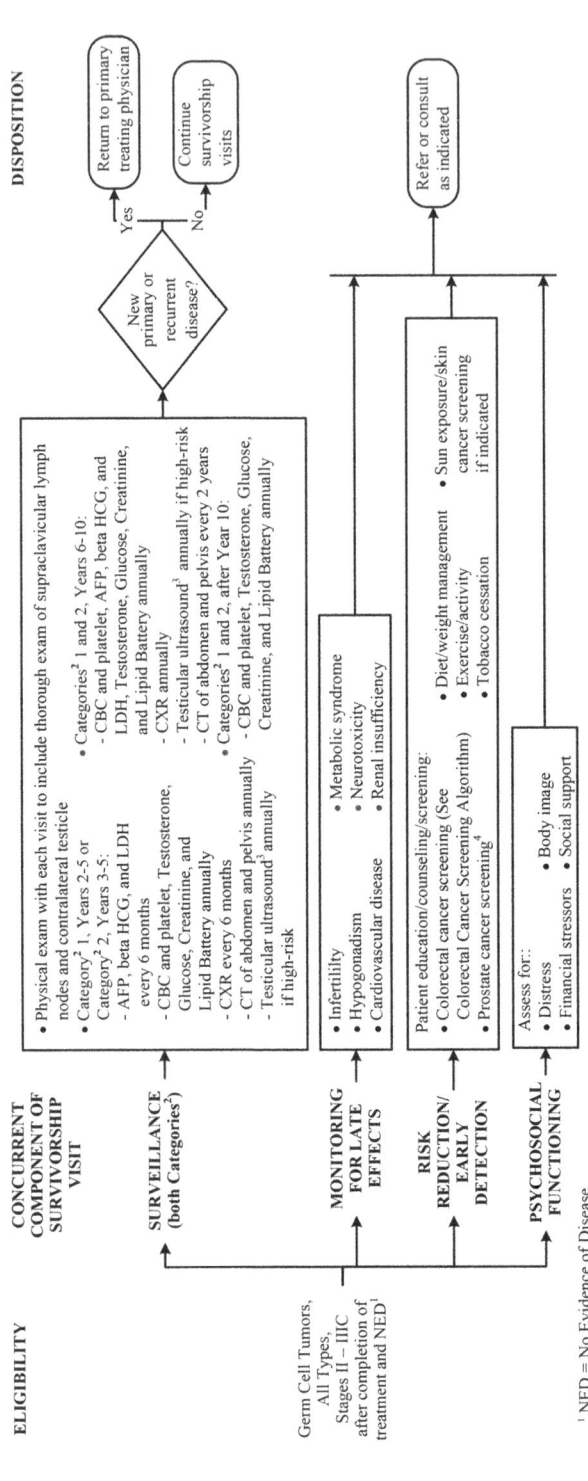

[1] NED = No Evidence of Disease

[2] Category 1: Germ cell tumors all types, Stages II – IIIA; no evidence of disease at 2 years
   Category 2: Germ cell tumors all types, Stages IIIB and IIIC; no evidence of disease at 3 years

[3] Annual ultrasound of contralateral testicle if one of the following is present: diagnosis of seminoma and less than 30 years old when diagnosed or testicular maldescent, or infertility.

[4] Beginning at age 50, men should discuss risks and benefits of prostate testing with their doctor.

Algorithm 7.9 Survivorship—testicular cancer, germ cell: all types, stages II-IIIC

Chapter 8
Gynecologic Cancer Survivorship Management

Diane C. Bodurka, Shannon N. Westin, and Charlotte C. Sun

Contents

Chapter Overview Over the past three decades, the number of gynecologic cancer survivors has grown substantially, most notably among women with early-stage disease. Cure of gynecologic cancers is possible with evidence-based and tailored combinations of surgery, chemotherapy, and radiation therapy. The ability to identify genetic predispositions to specific gynecologic malignancies has also positively affected gynecologic cancer survivors. Algorithms have been developed to provide appropriate survivorship care for patients with gynecologic malignancies. Each algorithm is geared toward care of survivors with a specific disease history. Surveillance tests and examinations, as well as risk reduction and early detection strategies, are recommended for survivors of each gynecologic malignancy. Monitoring schedules and testing methods for late effects and

L.E. Foxhall, M.A. Rodriguez (eds.), *Advances in Cancer Survivorship Management*, 125
MD Anderson Cancer Care Series, DOI 10.1007/978-1-4939-0986-5_8,
© The University of Texas M.D. Anderson Cancer Center 2015

psychosocial functioning (including referrals, when appropriate) are also provided. As the field of cancer survivorship develops and the number of gynecologic cancer survivors grows, these algorithms will become increasingly important. Many survivors suffer from long-term cancer- and treatment-related morbidities. We must recognize that the care of survivors extends far past their 5-year survival period, and that some late effects of treatment continue to worsen over time. Additionally, caregiver responsibilities, with subsequent benefits and stressors, must also be further evaluated and supported. The quality of life of each survivor affects and is affected by every member of her team, including her family caregivers.

Introduction

Advances in cancer treatment, especially for women with gynecologic malignancies, have turned this once uniformly fatal illness into a curable disease for some and a chronic illness for many. Today, an estimated one million gynecologic cancer survivors live in the United States. The National Cancer Institute Office of Cancer Survivorship estimates that approximately 9% of female cancer survivors (573,300 women) have uterine cancer; 4% (243,884 women) have cervical, vaginal, or vulvar cancer; and 3% (177,578 women) have ovarian, fallopian tube, or primary peritoneal cancer. Overall survival rates from gynecologic cancers have improved significantly over the past three decades. This improvement is most pronounced among women with early-stage uterine, ovarian, and cervical cancers, for whom cure is possible through administration of tailored combinations of surgery, chemotherapy, and radiation therapy. However, although these treatments have increased overall survival rates, they can lead to myriad health-related concerns for survivors. Addressing these needs is an essential step in the goal of eliminating cancer-related morbidity and mortality in the growing population of gynecologic cancer survivors.

Surveillance

Survivorship monitoring should occur yearly for all women who have survived gynecologic cancer, starting at a specified time point after completion of treatment (see below). If a new primary cancer or recurrent disease is suspected, appropriate cancer treatment algorithms should be consulted for further evaluation and treatment.

Endometrial Cancer

Endometrial cancer is the most common gynecologic cancer, as well as the most curable. Our cancer survivorship algorithm for endometrial cancer divides women into two groups for posttreatment surveillance: low-risk and high-risk. Low-risk endometrial cancer survivors are those who did not receive radiation therapy or chemotherapy as adjuvant treatment after the initial surgery, and survivorship begins three years after treatment is completed and the patient has no evidence of disease. High-risk endometrial cancer survivors are those who received radiation therapy or chemotherapy as adjuvant treatment after the initial surgery, and survivorship begins five years after treatment is completed and the patient has no evidence of disease. Although the posttreatment surveillance begins at different time points for the two groups, all patients, upon reaching that time point, undergo an annual physical examination including a pelvic examination, chest x-ray as clinically indicated, and CA 125 tests if levels were initially elevated (see the endometrial cancer survivorship algorithm presented at the end of this chapter).

Cervical/Vaginal/Vulvar Cancers

The cancer survivorship algorithm for cervical cancer is also used for survivors of vulvar and vaginal cancers. Survivorship begins three years after treatment is completed for women who have a history of vulvar cancer, underwent radiation therapy, and have no evidence of disease, and five years after treatment is completed for women with cervical cancer, vaginal cancer, or vulvar cancer treated with surgery and who have no evidence of disease. Women in both groups undergo a yearly physical examination with a Papanicolaou smear and pelvic examination, and they may also undergo a chest x-ray if clinically indicated (see the cervical cancer survivorship algorithm presented at the end of this chapter).

Ovarian/Fallopian Tube/Primary Peritoneal Cancers

The cancer survivorship algorithm for ovarian cancer is also used for patients with fallopian tube and primary peritoneal cancer, which behave similarly and are therefore treated in the same manner. All patients are examined annually starting five years after treatment for ovarian, fallopian tube, or primary peritoneal cancer is completed and the patient has no evidence of disease. Survivors undergo an annual physical examination, including a pelvic examination. In addition, complete blood count and chemistry profiles are performed as clinically indicated, CA 125 is tested if levels were initially elevated, and a computed tomographic scan of the chest, abdomen, and pelvis is performed as clinically indicated (see the ovarian cancer survivorship algorithm presented at the end of this chapter).

Risk Reduction and Early Detection of Second Primary Cancers

A second primary cancer has been defined as "the occurrence of a new cancer that is biologically independent of the original primary cancer" (Neugut et al. 1999). The precise etiology of a second primary cancer is not always clear. Although many

Table 8.1 Second primary cancers for which gynecologic cancer survivors are at increased risk

Location of second primary cancer	Endometrial cancer survivors	Cervical cancer survivors	Ovarian cancer survivors
Bladder	X	X	X
Breast	X	X	X
Colon	X	X	
Colon or rectum			X
Endometrium (uterine lining)			X
Kidney	X	X	
Leukemia			X
Lung or bronchus	X	X	
Ovary		X	
Pancreas		X	
Rectum or anus	X	X	
Ureter	X		
Urethra	X		
Uterus		X	
Vagina	X	X	
Vulva	X	X	

of these cancers are thought to be related to treatment, others are likely caused by environmental exposures. It has long been recognized that an individual who has had cancer in one paired organ is at increased risk of developing a second cancer in the contralateral organ. The underlying premise is that whatever predisposed an individual to develop the first cancer would also predispose that individual to develop a second cancer in the contralateral organ. Gynecologic cancer survivors are at risk for a variety of second primary cancers, many of which are not gynecologic in origin. The risk for second primary malignancies increases with age, and obesity, smoking, human papillomavirus infection, prior chemotherapy, prior radiation treatment, and use of hormonal therapy also increase the risk (Ng and Travis 2008). Early detection strategies include mammography, breast magnetic resonance imaging, fecal occult blood testing, colonoscopy, skin examination, and genetic counseling. Prevention strategies include smoking cessation, sun safety practices, prophylactic surgery, exercise, weight management, and energy balance (i.e., controlled caloric intake).

Endometrial Cancer

Endometrial cancer survivors are at risk for multiple second primary cancers, as illustrated in Table 8.1. The risk of developing a second primary cancer is highest in the breast and colon. The etiology of developing breast cancer after endometrial cancer is not thought to be related to treatment. Rather, the risk of a second primary breast cancer is thought to be related to the same risk factors as those for endometrial cancer. These include nulliparity, an increasing number of years of menstrual cycles, and postmenopausal obesity. Shared genetic factors are still another suspected cause, including hereditary non-polyposis colon cancer (HNPCC).

Screening efforts are tailored to each individual's medical history, family history, and prior treatment. Survivors are offered breast and colorectal cancer screening. Skin cancer screening is also offered, owing to the well-documented link between sun exposure and skin cancer. Referrals to the Smoking Cessation Clinic are also available, owing to the link between smoking and lung and oropharyngeal malignancies. Recent data have shown a relationship between obesity and the development of possible malignancies, including breast and colon cancers, as well as between obesity and medical comorbidities such as hypertension, coronary artery disease, and diabetes. Obesity is a well-established risk factor for endometrial cancer. Survivors who are physically inactive after a cancer diagnosis are at increased risk for a variety of problems, including cancer-related fatigue, weight gain, poor quality of life, and declines in physical functioning. Physically inactive survivors are also at an increased risk of developing second cancers and other chronic diseases such as diabetes, cardiovascular disease, and arthritis. Endometrial cancer survivors are more likely to die from diseases such as stroke or heart disease than from cancer.

Treatment with tamoxifen has also been identified as a risk factor for developing endometrial cancer. For women with breast cancer who still have a uterus, an annual gynecologic examination is recommended. Women should also be counseled about the early symptoms of endometrial cancer, including abnormal vaginal spotting, bleeding, or discharge, especially if the woman is postmenopausal. These symptoms should be reported promptly to a health care provider. The endometrium should be sampled and the specimen evaluated by a pathologist for possible malignancy.

Genetic counseling is offered to women who meet the criteria established for increased risk of Lynch syndrome, also called HNPCC, an inherited condition characterized by a mutation in one of the four key mismatch repair genes—MLH1, MSH2, MSH6, and PMS2. Carriers are already known to be at high risk of developing some cancers, particularly colon cancer, and are diagnosed with this cancer at younger ages than the general population. In addition to colon cancer, other cancers known to be associated with Lynch syndrome include uterine, ovarian, renal, stomach, and bladder malignancies. People with this disorder may also have increased risks for breast and pancreatic cancers. Screening criteria include a family member diagnosed with colorectal or endometrial cancer before the age of 50 years, cancer present in two or more generations, and three or more closely related family members with endometrial, colorectal, or other Lynch-associated cancers. These criteria are called the Amsterdam criteria. Not all families that meet the Amsterdam criteria have Lynch syndrome, and families that have Lynch syndrome may not meet all of the Amsterdam criteria. Therefore, an individual concerned about Lynch syndrome in her family should be referred to a genetic counselor for consultation.

Cervical/Vaginal/Vulvar Cancers

All survivors with a history of cervical, vaginal, and vulvar cancers are offered breast cancer screening and colorectal cancer screening as appropriate. Skin cancer screening is also offered. Smoking cessation is of high priority; many studies have shown a relationship between smoking and cervical and vulvar lesions. Diet and weight management assistance, as well as promotion of physical activity, are suggested as described above for endometrial cancer survivors.

Ovarian/Fallopian Tube/Primary Peritoneal Cancers

Each year an estimated 25,000 woman are diagnosed with ovarian cancer. The overall risk of developing a second cancer is approximately 20% greater in women with a history of ovarian cancer who survive at least five years. Risk for a second gynecologic malignancy is low because most women with ovarian cancer have been treated with hysterectomy. Treatment for ovarian cancer usually results in ablation of gonadal function, but this does not necessarily equate to a reduced risk of developing breast cancer. Although the elevated relative risk for a second primary cancer may partly be due to shared risk factors such as early menarche, late menopause, and nulliparity, mutations in the *BRCA1* and *BRCA2* genes substantially increase the risk of developing breast cancer. Individuals with *BRCA1*-associated cancers have a 50–80% lifetime risk of developing breast cancer, a 40–60% lifetime risk of developing a second primary breast cancer, and a 20–40% lifetime risk of developing ovarian cancer. Individuals with *BRCA2*-associated cancers have a 40–80% lifetime risk of developing breast cancer and a 10–25% lifetime risk of developing ovarian cancer. Therefore, survivors with a history of ovarian, fallopian tube, and primary peritoneal cancers are offered breast cancer screening.

Ovarian cancer has been observed in women with HNPCC mutations, which suggests that genetic determinants may influence the development of both ovarian and colorectal cancers. If the survivor has a personal history of ovarian or endometrial cancer diagnosed before the age of 60 years, colonoscopy is advised at age 40 years or at the time of diagnosis of endometrial cancer. Skin cancer screening and smoking cessation programs are offered to these patients, as in the groups of gynecologic cancer survivors described above.

We provide hereditary cancer genetic counseling and genetic testing services for women who have ovarian or endometrial cancer and a personal or family history that suggests a predisposition to inherited cancers. Genetic counseling is particularly recommended if a woman with ovarian cancer has ever had breast cancer, has any relatives who have had ovarian cancer, has any relatives who were diagnosed with breast cancer before the age of 50 years, has two or more relatives who had breast cancer at any age, or is of Ashkenazi (Eastern European) Jewish ancestry. Cancer survivors can benefit from genetic testing, even many years after diagnosis. Testing offers information about risk for other family members, including risks of developing second cancers. It is vital that the affected individual be tested first.

Survivors treated with some chemotherapeutic agents are at risk for second cancers associated with certain classes of chemotherapeutic agents. Women who received anthracyclines, including doxorubicin (Adriamycin), dactinomycin (Actinomycin-D), bleomycin, topoisomerase II inhibitors (Etoposide), and alkylating agents such as cyclophosphamide (Cytoxan), carboplatin, or cisplatin, are at increased risk of developing colorectal, breast, and bladder cancers, as well as myelodysplastic syndrome and leukemia.

As with endometrial cancer survivors, survivors of ovarian, fallopian tube, and primary peritoneal cancers derive benefits from diet and weight management and exercise and physical activity. For additional information regarding second primary cancers, please refer to Chap. 18.

Late Effects of Treatment

Survivor populations are unique by treatment and disease. Surgical interventions, radiation ports and doses, and chemotherapeutic interventions are also unique for each gynecologic malignancy. Interventions differ according to disease stage and biological and hormonal characteristics of each disease. Therefore, anticipated or potential side effects, both short- and long-term, are unique to each patient's initial disease presentation.

Surgery

Women who undergo surgery for gynecologic cancers are at risk for late effects specific to the type of procedure(s) performed. Endometrial cancer survivors are at increased risk of developing lower extremity lymphedema if they have had an extensive lymph node dissection. This is caused by destruction of the lymph system and stagnation of the lymph channel. Incidence rates range from 3.6% to 4.9% with radiation alone and 7% to 20% with pelvic node dissection (Maher and Denton 2008). The risk is increased if the patient required postoperative radiation treatment following lymph node dissection. Lymphedema can be triggered by injury or trauma, including insect bites, cuts, injections, sunburns, exposure to extreme temperatures, air travel, or cellulitis. Patients may require multiple hospitalizations for intravenous antibiotic therapy. Decongestive therapy may include the use of a compression bandage, manual lymph drainage massage, or lymphedema hosiery such as Jobst stockings. Good foot hygiene and skin care should be maintained. These interventions have been found to be useful as supportive care measures, but the edema rarely completely resolves once it develops. Risk reduction suggestions include maintenance of optimal body weight; avoidance of injury, extreme temperatures, and excessive sunlight; use of good shoes; and administration of early appropriate antibiotic prophylaxis for recurrent cellulitis.

Cervical cancer and vulvar cancer survivors are also at risk for lower extremity lymphedema owing to extensive lymph node dissection. This may also be compounded if postoperative radiation is administered. Lymphatic mapping is often performed in patients with vulvar cancer in an effort to determine the extent of groin lymph node dissection required, with the goal of decreasing the risk of future lymphedema.

Radiation Treatment

Some endometrial cancer survivors undergo surgery and others also receive postoperative radiation. Treatment options for cervical cancer survivors include surgery, surgery followed by chemotherapy and radiation therapy, or chemotherapy and radiation therapy without surgery. All endometrial cancer survivors who undergo pelvic and or para-aortic radiation therapy are at risk of developing radiation enteritis, which can involve any portion of the bowel from the small bowel to the rectum. Clinical manifestations include nausea and vomiting, abdominal pain and cramping, and weight loss. Other symptoms include frequent bowel movements, watery or bloody diarrhea, and fatty stools. Treatment strategies are based on nutritional therapy, including parenteral nutrition, and bowel rest. No data currently exist regarding the benefit of probiotics or antibiotics for chronic radiation enteritis. Cholestyramine can be useful to treat bile salt malabsorption.

Bowel obstruction caused by radiation fibrosis or adhesions, as well as bowel perforation, can also occur. If the small bowel is injured because of radiation fibrosis or perforation, the affected area can often be resected and remaining bowel anastomosed to a healthy piece of small bowel or to the colon because not all of the small bowel or colon is in the treatment field. If the colon is obstructed or perforated because of radiation injury, a colostomy is usually required because an anastomosis created in an irradiated field is extremely unlikely to heal. Patients may also require colostomy because of radiation proctitis, which can present as rectal bleeding and pain. Supportive care measures, including proctofoam and rowasa enemas, can be helpful; some patients may require blood transfusions. Hyperbaric oxygen may have a role, but it is very expensive. Patients should also understand that the colostomy may constrict because of radiation damage to the tissue.

Patients can also develop rectovaginal fistulae. Once recurrent disease has been ruled out, the extent of the fistula must be thoroughly evaluated, including the specific segments of involved bowel. Perineal irritation and pain usually indicate a small bowel component to the fistula. If the small bowel is involved in the fistula, two procedures are performed. The involved portion of small bowel is resected and reanastomosed to another portion of small bowel or to the colon. A colostomy is also created. The damaged piece of colon cannot be reanastomosed to a distal section of colon because the distal colon has been previously irradiated and the anastomosis will break down, causing leakage of stool and need for colostomy.

Cervical cancer survivors who receive postoperative radiation with or without chemotherapy are at risk for late effects similar to those described for endometrial cancer survivors who receive postoperative radiation, with or without chemotherapy.

As oncologists, we are aware that use of multiple treatment modalities, such as radiation therapy (with or without chemotherapy) following surgery, can significantly increase treatment-related morbidity. Therefore, we strive to recommend the single treatment modality associated with the longest survival and least morbidity. For example, if a patient has a high-risk cervical lesion that will presumably require postoperative chemotherapy and radiation (chemoradiation), it is usually preferable to treat the patient with chemoradiation rather than with radical hysterectomy followed by chemoradiation. The treatment option involving surgery followed by chemoradiation is clearly associated with more potential morbidity than the chemoradiation treatment alone because the patient faces risks associated with two rather than one treatment modality.

Patients who have been treated with radiation can also develop ureteral stenosis. This stenosis causes hydronephrosis and can impair the function of the involved renal unit. Although hydronephrosis is usually treated by stent or percutaneous nephrostomy tube placement, creation of a urinary conduit is occasionally required. Patients may also develop radiation cystitis, which is inflammation of the mucosal surface of the bladder or ureters. Late radiation cystitis can develop up to 20 years after completion of radiation therapy. Clinical manifestations include abdominal pressure, painful urination, urinary frequency and urgency, incontinence, nocturia, abnormal urine color, foul-smelling or strong urine odor, and hematuria. An underlying infection causing the hematuria must always be ruled out. Conservative management includes use of anticholinergic drugs such as oxybutynin (Ditropan), phenazopyridine hydrochloride (Pyridium/AZO Standard), and flavoxate hydrochloride (Urispas). Treatment for chronic hemorrhagic cystitis includes hydration, intravenous antibiotic treatment, and bladder irrigation with a three-way foley catheter. Patients may also require blood transfusions. Cystoscopy and cauterization of the bleeding areas, intravesical instillation of a variety of substances, hyperbaric oxygen treatment, or creation of a urinary conduit are additional therapeutic options. Patients may also develop ureterovaginal or vesicovaginal fistulae. Once the fistula has been appropriately evaluated, a urinary conduit is usually created.

Sexual dysfunction is defined as diminished or absent feeling of sexual interest or desire, absent sexual thoughts or fantasies, and lack of responsive desire. This is a very common complaint of cervical and vaginal cancer survivors owing to fibrosis and stenosis. The importance of vaginal dilatation in this group of women cannot be emphasized enough. We provide our patients with vaginal dilators and counsel them regarding appropriate use after radiation. Patients are encouraged to use the dilator or have vaginal intercourse three times per week after the completion of radiation therapy for 3 years. Generous lubrication is also recommended for the patient and her partner. The vagina is a potential space and vaginal dilatation is needed after radiation therapy to preserve patency and length. If the patient loses vaginal caliber and length, vaginal intercourse can become painful, sometimes to the extent that the patient avoids intercourse entirely. Although each couple copes with this scenario in their own way, sex therapists can often provide much-needed support and techniques that may help the couple achieve their desired level of intimacy and sexual functioning (Ratner et al. 2010).

Vulvar cancer survivors can develop painful labial edema caused by labial radiation. Although the pain can be temporized by medication, the edema may not resolve. These women also often experience sexual dysfunction. Late side effects include skin thickening and contractures, which worsen over time; changes in skin texture and color; fibrosis; shortening of the vaginal vault; decreased clitoral sensation; and painful intercourse. Please refer to Chap. 25 for more information regarding sexuality and survivorship.

Patients with recurrent ovarian cancer are occasionally treated with radiation, especially if the only site of recurrence is an unresectable mass. If the mass is near the rectum, the patient can develop a rectovaginal fistula. This is treated by colostomy. For additional information, please refer to Chap. 6 on colorectal cancer survivorship management and Chap. 7 on genitourinary cancer survivorship management; survivors of these cancers often experience similar late effects of treatment.

Chemotherapy

Treatment with chemotherapy causes different late effects than those caused by radiation therapy. Although many women develop neuropathy, resolution does not always occur. Despite treatment with neurontin or lyrica, some gynecologic cancer survivors are affected by severe neuropathy throughout the remainder of their lives. Other patients develop cognitive dysfunction, commonly referred to as "chemo brain." Survivors may have difficulty with short-term memory or learning or lose the ability to focus or multitask. A study evaluating long-term cognitive impairment in adult twins aged 65 years or older who were discordant for gynecologic cancer treatment revealed that cognitive impairment was associated with reduced scores on standardized mental and psychiatric tests, and that cognitive impairment was higher in women, especially in gynecologic cancer survivors (Kurita et al. 2011). These cognitive deficits can be so severe that they prevent survivors from functioning at their previous level at home or at work. Interventions include changing cognitive habits, treating fatigue and possible anemia, and physical activity. Modafinil can be helpful and erythropoietin has mixed effects, but methylphenidate demonstrated no effect on cognitive functioning (Fardell et al. 2011). Please refer to Chap. 20 for additional information regarding cognitive function.

Hormonal Therapy

Administration of hormone replacement therapy to gynecologic cancer survivors varies according to practice, physician preference, and geographic location. Premenopausal cervical cancer survivors treated with radiation undergo menopause during their treatment. We prescribe a combination of estrogen and progesterone because some viable endometrium may be present and we do not wish to increase the risk of endometrial cancer in these women. Many women treated for endometrial and ovarian cancers undergo surgical menopause. Endometrial cancer is related to an excess of estrogen. Some oncologists do not advocate hormonal therapy, whereas others feel comfortable prescribing hormones to patients with early-stage disease. No data have conclusively demonstrated that hormonal therapy increases the risk of endometrial cancer recurrence. Many women who undergo surgical menopause as a treatment for ovarian cancer receive hormonal therapy, especially to address quality of life issues such as vaginal dryness, osteoporosis, and hot flashes. Women with a history of granulosa cell tumor of the ovary do not receive estrogen because this tumor is known to be estrogen-dependent. We consult with each patient's oncologist if the patient has a history of breast cancer to determine whether hormonal therapy is a safe option for the patient. For women who experience hot flashes and other menopausal symptoms but cannot or do not wish to receive hormonal therapy, we offer several options, including treatment with venlafaxine (Effexor), clonidine, gabapentin, and bupropion. Although the estradiol vaginal ring (Estring) can provide local treatment with minimal systemic estrogen absorption, patients are counseled that vaginally administered conjugated estrogens (Premarin) have more systemic absorption than the estradiol vaginal ring. Options for nonhormonal vaginal lubricants are also discussed, including vitamin E suppositories, clitoral stimulators, and psychotherapy.

Each survivor has unique concerns. Some of our gynecologic cancer survivors who have a prior history of breast cancer or who are genetic mutation carriers experience such a poor quality of life that they are willing to undergo hormonal therapy in spite of the risks. If these survivors have received appropriate counseling regarding risks and benefits of hormonal therapy, we may prescribe the therapy for them.

Bone Health

Survivors who are postmenopausal or become postmenopausal because of their treatment also require bone health care. Our gynecologic bone health survivorship algorithm (presented at the end of this chapter) was developed for women aged 50 years or older or who are postmenopausal with any of the following risk factors: low body weight, prior bone fracture, family history of hip fracture, high-risk medical condition, rheumatoid arthritis, or history of steroid use lasting three months or longer. A baseline bone mineral density study and a test for 25-OH vitamin D levels are initially performed. Patients are then followed according to the algorithm.

Psychosocial Issues

The goals of psychosocial interventions are to maintain healthy relationships and a restored life for each cancer survivor. Cancer survivorship is a complicated process with both positive and negative aspects. Positive outcomes that have been reported include posttraumatic growth and benefit finding (Hodgkinson et al. 2007). Researchers are working to quantify the personal, psychological, spiritual, and social benefits survivors may report after experiencing a traumatic or stressful event. Such data help describe the extent and breadth of survivors' experiences and also provide a more balanced understanding of potentially achievable outcomes. High rates of anxiety, depression, sexual morbidity, and adjustment disorders have been well documented, as has the contribution of medical, psychosocial, and behavioral factors to psychosocial morbidity.

Few studies have explored the long-term psychosocial outcomes and supportive care needs of gynecologic cancer survivors. Additionally, the unique features associated with this group of cancers limit the validity of generalizations from other populations of cancer survivors. All cancer survivors face issues of uncertainty, financial and insurance concerns, reestablishment of life roles in the family and in the workplace, short- and long-term physical disabilities, reestablishment of autonomy, and possible development of second cancers. In addition to these general issues, gynecologic cancer survivors encounter sexual and often fertility issues, as well as body image issues. Women with gynecologic cancers face challenges directly related to the nature of their treatments, in addition to the general physical and psychological difficulties experienced by those with cancer. These challenges can negatively affect the quality of life not only of patients, but also of their caregivers. Therefore, we must consistently strive to understand survivors' support needs so we can assist them as they recover both physically and emotionally.

The working definition of quality of life for cancer patients is "the patient's appraisal and satisfaction with their current level of functioning as compared with what they perceive to be possible or ideal" (Cella and Cherin 1988). Quality of life includes five specific domains: physical, psychological, spiritual, social, and global. A study of long-term gynecologic cancer survivors revealed overall normal levels of quality of life and relationship adjustment (Hodgkinson et al. 2007). However, symptoms of anxiety were three times as high among gynecologic cancer survivors as in the community, and these levels were consistent with rates found in patients receiving treatment for cancer and among cancer patients during the first 12 months after diagnosis. One in five survivors also reported a symptom profile indicating posttraumatic stress disorder, characterized by hyperarousal, intrusive thoughts, and avoidance symptoms. Although these rates are considerably higher than prevalence rates found in other female cancer survivors, they are similar to rates found in breast cancer survivors who have undergone bone marrow transplantation and pediatric cancer patients and their parents.

Medical variables appear to play less of a role than psychological adjustment in predicting long-term psychological adjustment among gynecologic cancer survivors, which is consistent with recent findings for other cancer populations. Physical and mental quality of life, posttraumatic stress disorder, and total overall needs were most significantly related to levels of distress, indicating that current physical and mental functioning appear to be the biggest predictors of current levels of distress. Distress also significantly increased the likelihood of the survivor reporting at least one unmet need. These findings highlight the relationship between distress and supportive care needs, and the importance of addressing both of these issues in long-term survivors (Helgeson et al. 2004).

Interestingly, the number of years since diagnosis has not been found to be related to distress or need levels. Rather, long-term survivors have been found to have significantly higher rates of anxiety and poorer physical and mental quality of life than the general population, although no differences have been identified in other psychosocial or disease variables. These findings support the growing amount of data suggesting that longer survivorship periods are not necessarily associated with reduced levels of distress. Aging, declining physical quality of life, and compounding effects of treatment-related morbidities may exacerbate negative effects over time.

Survivors also frequently report needs related to the existential survivorship domain. This includes needs unique to survivors such as making decisions about life in the context of uncertainty, coping with changes to beliefs, and dealing with one's own and others' expectations of them as a "cancer survivor." Survivors have also expressed concerns about availability of and accessibility to health care services. Several investigators have reported that ovarian and cervical cancer survivors who are five or more years past the cancer diagnosis report persistent fears of disease recurrence and an unmet need for help to manage concerns about the cancer coming back (Wenzel et al. 2002). In contrast, elevated health care and information needs are typically the most frequently reported needs among other cancer populations. This significant difference in focus suggests the important need for assessment and intervention efforts specifically targeting gynecologic cancer survivorship issues. For additional information, please refer to Chap. 27 on patient–physician communication.

Caregivers

Although more than 65% of cancer patients survive for more than 5 years, quality of life issues continue and sometimes intensify for patients and their families after active treatment ends. Family caregivers are individuals who provide assistance or uncompensated care to a family member with cancer. Family caregivers are at risk of developing many side effects, including fatigue and sleep disturbances, slowed wound healing, reduced immune function, altered lipid profiles, and increased blood pressure. Positive effects of providing care include improved self-esteem, support, and satisfaction, which may serve as a buffer to residual negative effects of caregiving (Given et al. 2011).

Caregivers report having their own unmet needs at five years after the cancer survivor has completed treatment. The prevalence of medical support needs among caregivers was 28% at five years, whereas 36% of caregivers identified unmet psychosocial needs at five years (Yabroff and Kim 2009). Among caregivers whose financial needs were not met at the time of active treatment, 19% also reported financial needs at five years after treatment.

Unmet needs can vary from assisting patients with residual symptoms such as fatigue, pain, cognitive deficits, depression, and sleep disturbance to dealing with late effects of treatment, including lymphedema, diarrhea, constipation, pulmonary fibrosis, cardiac changes, incontinence, and anorexia (Kurtz et al. 2004). The severity of a patient's functional impairment or disability can increase demands on caregivers and restrict caregiver activities. As the number and severity of long-term late effects increases, the survivor can become more and more dependent upon her caregiver. This can significantly increase the caregiver's level of distress, as well as incidence of the symptoms mentioned above (Andrews 2001).

As treatments improve and become more tailored to specific patients and diseases, the number of gynecologic cancer survivors continues to grow. All members of the patient and caregiver care team need to be cognizant of the significant medical, psychosocial, and supportive care needs that may potentially occur many years after the successful treatment of a gynecologic malignancy, as well as the fact that these needs may not decrease over time. The importance of routine and ongoing psychosocial assessment and intervention cannot be overemphasized and should be included as part of the survivor's surveillance program. Patients and their caregivers require both medical and psychosocial preparation for the survivorship period, as well as improved access to supportive care services. Health policy changes with regard to family caregiving need to be evidence-based and linked to the continuing problems faced by survivors. Including the caregiver and supporting a clear survivorship plan for both the patient and her caregivers should be a standard component of quality cancer care. As cancer care becomes more personalized, research must also be directed toward identifying women at increased risk for treatment-related toxicities, in an effort to provide the best clinical outcome and least morbidity for each gynecologic cancer survivor.

Key Practice Points

- The number of gynecologic cancer survivors continues to increase.
- Gynecologic cancer survivors are at significant risk of developing specific second primary cancers, especially among women who carry genetic mutations.
- Late treatment-related effects can develop and intensify over time.
- Although specific interventions are available for some treatment-related effects, such as radiation enteritis and lymphedema, the morbidity of these interventions can be substantial.
- Sexual and cognitive functioning, in addition to other late effects, are minimally understood and require more evaluation and development of appropriate interventions.
- Quality of life is linked to survival and is important to patients and their caregivers.
- Survivor and caregiver issues, including distress, quality of life, finances, and employment, need to be further understood and appropriate interventions and support systems developed.

Suggested Readings

Andrews S. Caregiver burden and symptom distress in people with cancer receiving hospice care. *Oncol Nurs Forum* 2001;28:1469–1474.

Carmack CL, Basen-Engquist K, Gritz ER. Survivors at higher risk for adverse late outcomes due to psychosocial and behavioral risk factors. *CEBP FOCUS Cancer Epidemiol Biomarkers Prev* 2011;20(1):2068–2077.

Cella DF, Cherin EA. Quality of life during and after treatment. *Compr Ther* 1988;14:69–75.

Fardell JE, Vardy J, Johnston IN, Winocur G. Chemotherapy and cognitive impairment: treatment options. *Clin Pharmacol Ther* 2011;90(3):366–376.

Given BA, Sherwood P, Given CW. Support for caregivers of cancer patients: transition after active treatment. *CEBP FOCUS Cancer Survivorship Research* 2011;20(10):2015–2019.

Helgeson VS, Snyder P, Seltman H. Psychological and physical adjustment to breast cancer over 4 years: identifying distinct trajectories of change. *Health Psychol* 2004;23:3–15.

Hodgkinson K, Butow P, Fuchs A, et al. Long-term survival from gynecologic cancer: psychosocial outcomes, supportive care needs and positive outcomes. *Gynec Oncol* 2007;104: 381–389.

Kurita K, Meyerowitz BE, Hall P, Gatz M. Long-term cognitive impairment in older adult twins discordant for gynecologic cancer treatment. *J Gerontol A Biol Sci Med Sci* 2011;66(12): 1343–1349.

Kurtz M, Kurtz J, Given C, Given B. Depression and physical health among family caregivers of geriatric patients with cancer—a longitudinal view. *Med Sci Monit* 2004;10:CR447-CR456.

Maher, EJ, Denton, A. Survivorship, late effects and cancer of the cervix. *Clin Oncol* 2008;20: 479–487.

Mahon SM. Tertiary prevention. Implications for improving the quality of life of long-term survivors of cancer. *Semin Oncol Nurs* 2005;21(4):260–270.

Matei D, Miller AM, Monahan P, et al. Chronic physical effects and health care utilization in long-term ovarian germ cell tumor survivors: a Gynecologic Oncology Group study. *J Clin Oncol* 2009;(27)25:4142–4149.

Ng, AK, Travis, LB. Subsequent malignant neoplasms in cancer survivors. *Cancer J* 2008;14(6): 429–434.

Neugut AI, Weinberg MD, Ahsan H, Rescigno J. Carcinogenic effects of radiotherapy for breast cancer. Oncology (Williston Park) 1999;13(9):1245–1256.

Ratner ES, Foran KA, Schwartz PE, Minkin MJ. Sexuality and intimacy after gynecological cancer. *Maturitas* 2010;66:24–26.

Wenzel LB, Donnelly JP, Fowler JM, et al. Resilience, reflection, and residual stress in ovarian cancer survivorship: a Gynecologic Oncology Group study. *Psycho-Oncol* 2002;11:142–153.

Yabroff KR, Kim Y. Time costs associated with informal caregiving for cancer survivors. *Cancer* 2009;115(18):4362–4373.

Survivorship Algorithms

These cancer survivorship algorithms have been specifically developed for MD Anderson using a multidisciplinary approach and taking into consideration circumstances particular to MD Anderson, including the following: MD Anderson's specific patient population, MD Anderson's services and structure, and MD Anderson's clinical information. These algorithms are provided for informational purposes only and are not intended to replace the independent medical or professional judgment of physicians or other health care providers. Moreover, these algorithms should not be used to treat pregnant women.

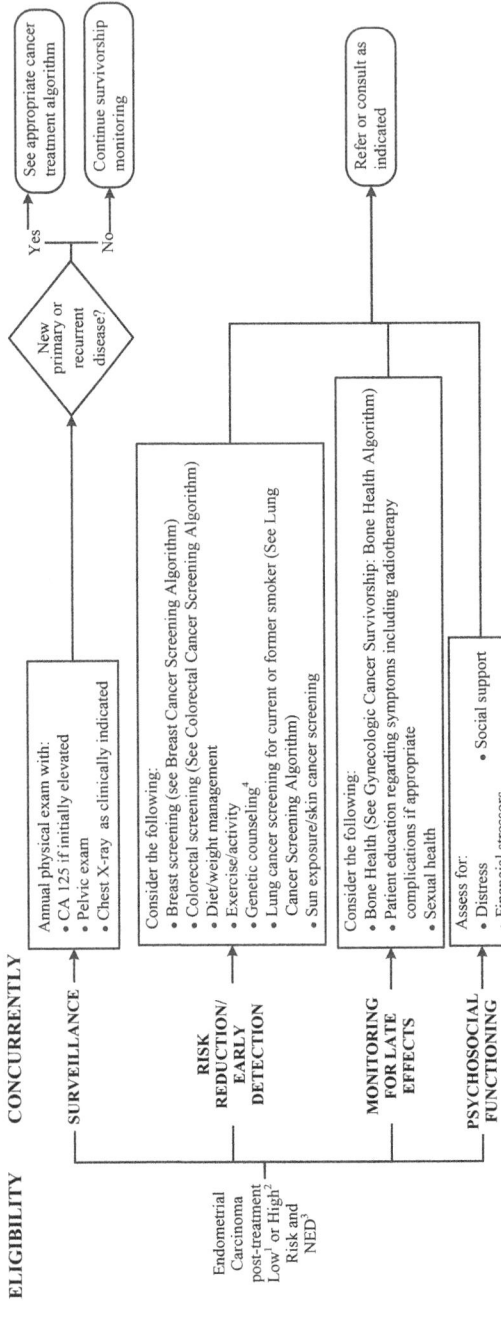

ELIGIBILITY **CONCURRENTLY**

SURVEILLANCE

Annual physical exam with:
- CA 125 if initially elevated
- Pelvic exam
- Chest X-ray as clinically indicated

RISK REDUCTION/ EARLY DETECTION

Consider the following:
- Breast screening (see Breast Cancer Screening Algorithm)
- Colorectal screening (See Colorectal Cancer Screening Algorithm)
- Diet/weight management
- Exercise/activity
- Genetic counseling [4]
- Lung cancer screening for current or former smoker (See Lung Cancer Screening Algorithm)
- Sun exposure/skin cancer screening

MONITORING FOR LATE EFFECTS

Consider the following:
- Bone Health (See Gynecologic Cancer Survivorship: Bone Health Algorithm)
- Patient education regarding symptoms including radiotherapy complications if appropriate
- Sexual health

PSYCHOSOCIAL FUNCTIONING

Assess for:
- Distress
- Financial stressors
- Social support

Endometrial Carcinoma post-treatment Low[1] or High[2] Risk and NED[3]

New primary or recurrent disease?

Yes → See appropriate cancer treatment algorithm

No → Continue survivorship monitoring

Refer or consult as indicated

[1] Low risk endometrial cancer is defined as any patient who did not receive chemotherapy or radiotherapy as adjuvant treatment after their initial surgery. Survivorship begins 3 years post-treatment and NED.
[2] High risk defined as women who did receive chemotherapy or radiotherapy as adjuvant treatment after their surgery. Survivorship begins 5 years post-treatment and NED.
[3] NED = No Evidence of Disease
[4] Consider genetic counseling if there has been a significant family history change since the last genetic consult, or if the patient has not previously had genetic counseling and has Lynch Syndrome risk factors. Lynch Syndrome risk factors: personal history of colon or rectal cancer; immediate family (first degree relatives such as parent, child, or sibling) with colorectal or endometrial cancer; immediate or extended family (first, second or third degree relatives including parent, child, sibling, aunt, uncle, nieces, nephews, grandparents, and first cousins) diagnosed before age 50 with colon, rectal or uterine cancer; any relatives tested positive for a Lynch Syndrome mutation (MLH1, MSH2, MSH6, PMS2 genes).

Algorithm 8.1 Survivorship—endometrial cancer

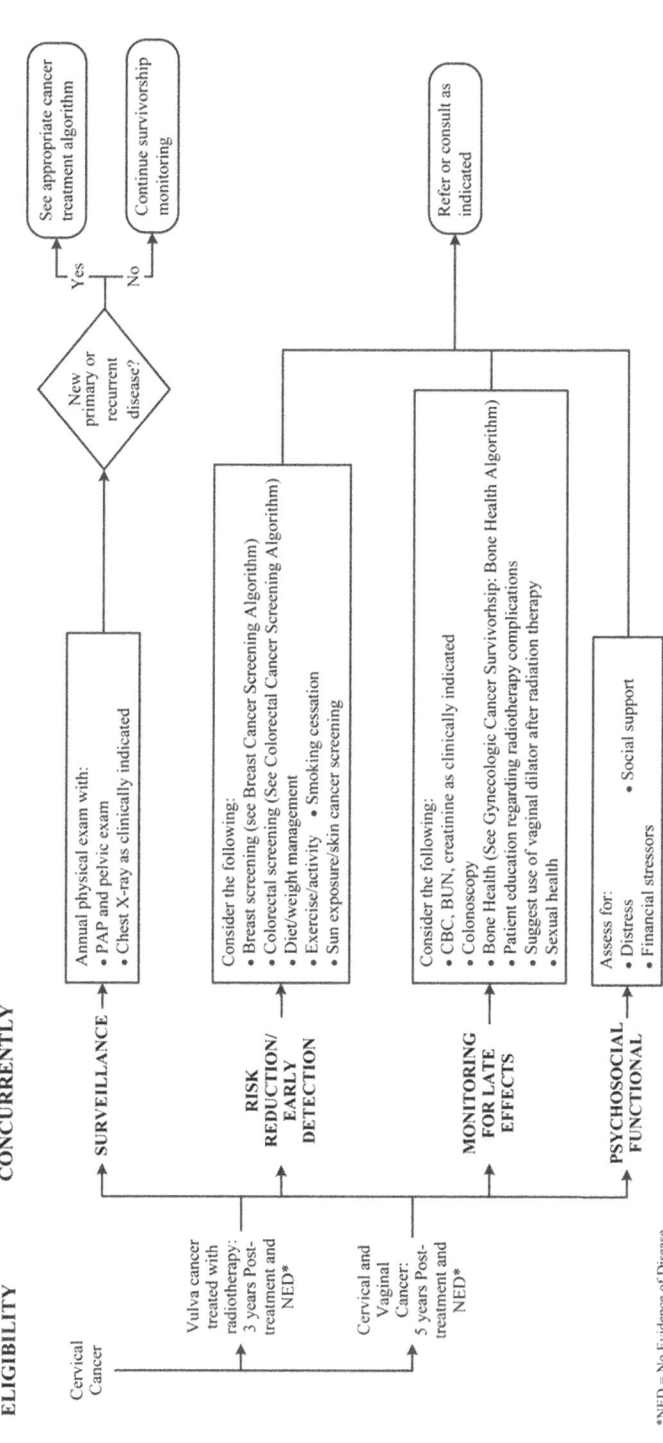

Algorithm 8.2 Survivorship—cervical cancer (includes vulva and vagina)

Copyright 2011 The University of Texas M.D. Anderson Cancer Center

*NED = No Evidence of Disease

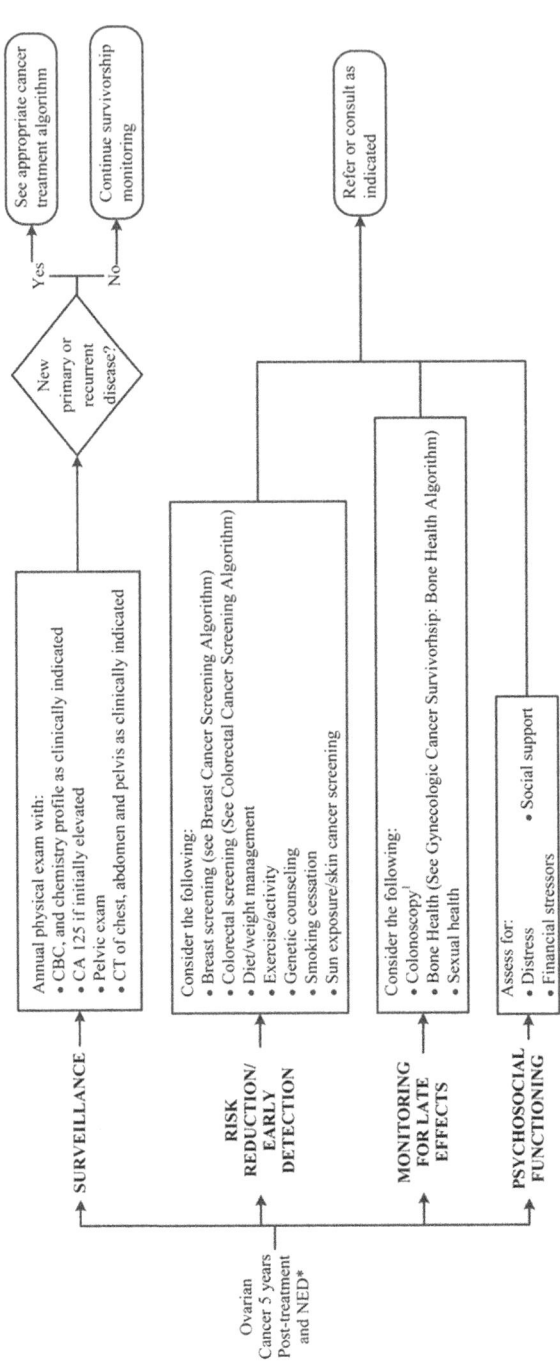

ELIGIBILITY   CONCURRENTLY

Ovarian Cancer 5 years Post-treatment and NED*

SURVEILLANCE

Annual physical exam with:
- CBC, and chemistry profile as clinically indicated
- CA 125 if initially elevated
- Pelvic exam
- CT of chest, abdomen and pelvis as clinically indicated

RISK REDUCTION/ EARLY DETECTION

Consider the following:
- Breast screening (see Breast Cancer Screening Algorithm)
- Colorectal screening (See Colorectal Cancer Screening Algorithm)
- Diet/weight management
- Exercise/activity
- Genetic counseling
- Smoking cessation
- Sun exposure/skin cancer screening

MONITORING FOR LATE EFFECTS

Consider the following:
- Colonoscopy[1]
- Bone Health (See Gynecologic Cancer Survivorship: Bone Health Algorithm)
- Sexual health

PSYCHOSOCIAL FUNCTIONING

Assess for:
- Distress
- Financial stressors
- Social support

New primary or recurrent disease?

Yes → See appropriate cancer treatment algorithm

No → Continue survivorship monitoring

Refer or consult as indicated

*NED = No Evidence of Disease
[1] If personal history of ovarian or endometrial cancer diagnosed at age less than 60 years, begin colonoscopy at age 40 or at diagnosis of endometrial cancer. (NCCN) All others should begin colonoscopy at age 50. (ACS)

Copyright 2011 The University of Texas M.D. Anderson Cancer Center

Algorithm 8.3 Survivorship—ovarian cancer (includes fallopian tube and peritoneal primary)

Department of Clinical Effectiveness V3
Approved by the Executive Committee of the Medical Staff 03/29/2011

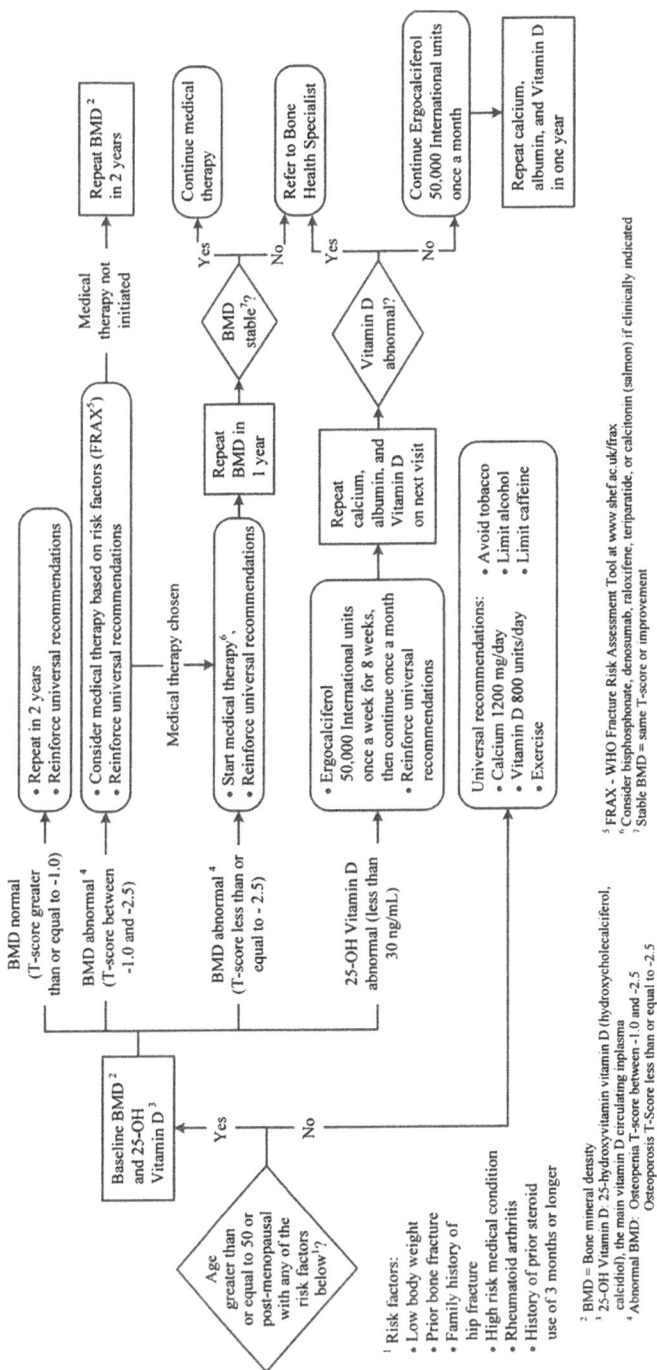

Algorithm 8.4 Gynecologic cancer survivorship: bone health

Chapter 9
Head and Neck Cancer Survivorship Management

Katherine A. Hutcheson and Carol M. Lewis

Contents

Chapter Overview Head and neck cancer (HNC) survivors present with unique needs related to the long-term effects of cancer therapy on upper aerodigestive tract functions. Management of HNC varies depending on the patient's individual stage and subsite of HNC, cancer treatment history, and psychosocial needs. In general, long-term functioning is optimized by multidisciplinary treatment planning with consideration of both acute and late adverse effects. Risk-reduction strategies such as oral care, targeted exercise, swallowing therapy, nutritional counseling, and audiologic monitoring are best implemented early in the HNC treatment trajectory. Posttreatment surveillance facilitates detection of recurrences and second primary tumors, as well as monitoring of long-term functional rehabilitation needs.

L.E. Foxhall, M.A. Rodriguez (eds.), *Advances in Cancer Survivorship Management*,
MD Anderson Cancer Care Series, DOI 10.1007/978-1-4939-0986-5_9,
© The University of Texas M.D. Anderson Cancer Center 2015

Introduction

Head and neck cancer (HNC) accounts for roughly 5% of all cancers. In 2010, 36,540 cases of oral cavity and oropharyngeal cancers and 12,720 cases of laryngeal cancer were diagnosed in the United States. Oral cavity and oropharyngeal cancers comprised 3% of all cancers in men (Jemal et al. 2010). More than 85% of cases of HNC are squamous cell carcinoma (Mehanna et al. 2010b), which will be the focus of this chapter.

The upper aerodigestive tract (UADT) is separated into different subsites; the treatment of cancer in each of these subsites requires specific anatomic and functional considerations. The nasopharynx is posterior to the nasal cavity, superior to the palate, and inferior to the skull base. The oral cavity starts at and includes the lips and ends posteriorly at the soft palate. The oropharynx includes the soft palate and posterior pharyngeal wall and is limited inferiorly by the level of the hyoid bone. The hypopharynx starts at the level of the hyoid bone and extends to the inferior aspect of the cricoid bone. The larynx encompasses the epiglottis, arytenoids, and aryepiglottic folds superiorly and extends inferiorly to 1 cm below the true vocal folds (TVFs).

The management of cancer arising in these subsites requires multidisciplinary planning. The head and neck oncology team should consist of a head and neck surgeon, medical oncologist, radiation oncologist, dentist, speech pathologist, dietitian, and social worker at the very minimum, and treatment plans should be formulated through multidisciplinary discussion.

Overview of Treatment Modalities

Chemotherapy

Eradication of systemic disease is the goal of chemotherapy, although in HNC, chemotherapy functions as an adjuvant to surgery and radiation therapy (RT) to improve local and regional control. Chemotherapy also serves a palliative role in patients with distant metastases or locoregional recurrence for whom surgery or RT are no longer reasonable options. In the latter group, approximately one-third of patients will obtain a 3- to 6-month survival benefit from chemotherapy (Brockstein and Volkes 2006).

As an adjuvant treatment, chemotherapy can be given as induction therapy prior to definitive surgery or RT or concurrently with postoperative or definitive RT. The advantages of induction therapy include the potential to decrease tumor burden, predict response to subsequent treatment, and decrease morbidity by facilitating less extensive definitive treatment. Perhaps the most well-known example of induction chemotherapy in HNC is the Department of Veterans Affairs Laryngeal Cancer

Study Group, which demonstrated identical 2-year overall survival rates in patients receiving induction chemotherapy and definitive RT (with salvage surgery as indicated) and, for patients who did not respond to induction chemotherapy, in those who underwent surgery with postoperative RT. In the former group of patients, 64% had laryngeal preservation, and 39% of the patients with laryngeal preservation were disease-free with an intact larynx (Department of Veterans Affairs Laryngeal Cancer Study Group 1991).

When given concurrently with RT, chemotherapy acts to enhance the efficacy of RT. Although concurrent chemoradiation has never been compared with surgery in a randomized fashion, the reported rates of overall survival for certain cancers rival those published for surgical management (Forastiere et al. 2003). In patients undergoing surgery for disease with adverse features, such as extracapsular spread (wherein the tumor grows outside the capsule of the lymph node), concurrent postoperative chemoradiation has been shown to improve locoregional control and overall survival (Cooper et al. 2004).

Radiation Therapy

RT may take the form of external beam RT, conformal RT, or brachytherapy. External beam RT, or standard RT, is delivered with beam energy specific to the depth of the tumor. Conformal RT, or intensity-modulated radiation therapy, customizes the high-dose region to the tumor, or target volume. Conformal fields are composed of numerous smaller beams, each with a target dose and acceptable range of doses, as determined by its mark. In brachytherapy, the radioactive source is placed in close proximity to the target volume. It can be placed into the tumor itself (interstitial) or superficially, and radiation is delivered at a continuously low rate. Because the radiation is confined, there is less risk to surrounding structures, but this method is limited by the volume of the tumor and the extent of needed coverage. RT can be given as definitive, adjuvant, or palliative treatment. Definitive treatment doses are generally 66–70 Gy (over 6–7 weeks). Postoperative doses are generally 60–66 Gy.

Surgery

The role of surgery is recognized in current American Joint Cancer Committee staging for various subsites of HNC. Stage T4b represents unresectable disease; this is defined anatomically and includes encasement of the carotid, intracranial extension, or invasion of the prevertebral fascia, skull base, pterygoid plates, masticator space, or mediastinal structures. Surgical planning must account for anticipated functional effects to limit treatment morbidity.

Overview of Head and Neck Cancer

The incidence of HNC increases with age and is more common in men, with male to female ratios ranging from 2:1 to 15:1, depending on the site of HNC (Mehanna et al. 2010a). The major risk factors are alcohol and tobacco, including smokeless forms. Alcohol and tobacco account for 75% of cases of HNC, and are both independent and synergistic risk factors (Conway et al. 2009). Quitting smoking for 1–4 years reduces the risk of HNC, with further benefit at 20 years, at which point the risk is similar to that associated with never smoking. Similarly, quitting alcohol for 20 or more years confers the same benefit as never drinking (Marron et al. 2010). A genetic predisposition is suggested: HNC in a first-degree relative confers a 1.7-fold increased risk (Conway et al. 2009). This may be related to the metabolism of tobacco and alcohol (Mehanna et al. 2010a).

Another risk factor of HNC is viral infection. Eighty percent to 90% of patients with non-keratinizing nasopharyngeal cancer have been found to have abnormally elevated antibody titers to Epstein Barr virus proteins. More recently, human papilloma virus (HPV) has been associated with oropharyngeal carcinoma; patients whose tumors are HPV-positive have a significantly higher overall survival rate than those whose tumors are not (Ang et al. 2010).

Treatment and Survival

Oral Cavity

Oral cavity cancer is a surgical disease. Surgery is the mainstay of treatment for all stages and postoperative RT is recommended for histologic evidence of perineural invasion, lymphovascular invasion, positive margins, cartilage or bone invasion, or nodal disease. If there is extracapsular extension, then postoperative chemoradiation is recommended. Reconstruction may range from healing by secondary intent to free flap reconstruction, depending on the extent of resection. If the patient cannot have surgery (e.g., because of comorbid illness), definitive RT may be considered, with chemotherapy for advanced disease. The 5-year overall survival rates for patients with stages I-IV disease are 75–95%, 65–85%, 45–65%, and 10–35%, respectively.

Oropharynx

In recent decades, treatment of oropharyngeal cancer has trended towards definitive RT, largely because of similar survival outcomes between patients who undergo surgery and those who undergo definitive RT, with the expectation of superior function after nonsurgical organ preservation. Chemotherapy is given in the neoadjuvant setting for bulky or low cervical adenopathy, or for large tumors. Concurrent chemoradiation is indicated for large (T3 or T4) tumors or N2 or N3 adenopathy. The role of surgery was largely salvage until recent endoscopic and robotic advances enabled minimally invasive approaches to select early-stage tumors. The 5-year overall survival rates for patients with stages I-IV disease are 67%, 46%, 31%, and 32%, respectively (Seikaly and Rassekh 2001). Patients with HPV-positive tumors have better prognoses, with 3-year overall survival rates of 82.7% compared with 57.1% in patients with HPV-negative tumors (Ang et al. 2010).

Nasopharynx

The primary treatment for nasopharyngeal cancer is definitive RT, with concurrent chemotherapy for large primary tumors or N2/N3 cervical adenopathy. Induction chemotherapy is considered for patients with large primary tumors or bulky or low adenopathy. The role of surgery is largely salvage. For patients with stage I-IV disease, 5-year overall survival rates are approximately 70%, 60%, 60%, and 40%, respectively.

Hypopharynx/Larynx

The management of hypopharyngeal and laryngeal cancers largely depends on what treatment will best maintain function. Early-stage tumors are generally managed with single-modality treatment (definitive RT or surgery) and late-stage tumors are managed with either concurrent chemoradiation or surgery with postoperative RT. Induction chemotherapy is considered for bulky tumors or adenopathy. Five-year disease-free survival rates for patients with stage I-IV laryngeal cancer are 84–90%, 83–85%, 73–75%, and roughly 45%, respectively.

Posttreatment Surveillance

Posttreatment surveillance serves the purpose of detecting recurrences and second primary tumors. In addition, it benefits patients' psychological and emotional well-being and addresses functional rehabilitation (Manikantan et al. 2009). Overall, HNC recurrences are reported for 33–49% of patients (Boysen et al. 1992; de Visscher and Manni 1994), with 76% and 87% of recurrences presenting within the first 2 and 3 years after treatment, respectively (Boysen et al. 1992). The rate of second primary tumors is roughly 15% (de Visscher and Manni. 1994); most arise within the UADT, more commonly in the oral cavity, oropharynx, and hypopharynx than in the larynx, although lung second primary tumors are also prevalent.

The National Comprehensive Cancer Network recommends a history and physical examination every 1–3 months for the first year, every 2–4 months for the second year, every 4–6 months for years 3–5, and every 6–12 months thereafter. At MD Anderson, we follow HNC patients every 3 months for the first year, every 4 months for the second year, and every 6 months for the third year. For patients in whom recurrence is of particular concern, closer monitoring is undertaken. Posttreatment imaging, when indicated, is obtained within 3 months of completing treatment and at indicated intervals thereafter. If the patient has been irradiated, thyroid function studies are drawn with every visit because post-RT hypothyroidism may occur any time between 4 weeks and 10 years after treatment. Chest imaging is obtained at least annually for detection of second primary tumors or distant metastases. Because the overwhelming majority of recurrences occur within the first 3 years of treatment, patients are referred to a HNC survivorship program after 3 years of uneventful surveillance.

The foundation of long-term surveillance is composed of symptom management and complete physical examination. This involves the examination of both ears, looking specifically for middle ear fluid, and a full cranial nerve examination. Direct inspection of the oral cavity (all sides of the oral tongue, floor of mouth, hard palate, and buccal, gingival, and labial surfaces), soft palate, and tonsillar fossae should be performed. The tongue base, tonsillar fossae, and any concerning findings should be palpated. If the examining physician is comfortable with indirect mirror laryngoscopy or nasopharyngoscopy, one of these should be undertaken. Cervical palpation for adenopathy or thyroid masses must be included. Worsening pain, dysphagia, or dysphonia are symptoms that warrant further investigation or referral to the treating team. Axial imaging may be helpful in cases in which the region of concern cannot be examined or in which anatomy has been so altered as to render adequate examination difficult.

Upper Aerodigestive Tract Function and Head and Neck Cancer

Normal Function

HNC has the potential to adversely affect a number of complex UADT functions, including respiration, speech, and swallowing. During normal respiration, the laryngopharynx serves as a conduit for air exchange between the upper and lower airways. Pulmonary airflow through the larynx also serves as the power source to generate vibratory sound production as the TVFs adduct during phonation. This phonatory signal resonates throughout the vocal tract and is shaped into words by the articulators in the oral cavity (i.e., the lips, tongue, and teeth). Normal deglutition is commonly described in four phases: (1) oral preparatory, (2) oral, (3) pharyngeal, and (4) esophageal. In the oral preparatory phase of swallowing, food or liquid is taken into the mouth and manipulated into a cohesive bolus that is then propelled posteriorly to the pharynx by the tongue during the oral phase of swallowing. Two primary actions occur in the pharyngeal phase of swallowing: (1) laryngeal closure to prevent tracheal aspiration, and (2) bolus propulsion to the esophagus via tongue base retraction and pharyngeal contraction.

Long-Term Effects of Treatment

Long-term effects of treatment for HNC vary depending on the primary site of disease and treatment regimen. In general, surgical resection affects function by anatomically or structurally altering the UADT. The local effects of surgical resection are related to the normal function of the resected structures and the volume of the resection. For instance, the lingual defect after glossectomy impairs articulation, bolus formation, and lingual pressures to assist with bolus propulsion during swallowing. Resection of the supraglottic larynx disrupts normal airway closure during swallowing and increases the risk of aspiration, whereas total laryngectomy results in complete loss of voice (aphonia), requiring various methods of alaryngeal voice restoration. In addition, emerging experience suggests a functional advantage of using minimally invasive approaches, such as endoscopic or robotic resection, rather than traditional open approaches that disrupt adjacent normal tissue will leave patients with better function.

Fibrosis has long been considered a primary source of late functional complications after RT. The fibrotic process is self-inducing and may spread to adjacent regions, causing chronic, often progressive symptoms. In addition, denervation of oral, pharyngeal, or laryngeal structures may occur as a result of direct neural infiltration by the tumor, chemotoxicity, iatrogenic surgical injury, or as a late effect of RT. Roughly half of survivors who present with late, refractory radiation-associated dysphagia have de novo cranial neuropathies, most commonly X and XII, years after treatment. In addition, preliminary data from the National Institutes of Health Laryngeal Study Section found at least partial denervation of suprahyoid musculature on electromyography in most (>90%) nonsurgical HNC patients with chronic dysphagia after RT or chemoradiation (Martin et al. 2010). The pathophysiology of peripheral motor neuropathy after RT is not fully understood, but devascularization and compressive injury from adjacent fibrosis is most commonly suggested.

Lymphatic insufficiency is a common consequence of surgery and RT. Blockage, damage, or removal of lymph vessels results in abnormal accumulation of interstitial fluid or lymphedema. In early stages, lymphedema is associated with a soft swelling. Lymphedema can progress in later stages to a hard, fibrotic process. This under-recognized complication of treatment for HNC is often thought to be a cosmetic issue, but the potential functional implications of chronic lymphedema are increasingly recognized (Smith and Lewin 2010).

Dysphagia

Denervation and fibrosis of the oral, laryngeal, and pharyngeal musculature may occur or persist long after the completion of treatment for HNC. These late effects ultimately impair range of motion of key swallowing structures and have been implicated as the primary mechanisms of chronic dysphagia in HNC survivors. In severe cases of chronic dysphagia, dietary restrictions and malnutrition mandate lifelong gastrostomy tube dependence. HNC survivors may also experience aspiration of food and liquids, posing a risk for potentially life-threatening aspiration pneumonia (Rosenthal et al. 2006). A variety of metrics are used to estimate the burden of dysphagia in HNC survivors, and rates depend greatly on the specific subsite of disease and treatment modality. The prevalence of aspiration in long-term HNC survivors reported in the literature ranges from 23% (stage III/IV HNC treated with chemoradiation) to 44% (all sites, stages, and treatment modalities; Campbell et al. 2004; Rütten et al. 2011), whereas rates of chronic gastrostomy dependence (>2 years after treatment) are typically lower (6–22%; Ang et al. 2005; Cheng et al. 2006). Neither aspiration nor gastrostomy rates should be considered sensitive indicators of the presence of dysphagia; many HNC survivors maintain oral intake despite significant physiologic swallowing impairment and aspiration.

Instrumental examinations are considered the gold standard assessment of swallowing function in HNC survivors. Instrumental assessment is particularly important in HNC survivors with chronic dysphagia because high rates of silent aspiration and physiologic impairment are observed in this population (Rosenthal et al. 2006). The primary options for instrumental swallowing assessment include flexible fiberoptic endoscopic evaluation of swallowing (FEES) and radiographic evaluation using the modified barium swallow (MBS) study. Detailed comparisons of these examinations have been published previously (Langmore 2003). At MD Anderson, the MBS study is typically chosen for the following reasons: (1) swallowing physiology and aspiration events that occur during the swallow can be observed directly (peak swallow is obscured by peak white-out on FEES), and (2) the extent of the upper esophageal sphincter opening can be assessed. On the other hand, FEES can be extremely useful for biofeedback when training compensatory swallowing maneuvers.

HNC survivors with chronic dysphagia are followed by speech pathologists who tailor dysphagia management on the basis of the findings of instrumental examination, as well as the compensatory abilities, comorbidities, and pulmonary status of the individual. In general, compensatory swallowing strategies become a primary focus of dysphagia management in the years after treatment for HNC. Strategies may be used to facilitate more efficient swallowing (i.e., increase speed and ease of oral intake) or to improve airway protection (i.e., decrease the risk of aspiration). These techniques include but are not limited to positional changes (e.g., chin tuck or head rotation), maneuvers (e.g., supraglottic swallow), or diet modifications (e.g., thickened liquid or pureed food). Swallowing exercise may also be prescribed in an effort to prevent the progression of chronic dysphagia. Intensive paradigms or progressive, resistive therapy are likely needed to rehabilitate patients with chronic or late radiation-associated dysphagia. Increasing evidence suggests that early, preventive swallowing exercise is beneficial for HNC patients treated with RT-based regimens (Carnaby-Mann et al. 2012). At MD Anderson, HNC patients are referred to a speech pathologist prior to treatment for baseline assessment and training in targeted preventive swallowing exercise. The motto "use it or lose it" underlies risk-reduction strategies during RT for HNC. Therapy goals are designed to encourage ongoing use and exercise of UADT musculature.

Stricture is a less common (<10% incidence; Francis et al. 2010) but important contributor to chronic dysphagia in HNC survivors. Particular subgroups of HNC survivors, including those with a history of hypopharyngeal cancer, have an elevated risk of stricture. When stricture is identified, esophageal dilatation may be offered by the head and neck surgeon or gastroenterologist. Multidisciplinary evaluation including an MBS study is essential to provide realistic expectations of the dilatation procedure. In the absence of adequate pharyngeal propulsion and airway protection, substantial dysphagia may persist despite a successful dilatation.

Laryngeal Dysfunction

The larynx is a critical structure for normal speech, respiration, and swallowing. Laryngeal dysfunction may take on various forms in long-term HNC survivorship, including (1) glottic insufficiency related to TVF immobility; (2) airway obstruction owing to laryngeal edema, fibrosis, or TVF immobility; or (3) laryngeal chondroradionecrosis. Delayed onset of any of these complications or symptoms warrants careful physical examination and imaging to rule out recurrent cancer. Imaging should assess for locoregional recurrence, as well as distant metastases; positron emission tomography or computed tomography of the head, neck, and chest suffice. At MD Anderson, workup also includes detailed functional assessment via laryngeal videostroboscopy. This endoscopic office procedure provides critical data regarding TVF mobility, approximation, symmetry, vibration, and pathology.

Delayed onset of TVF immobility in HNC survivors is most often a long-term complication of RT (Tirado et al. 2010). The primary symptom of unilateral TVF immobility is dysphonia, although glottic insufficiency may also elevate the risk of aspiration and, consequently, pneumonia. Aspiration risk is a particular concern in HNC survivors who have coexisting pharyngeal dysfunction related to prior treatments. Although management of TVF paralysis may improve glottic closure during the swallow and the effectiveness of the cough to clear aspirate, it will not improve other components of dysphagia such as diminished hyolaryngeal excursion or reduced pharyngeal contraction. As such, an MBS study is typically recommended for HNC survivors found to have late-onset TVF immobility. The MBS study is used to determine the extent and etiology of coexisting dysphagia, and to assess the potential impact of TVF management on swallowing function. After multidisciplinary evaluation by the head and neck surgeon and speech pathologist, TVF management may be offered in the form of injection laryngoplasty or medialization thyroplasty. The efficacy of in-office injection laryngoplasty in the previously irradiated larynx has been previously reported (Tirado et al. 2010), but the effects are typically temporary. Medialization thyroplasty can be considered as a surgical alternative for long-term management of unilateral TVF immobility.

Laryngeal edema, fibrosis, scarring or webbing, radionecrosis, or laryngeal fixation may contribute to airway distress after treatment for HNC. Severe laryngeal edema and soft tissue necrosis are rare (<5% incidence) but potentially life-threatening late effects that are commonly associated with continued smoking after treatment for HNC. Treatments are largely symptom-based because previous treatments can alter anatomy and confound clinical examination. Tracheotomy is indicated when the patient can no longer comfortably complete activities of daily living because of dyspnea. Hyperbaric oxygen may be a consideration for radionecrosis once recurrence has been confidently ruled out. Ultimately, an elective total laryngectomy may be offered for definitive surgical management of radionecrosis, airway obstruction, or refractory laryngeal dysfunction to restore the airway and prevent aspiration (Hutcheson et al. 2012). Rehabilitative potential after elective laryngectomy is evaluated by the multidisciplinary team and should be discussed candidly with the patient.

Oral Complications

HNC survivors are at risk for lifelong oral health complications owing to chronic salivary dysfunction, surgical ablation, and local radiation-induced cellular injury. Oral health complications commonly encountered in long-term HNC survivorship include xerostomia, trismus, and osteoradionecrosis (ORN).

Xerostomia, or dry mouth, occurs in most HNC survivors treated with RT as the result of damage to major and minor salivary glands in the field of radiation. The extent of salivary dysfunction depends on RT dose and the volume of the salivary glands exposed. Glandular damage reduces salivary flow but also changes the composition of saliva and alters the oral microflora. For this reason, xerostomia predisposes patients to oral discomfort, loss of appetite, changes in taste, weight loss, dental caries, oral infections, and ORN of the mandible. In addition to stringent oral care, management of xerostomia may include use of topical saliva substitutes or pharmacotherapy as directed by the dental team (Chambers et al. 2004).

Trismus results in reduced oral opening after treatment for HNC and may be associated with impaired mastication, nutritional deficiencies, and reduced access for oral care. Trismus occurs when the masticatory muscles (pterygoids, masseter) or temporomandibular joint are injured as a result of tumor involvement, surgery, neuropathy, or postradiation fibrosis. Definitions and diagnostic criteria for trismus vary widely in the literature; however, an interincisal opening of ≤35 mm is considered abnormal by many sources. Summary estimates from the International Society of Oral Oncology suggest that the prevalence of trismus varies greatly by treatment modality (weighted prevalence: 5% after intensity-modulated RT, 25% after conventional RT, and 31% after combined chemoradiation). The risk of trismus is elevated after combined-modality therapies. A variety of interventions (pentoxifyl-

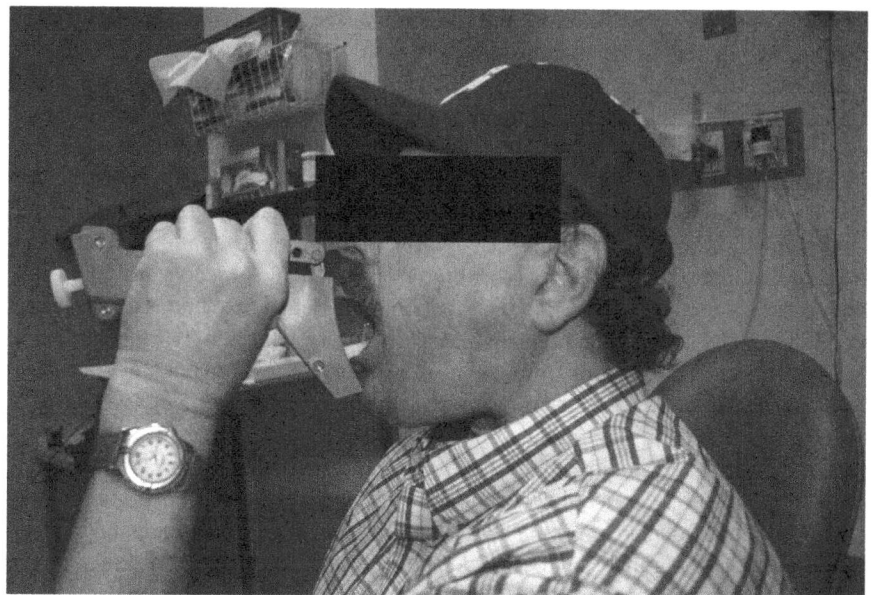

Fig. 9.1 Range of motion exercise for the treatment of trismus using the TheraBite device

line, botulinum toxin) and devices (e.g., tongue blades, intraincisal corkscrews, TheraBite, DynaSplint) have been proposed to facilitate improved oral opening. Current data suggest a clinical benefit from passive range of motion exercise against an external force (e.g., TheraBite, DynaSplint; Bensadoun et al. 2010). At MD Anderson, passive range of motion exercise (Fig. 9.1) is introduced early under the direction of the oncologic dentist because experience suggests that limitations in oral opening may slowly progress after treatment for HNC.

ORN can be a significant late effect of radiotherapy in HNC survivors. ORN typically affects the mandible. A comprehensive review suggests an overall incidence of less than 10% in HNC survivors (Chrcanovic et al. 2010). However, a disproportionate number of those who develop ORN have a history of oral malignancies, stage IV disease, or RT doses in excess of 60 Gy. The diagnosis of ORN is obtained by clinical signs and symptoms, including prolonged bone exposure with mucosal ulceration or necrosis in the absence of recurrent disease. ORN may also be associated with pain and trismus, and it has the potential to progress to pathologic fracture or orocutaneous fistula if left untreated. ORN may present spontaneously or as a result of trauma (e.g., surgery, extraction, prosthetic irritation) in the irradiated field. At MD Anderson, treatment for ORN begins with conservative nonsurgical therapy, including daily irrigation and antibiotic coverage. Additional management is required for most individuals and may include surgical sequestrectomy, debridement, or hyperbaric oxygen therapy. A 15-year review of MD Anderson data found that approximately 40% of patients had resolution of ORN with these conservative therapies. Radical resection and free flap reconstruction is typically reserved for cases of ORN that fail to respond to conservative management or that present with pathologic fracture, fistula, pain, or trismus (Oh et al. 2009).

Optimal oral care in HNC survivors begins before cancer treatment. Risk-reduction strategies include stringent oral hygiene, adequate nutritional intake, and lifelong prophylaxis to prevent dental caries (topical stannous fluoride daily). At MD Anderson, all HNC patients are evaluated by an oncologic dentist before delivery of therapy for baseline evaluation of oral status (mucosa, periodontium, and teeth) and initiation of an oral care regimen. The baseline dental evaluation is scheduled as early as possible to allow time for the patient to receive and heal from any necessary pretreatment dental intervention (e.g., dental extraction). Patients are then followed by an oncologic dentist in the early survivorship period, for a minimum of 1 year after the completion of therapy, after which HNC survivors may transition care back to their routine dentist for standard nonsurgical management. Elective oral surgical procedures in the irradiated field (e.g., extractions, soft tissue surgery) are generally contraindicated owing to the elevated risk of complications. When medically indicated, oral surgical intervention after RT requires careful planning by the oncologic dentist to make recommendations regarding presurgical hyperbaric oxygen therapy, oral care regimens, and antibiotic coverage (Chambers et al. 2004).

Oncologic dentists and maxillofacial prosthodontists also aid select HNC survivors in prosthetic rehabilitation. A variety of intraoral (palatal, maxillary) and facial (orbital, auricular, nasal) prostheses can be fabricated for functional and cosmetic restoration after surgery. Initial prosthetic management typically occurs early in survivorship; however, periodic revision of prosthetic devices may be required in long-term follow-up.

Lymphedema

As many as 40–50% of HNC survivors are estimated to experience lymphedema as a consequence of therapy. The cosmetic and functional effects are often significant when the UADT is edematous. Head and neck lymphedema may adversely impact secretion management, deglutition, and communication. In extreme cases, distal neck edema may obstruct the postlaryngectomy airway and orbital edema may impair vision. Thus, management of lymphedema is encouraged to improve both the cosmetic and functional status of HNC survivors (Fig. 9.2; Smith and Lewin 2010).

A comprehensive head and neck lymphedema program is offered at MD Anderson. The treatment paradigm follows the model of Complete Decongestive Therapy (CDT). CDT is the international standard of care for treating lymphedema. CDT combines manual lymphatic drainage massage, compression bandaging, targeted exercise, and skin care. The therapy is designed to decongest and prevent refilling of the edematous region by promoting drainage to adjacent areas with intact lymphatic vessels. CDT is traditionally provided by a certified lymphedema therapist in two phases: an intensive phase of outpatient treatment provided 3–5

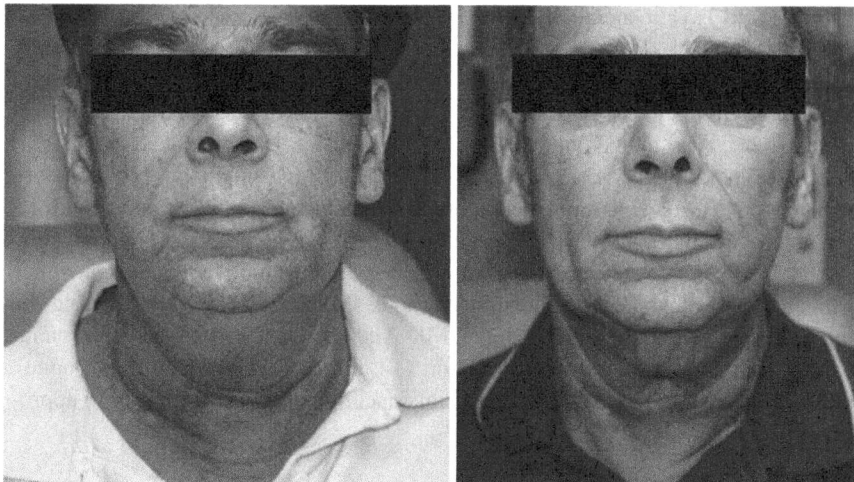

Fig. 9.2 Lymphedema in the neck and submental region after chemoradiation for nasopharyngeal carcinoma (*left*); lymphedema improved after therapy (*right*)

days per week over 2–4 weeks, followed by a maintenance phase of daily self-administered CDT in the home. At MD Anderson, we offer both outpatient clinician-administered CDT and a home-based treatment program administered by the patient or caregiver after one or two training sessions in the clinic. Institutional data suggest a benefit from both methods of CDT, although superior outcomes have been reported with traditional outpatient delivery (Smith and Lewin 2010).

Ototoxicity

HNC survivors with a history of ototoxic drug exposure (e.g., cisplatin >100 mg/m^2) are at risk for chronic, potentially progressive sensorineural hearing loss (Hitchcock et al. 2009). Ototoxic agents first affect the high-frequency range (frequencies above those needed for speech processing). For this reason, hearing loss may not be detected until it progresses to the lower frequency range and interferes with routine communication. At MD Anderson, HNC survivors treated with potentially ototoxic therapies receive audiologic monitoring annually after the first year of treatment (American Speech-Language-Hearing Association 1994). The audiologic examination includes tympanometry, pure tone testing (air conduction and bone conduction), speech reception threshold and word recognition testing, and distortion product otoacoustic emissions (Lonsbury-Martin and Martin 2001; Fausti 2006). Audiologic intervention is tailored on the basis of results from annual monitoring and may include education to reduce noise exposure or fitting of hearing aids.

Systemic and Psychosocial Effects

Systemic late effects in HNC survivors include micronutrient deficiencies, weight loss, hypothyroidism, pain, and fatigue. Dysphagia, xerostomia, and dental extractions have been associated with dietary adaptations after HNC that lead to a disproportionate intake of low-fiber, low-antioxidant, and high-fat foods. Inflammatory mediators have also been implicated as possible mechanisms of more general effects such as fatigue. In addition, HNC survivors suffer from high levels of anxiety, distress, and body image concerns that may adversely impact motivation and adherence to medical and rehabilitation recommendations (Murphy et al. 2007). During the long-term phase of HNC survivorship at MD Anderson, patients are screened annually for nutritional status, thyroid function (T4 and thyroid-stimulating hormone), pulmonary function, pain, and psychosocial concerns to facilitate referrals to appropriate specialists.

Key Practice Points

- HNC comprises distinct subsites of disease. The subsite and stage of disease greatly influence the selection of therapy, survival probability, and long-term functional outcomes.
- Surgery and radiotherapy are the primary modalities for definitive treatment of HNC.
- Prevention of severe late effects begins at the time of multidisciplinary treatment planning with pretreatment referral to key specialists (e.g., oncologic dentist, speech pathologist, audiologist, dietitian, social workers). Multidisciplinary coordination remains a key aspect of long-term HNC survivorship care.
- Although many HNC survivors can transition to a structured survivorship program after 3 years, any physician overseeing the long-term care of HNC survivors must be familiar with symptom management and understand the importance of investigating whether worsening pain, dysphonia, or dysphagia are a result of recurrence or a second primary tumor, as well as how to treat these symptoms with the goal of maximizing functional outcomes for the survivor.

Suggested Readings

American Speech-Language-Hearing Association. Audiologic management of individuals receiving cochleotoxic drug therapy. http://www.asha.org/policy/GL1994-00003/. Published 1994. Accessed July 5, 2013.

Ang KK, Harris J, Garden AS, et al. Concomitant boost radiation plus concurrent cisplatin for advanced head and neck carcinomas: radiation therapy oncology group phase II trial 99–14. *J Clin Oncol* 2005;23:3008–3015.

Ang KK, Harris J, Wheeler R, et al. Human papillomavirus and survival of patients with oropharyngeal cancer. *N Engl J Med* 2010;363:24–35.

Bensadoun RJ, Riesenbeck D, Lockhart PB, Elting LS, Spijkervet FK, Brennan MT. A systematic review of trismus induced by cancer therapies in head and neck cancer patients. *Support Care Cancer* 2010;18:1033–1038.

Boysen M, Lovdal O, Tausjo J, Winther F. The value of follow-up in patients treated for squamous cell carcinoma of the head and neck. *Eur J Cancer* 1992;28(2–3):426–430.

Brockstein BE, Vokes EE. Principles of chemotherapy in the management of head and neck cancer. In: Newlands SD, ed. *Head and Neck Surgery - Otolaryngology*. 4th ed. Philadelphia: Lippincott Williams and Wilkins; 2006:1427–1440.

Campbell BH, Spinelli K, Marbella AM, Myers KB, Kuhn JC, Layde PM. Aspiration, weight loss, and quality of life in head and neck cancer survivors. *Arch Otolaryngol Head Neck Surg* 2004;130:1100–1103.

Carnaby-Mann G, Crary MA, Schmalfuss I, Amdur R. "Pharyngocise": Randomized controlled trial of preventative exercises to maintain muscle structure and swallowing function during head-and-neck chemoradiotherapy. *Int J Radiat Oncol Biol Phys* 2012;83:210–219.

Chambers MS, Garden AS, Kies MS, Martin JW. Radiation-induced xerostomia in patients with head and neck cancer: pathogenesis, impact on quality of life, and management. *Head Neck* 2004;26:796–807.

Cheng SS, Terrell JE, Bradford CR, et al. Variables associated with feeding tube placement in head and neck cancer. *Arch Otolaryngol Head Neck Surg* 2006;132:655–661.

Chrcanovic BR, Reher P, Sousa AA, Harris M. Osteoradionecrosis of the jaws—a current overview—part 1: physiopathology and risk and predisposing factors. *Oral Maxillofac Surg* 2010; 14:3–16.

Conway DI, Hashibe M, Boffetta P, et al. Enhancing epidemiologic research on head and neck cancer: INHANCE - the international head and neck cancer epidemiology consortium. *Oral Oncol* 2009;45:743–746.

Cooper JS, Pajak TF, Forastiere AA, et al. Postoperative concurrent radiotherapy and chemotherapy for high-risk squamous-cell carcinoma of the head and neck. *N Engl J Med* 2004;350:1937–1944.

Department of Veterans Affairs Laryngeal Cancer Study Group. Induction chemotherapy plus radiation compared with surgery plus radiation in patients with advanced laryngeal cancer. *N Engl J Med* 1991;324:1685–1690.

Fausti S. Audiologic monitoring for ototoxicity and patient management. In: Campbell KC, ed. *Pharmacology and Ototoxicity for Audiologists*. Clifton Park, NY: Thompson Delmar Learning; 2006:230–251.

Forastiere AA, Goepfert H, Maor M, et al. Concurrent chemotherapy and radiotherapy for organ preservation in advanced laryngeal cancer. *N Engl J Med* 2003;349:2091–2098.

Francis DO, Weymuller EA, Jr, Parvathaneni U, Merati AL, Yueh B. Dysphagia, stricture, and pneumonia in head and neck cancer patients: does treatment modality matter? *Ann Otol Rhinol Laryngol* 2010;119:391–397.

Hitchcock YJ, Tward JD, Szabo A, Bentz BG, Shrieve DC. Relative contributions of radiation and cisplatin-based chemotherapy to sensorineural hearing loss in head-and-neck cancer patients. *Int J Radiat Oncol Biol Phys* 2009;73:779–788.

Hutcheson KA, Alvarez CP, Barringer DA, Kupferman ME, Lapine PR, Lewin JS. Outcomes of elective total laryngectomy for laryngopharyngeal dysfunction in disease-free head and neck cancer survivors. *Otolaryngol Head Neck Surg* 2012;146:585–590.

Jemal A, Siegel R, Xu J, Ward E. Cancer statistics, 2010. *CA Cancer J Clin* 2010;60:277–300.

Langmore SE. Evaluation of oropharyngeal dysphagia: which diagnostic tool is superior? *Curr Opin Otolaryngol Head Neck Surg* 2003;11:485–489.

Lonsbury-Martin B, Martin GK. Evoked otoacoustic emissions as objective screeners for ototoxicity. *Semin Hear* 2001;22:377–392.

Manikantan K, Khode S, Dwivedi RC, et al. Making sense of post-treatment surveillance in head and neck cancer: when and what of follow-up. *Cancer Treat Rev* 2009;35:744–753.

Marron M, Boffetta P, Zhang ZF, et al. Cessation of alcohol drinking, tobacco smoking and the reversal of head and neck cancer risk. *Int J Epidemiol* 2010;39:182–196.

Martin S, Chung B, Bratlund C, et al. Eighteenth Annual Dysphagia Research Society Meeting Scientific Paper Sessions: Movement trajectories during percutaneous stimulation at rest of the hyolaryngeal muscles in head and neck cancer patients treated with radiation therapy. *Dysphagia* 2010;25:358–359.

Mehanna H, Paleri V, West CM, Nutting C. Head and neck cancer—Part 1: Epidemiology, presentation, and prevention. *BMJ* 2010a;341:c4684.

Mehanna H, West CM, Nutting C, Paleri V. Head and neck cancer—Part 2: Treatment and prognostic factors. *BMJ* 2010b;341:c4690.

Murphy BA, Gilbert J, Cmelak A, Ridner SH. Symptom control issues and supportive care of patients with head and neck cancers. *Clin Adv Hematol Oncol* 2007;5:807–822.

Oh HK, Chambers MS, Martin JW, Lim HJ, Park HJ. Osteoradionecrosis of the mandible: treatment outcomes and factors influencing the progress of osteoradionecrosis. *J Oral Maxillofac Surg* 2009;67:1378–1386.

Rosenthal DI, Lewin JS, Eisbruch A. Prevention and treatment of dysphagia and aspiration after chemoradiation for head and neck cancer. *J Clin Oncol* 2006;24:2636–2643.

Rütten H, Pop LA, Janssens GO, et al. Long-term outcome and morbidity after treatment with accelerated radiotherapy and weekly cisplatin for locally advanced head-and-neck cancer: results of a multidisciplinary late morbidity clinic. *Int J Radiat Oncol Biol Phys* 2011;81: 923–929.

Seikaly H, Rassekh CH. Oropharyngeal cancer. In: Calhoun KH, ed. *Head and Neck Surgery - Otolaryngology*. 3rd ed. Philadelphia: Lippincott Williams and Wilkins; 2001:1413–1441.

Smith BG, Lewin JS. Lymphedema management in head and neck cancer. *Curr Opin Otolaryngol Head Neck Surg* 2010;18:153–158.

Tirado Y, Lewin JS, Hutcheson KA, Kupferman ME. Office-based injection laryngoplasty in the irradiated larynx. *Laryngoscope* 2010;120:703–706.

de Visscher AV, Manni JJ. Routine long-term follow-up in patients treated with curative intent for squamous cell carcinoma of the larynx, pharynx, and oral cavity. Does it make sense? *Arch Otolaryngol Head Neck Surg* 1994;120:934–939.

Survivorship Algorithms

These cancer survivorship algorithms have been specifically developed for MD Anderson using a multidisciplinary approach and taking into consideration circumstances particular to MD Anderson, including the following: MD Anderson's specific patient population, MD Anderson's services and structure, and MD Anderson's clinical information. These algorithms are provided for informational purposes only and are not intended to replace the independent medical or professional judgment of physicians or other health care providers. Moreover, these algorithms should not be used to treat pregnant women.

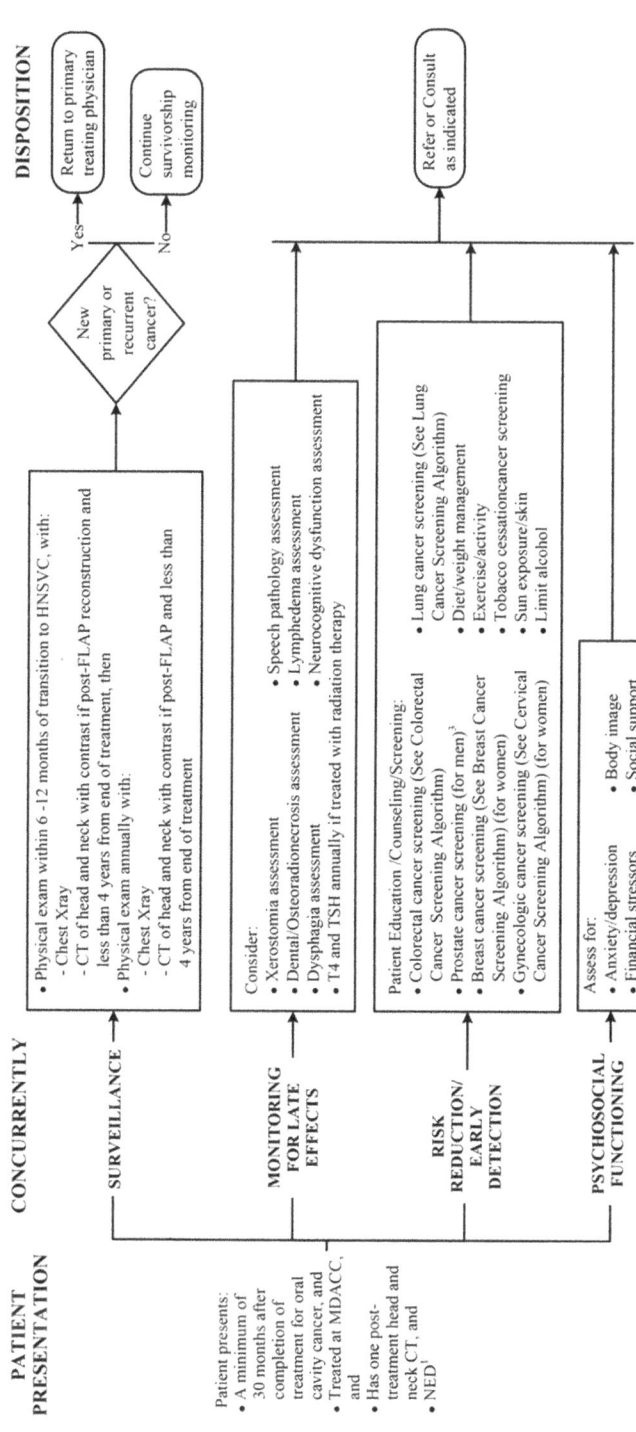

Algorithm 9.1 Head and neck survivorship: oral cavity cancer

¹ NED = No evidence of disease
² HNSVC = Head and Neck Survivorship Clinic
³ Based on American Cancer Society Prostate Cancer Screening Guidelines

Copyright 2013 The University of Texas MD Anderson Cancer Center

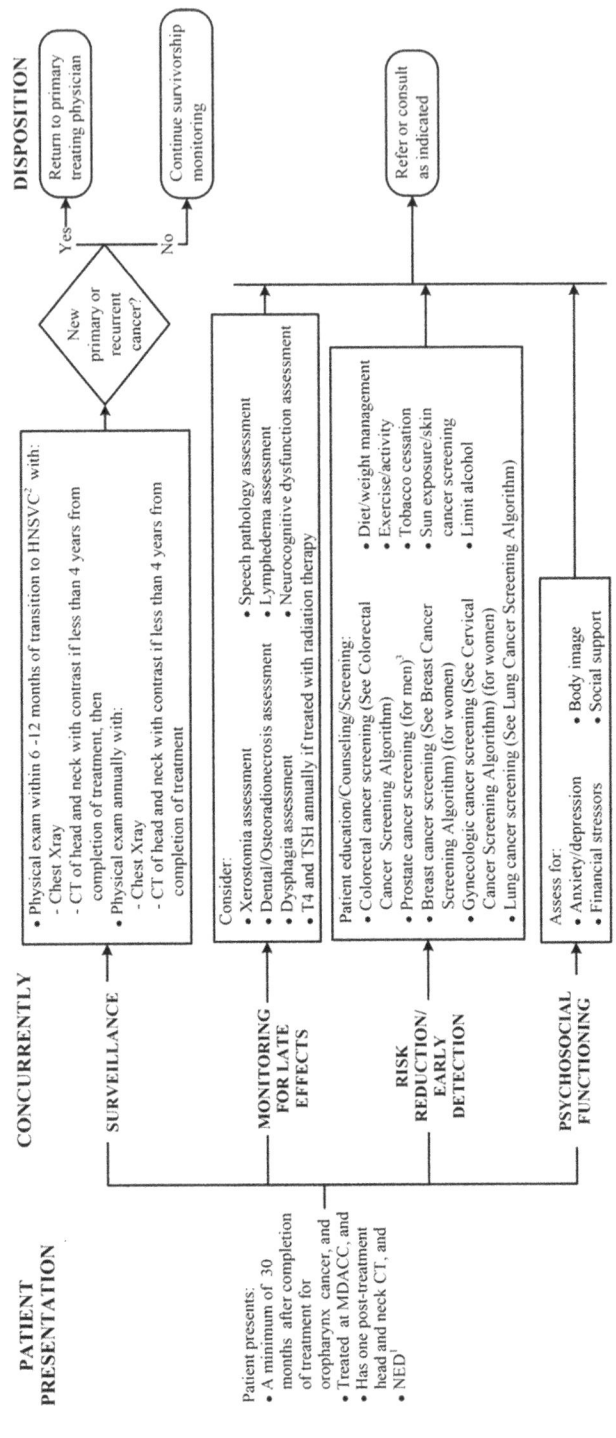

Algorithm 9.2 Head and neck survivorship: oropharynx cancer

Department of Clinical Effectiveness V2
Approved by the Executive Committee of the Medical Staff on 09/24/2013

[1] NED = No evidence of disease
[2] HNSVC = Head and Neck Survivorship Clinic
[3] Based on American Cancer Society Prostate Cancer Screening Guidelines

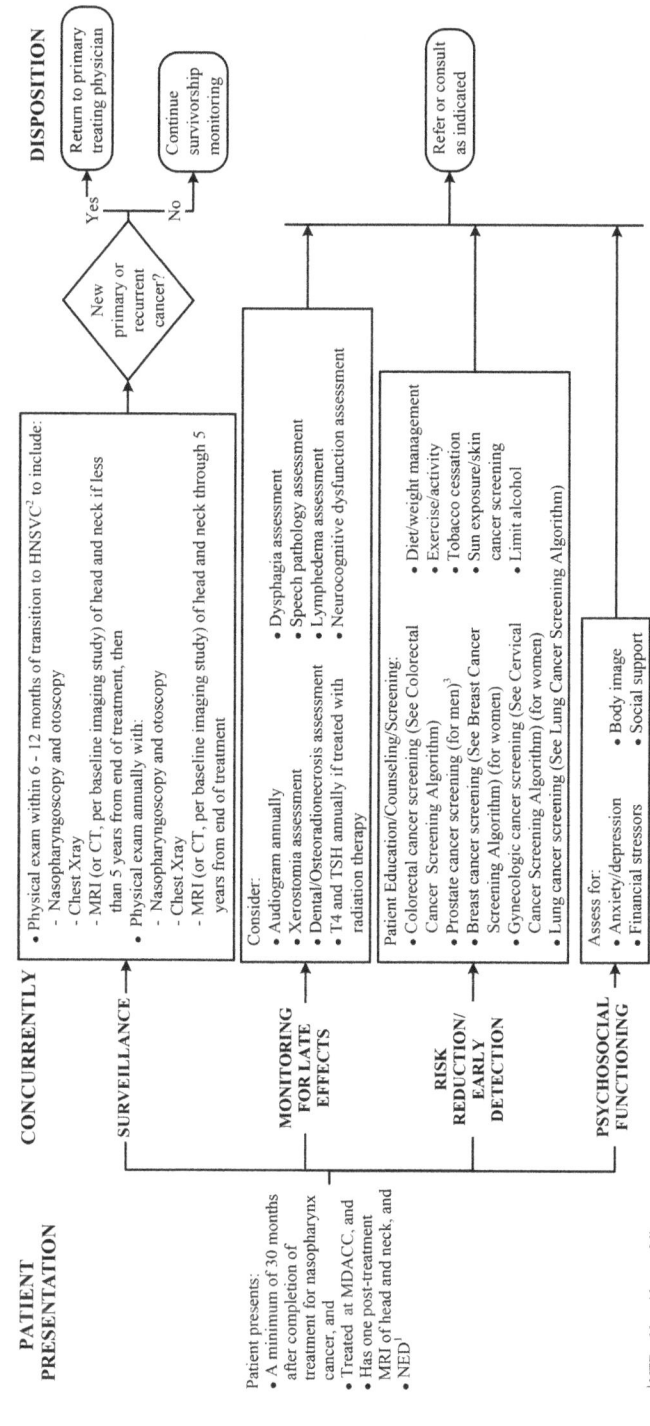

PATIENT PRESENTATION

Patient presents:
- A minimum of 30 months after completion of treatment for nasopharynx cancer, and
- Treated at MDACC, and
- Has one post-treatment MRI of head and neck, and
- NED[1]

CONCURRENTLY

SURVEILLANCE →
- Physical exam within 6 - 12 months of transition to HNSVC[2] to include:
  - Nasopharyngoscopy and otoscopy
  - Chest Xray
  - MRI (or CT, per baseline imaging study) of head and neck if less than 5 years from end of treatment, then
- Physical exam annually with:
  - Nasopharyngoscopy and otoscopy
  - Chest Xray
  - MRI (or CT, per baseline imaging study) of head and neck through 5 years from end of treatment

MONITORING FOR LATE EFFECTS →
Consider:
- Audiogram annually
- Xerostomia assessment
- Dental/Osteoradionecrosis assessment
- T4 and TSH annually if treated with radiation therapy
- Dysphagia assessment
- Speech pathology assessment
- Lymphedema assessment
- Neurocognitive dysfunction assessment

RISK REDUCTION/ EARLY DETECTION →
Patient Education/Counseling/Screening:
- Colorectal cancer screening (See Colorectal Cancer Screening Algorithm)
- Prostate cancer screening (for men)[3]
- Breast cancer screening (See Breast Cancer Screening Algorithm) (for women)
- Gynecologic cancer screening (See Cervical Cancer Screening Algorithm) (for women)
- Lung cancer screening (See Lung Cancer Screening Algorithm)
- Diet/weight management
- Exercise/activity
- Tobacco cessation
- Sun exposure/skin cancer screening
- Limit alcohol

PSYCHOSOCIAL FUNCTIONING →
Assess for:
- Anxiety/depression
- Financial stressors
- Body image
- Social support

DISPOSITION

New primary or recurrent cancer?
- Yes → Return to primary treating physician
- No → Continue survivorship monitoring

Refer or consult as indicated

[1] NED = No evidence of disease
[2] HNSVC = Head and Neck Survivorship Clinic
[3] Based on American Cancer Society Prostate Cancer Screening Guidelines

Department of Clinical Effectiveness V2
Approved by the Executive Committee of the Medical Staff on 09/24/2013

Copyright 2013 The University of Texas MD Anderson Cancer Center

Algorithm 9.3 Head and neck survivorship: nasopharynx cancer

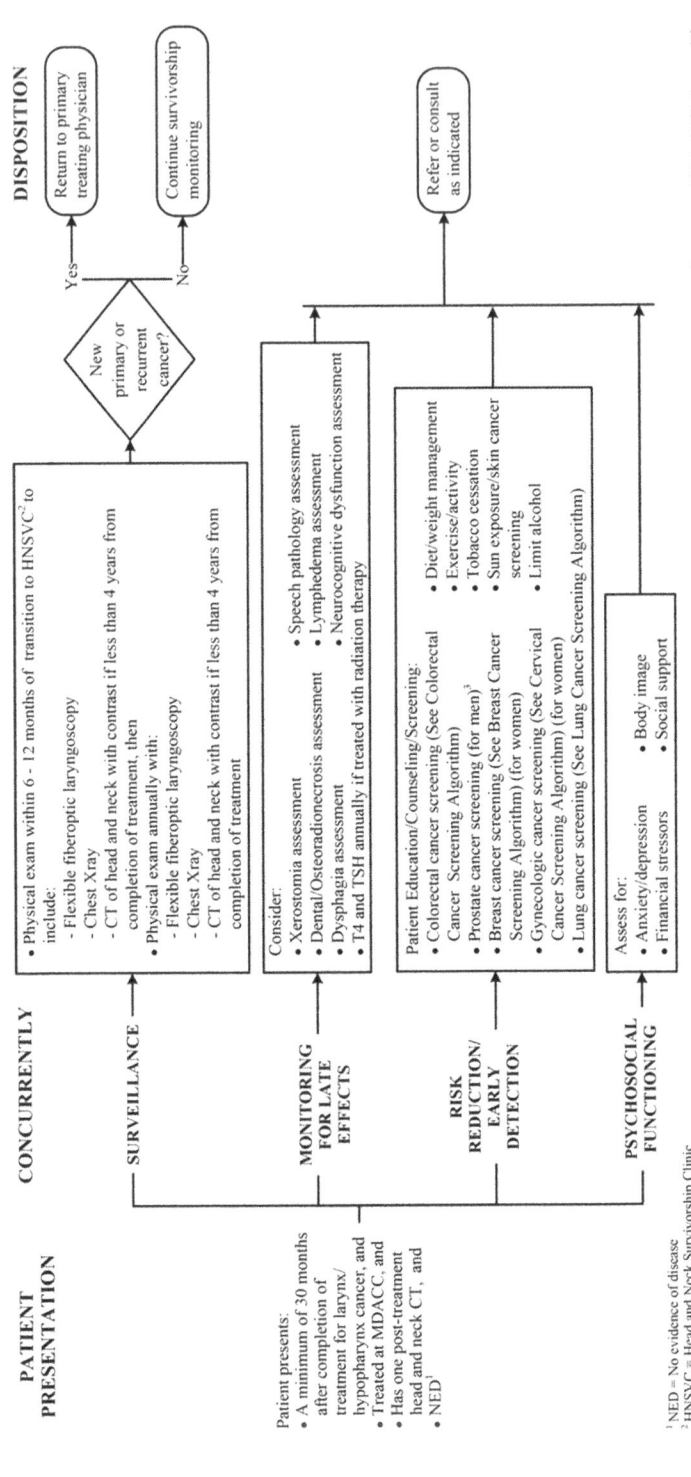

Algorithm 9.4 Head and neck survivorship: larynx/hypopharynx cancer

[1] NED = No evidence of disease
[2] HNSVC = Head and Neck Survivorship Clinic
[3] Based on American Cancer Society Prostate Cancer Screening Guidelines
Copyright 2013 The University of Texas MD Anderson Cancer Center

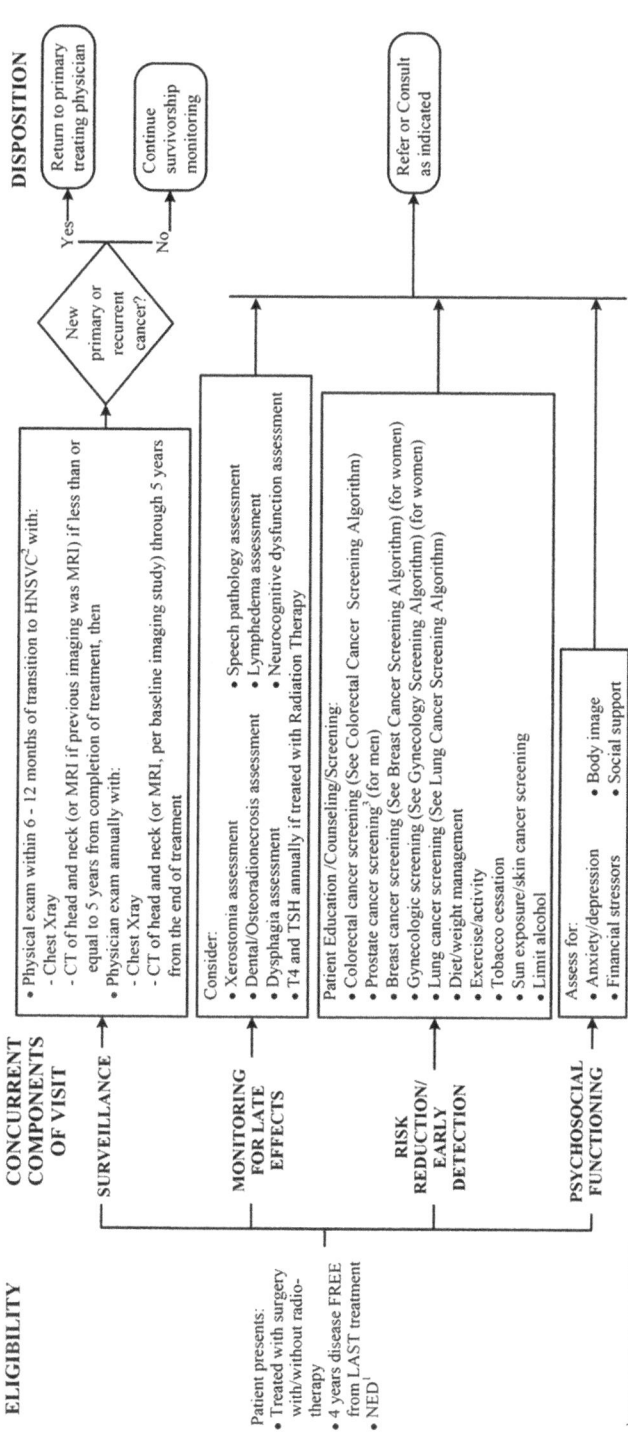

Algorithm 9.5 Head and neck survivorship: salivary cancer

[1] NED = No Evidence of Disease
[2] HNSVC = Head and Neck Survivorship Clinic
[3] Based on American Cancer Society Prostate Cancer Screening Guidelines

Copyright 2013 The University of Texas MD Anderson Cancer Center

Department of Clinical Effectiveness V2
Approved by the Executive Committee of the Medical Staff on 09/24/2013

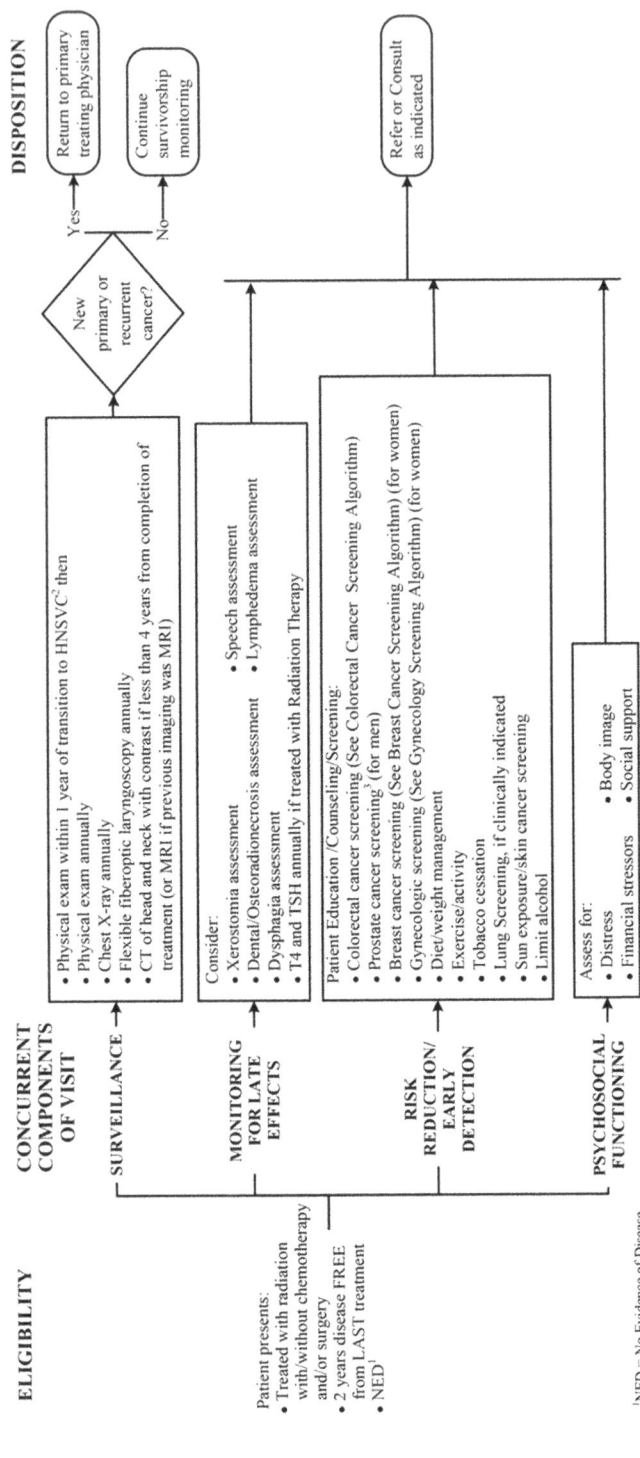

DISPOSITION

Return to primary treating physician

Continue survivorship monitoring

New primary or recurrent cancer?

Yes

No

Refer or Consult as indicated

ELIGIBILITY

Patient presents:
• Treated with radiation with/without chemotherapy and/or surgery
• 2 years disease FREE from LAST treatment
• NED[1]

CONCURRENT COMPONENTS OF VISIT

SURVEILLANCE

• Physical exam within 1 year of transition to HNSVC[2] then
• Physical exam annually
• Chest X-ray annually
• Flexible fiberoptic laryngoscopy annually
• CT of head and neck with contrast if less than 4 years from completion of treatment (or MRI if previous imaging was MRI)

MONITORING FOR LATE EFFECTS

Consider:
• Xerostomia assessment
• Dental/Osteoradionecrosis assessment
• Dysphagia assessment
• T4 and TSH annually if treated with Radiation Therapy
• Speech assessment
• Lymphedema assessment

RISK REDUCTION/ EARLY DETECTION

Patient Education /Counseling/Screening:
• Colorectal cancer screening (See Colorectal Cancer Screening Algorithm)
• Prostate cancer screening[3] (for men)
• Breast cancer screening (See Breast Cancer Screening Algorithm) (for women)
• Gynecologic screening (See Gynecology Screening Algorithm) (for women)
• Diet/weight management
• Exercise/activity
• Tobacco cessation
• Lung Screening, if clinically indicated
• Sun exposure/skin cancer screening
• Limit alcohol

PSYCHOSOCIAL FUNCTIONING

Assess for:
• Distress
• Financial stressors
• Body image
• Social support

[1]NED = No Evidence of Disease
[2]HNSVC = Head and Neck Survivorship Clinic
[3]Based on American Cancer Society Prostate Cancer Screening Guidelines

Department of Clinical Effectiveness V1
Approved by the Executive Committee of the Medical Staff on 12/18/2012

Algorithm 9.6 Head and neck survivorship: unknown primary

Chapter 10
Hematologic Cancer Survivorship Management: Transplantation

Karen Stolar, Amin Alousi, Joyce Neumann, and Richard Champlin

Contents

Chapter Overview This chapter will review the late effects of treatment impacting hematopoietic stem cell transplantation (HSCT) survivors. In general, HSCT patients receive high doses of chemotherapy with or without radiation therapy to eradicate their malignancy, together with an infusion of their own (autologous) or another person's (allogeneic) stem cells to restore hematopoiesis (the blood and immune system). Allogeneic cells may be from bone marrow, peripheral blood, or umbilical cord blood obtained from a related or unrelated donor. Patients experience the toxic effects of the cytotoxic treatment and are at high risk for infections owing to posttransplant immune deficiency. Late effects for HSCT survivors are commonly compounded by the toxic effects of their previous cancer treatment. This chapter

L.E. Foxhall, M.A. Rodriguez (eds.), *Advances in Cancer Survivorship Management*,   167
MD Anderson Cancer Care Series, DOI 10.1007/978-1-4939-0986-5_10,
© The University of Texas M.D. Anderson Cancer Center 2015

will cover physiologic and psychological aspects of survivorship for HSCT patients, as well as graft-versus-host disease, a common and frequently chronic condition that occurs after allogeneic HSCT.

Unique Needs of Hematopoietic Stem Cell Transplantation Survivors

Multiple factors contribute to the development of late effects of disease or treatment for hematopoietic stem cell transplantation (HSCT) survivors. One of these factors is the accompanying treatment plan (chemotherapy and/or radiation). Recently, nonmyeloablative or reduced-intensity preparative regimens have been used; these regimens produce fewer acute toxic effects and can be used in elderly patients and those with comorbidities. The incidence and severity of late effects depend on cumulative exposure to cytotoxic therapies, infectious complications, and, with allogeneic transplants, the effects of graft-versus-host disease (GVHD). Age and the presence of comorbid conditions also impact late effects. For these reasons, HSCT survivors deserve early and ongoing education about known late effects, guidance about prevention and healthy lifestyle behaviors, lifelong monitoring, and immediate evaluation and management of potential late effects.

At MD Anderson, we have initiated a survivorship program designed to address the unique needs of HSCT survivors, including disease surveillance, monitoring for late effects, risk reduction, early detection, and attention to psychosocial functioning. HSCT survivors are also at risk to develop other medical problems that may be independent of their cancer treatment, such as new cancers or cardiovascular or degenerative diseases. An HSCT survivorship program nurse practitioner visit accompanies follow-up with the primary HSCT physician. Visits are scheduled for the same or next day as the survivor's HSCT physician follow-up appointment and occur at critical points along the survivorship continuum, beginning at around 100 days after infusion of stem cells and then at 6, 12, 18, and 24 months, and annually thereafter. The deliberately separate clinic visit shifts the focus of the survivorship clinic visit from disease management to "survivorship." At the identified time point above, HSCT survivors are screened and if indicated receive treatment and guidance from experts in nutrition, behavioral science, neurocognitive science, vocational counseling, psychiatry, sexuality, fertility, cancer prevention services, bone health, infectious disease, endocrinology, pulmonology, cardiology, nephrology, and other organ systems. HSCT survivors have a lifelong need for monitoring of potential late effects as an integral part of the education and planning that they receive, and individualized survivorship plans will soon to be available electronically in each survivor's medical record. These plans can guide all health care providers regarding lifelong survivorship care. A review of the most common late effects that may impact the health of survivors and our plan for monitoring follows.

Physiologic Late Effects

Secondary Malignancy

HSCT survivors are at high risk of developing secondary malignancies, most commonly myelodysplastic syndrome (MDS) and acute myeloid leukemia (AML), solid tumors, and posttransplant lymphoproliferative disorders.

The risk for secondary malignancies is significantly higher than in the general population for both autologous and allogeneic HSCT survivors (Tichelli et al. 2009). This is related to the cumulative exposure to cytotoxic agents. Exposure to radiation, either through total body irradiation (TBI) or limited-field radiation therapy, is the most significant risk factor for secondary malignancies occurring more than 5 years after completion of treatment.

Risk factors for MDS/AML include pretransplant treatment with alkylating agents (e.g., cyclophosphamide, melphalan, carmustine, busulfan, dacarbazine, thiotepa, and temozolomide), treatment with topoisomerase II inhibitors (e.g., doxorubicin, epirubicin, etoposide, mitoxantrone, and amsacrine), limited-field radiation therapy, TBI, and autologous HSCT. Development of MDS/AML most frequently occurs 2–5 years after autologous HSCT (Majhail 2008). Therapy-related MDS/AML is rare after allogeneic HSCT.

Common solid tumors occurring after HSCT include thyroid cancers; squamous cell cancers of the head, neck, and vulva; breast cancer; melanoma; and non-melanoma skin cancer. The most common of these are basal-cell skin cancers and central nervous system tumors (Schwartz et al. 2009). The incidence of solid tumors is calculated to be 1% in allogeneic HSCT survivors living 10 years after HSCT and 2.2% in allogeneic HSCT survivors living 15 years after HSCT (Majhail et al. 2011). Risk factors for solid tumors include TBI, chronic GVHD, and prolonged immunosuppression. Cutaneous melanoma generally has a latent period of 1 year or less, and radiation therapy and T-cell depletion are cited as contributing factors (Rizzo et al. 2009).

Posttransplant lymphoproliferative disorders are related to Epstein-Barr virus infection and usually occur within the first 6 months after HSCT. The incidence is 1–6%, and the disorders tend to occur in the most severely immunocompromised patients; risk factors include T-cell–depleted grafts, use of antithymocyte globulin, and unrelated or human leukocyte antigen (HLA)-mismatched donor grafts (Majhail 2008; Rizzo et al. 2009).

The risk for secondary malignancies continues as survivors age. Each survivor should be well educated about self-examination and the importance of yearly physical examinations and frequent dental examinations, which screen for head and neck cancers. Careful examination of oral mucosal surfaces with each dental evaluation and at yearly follow-up visits with a health care professional should be performed. Annual physical examinations should include a complete blood count, as well as palpation of the neck, thyroid, and lymph nodes and examination and palpation of the skin, breast, and testicles. Adherence to the American Cancer Society and

American Society for Blood and Marrow Transplantation cancer screening guidelines is recommended, and some may recommend starting screening at an early age, such as beginning annual mammograms at an earlier age in patients who have received radiation therapy to the chest (Majhail et al. 2011).

Ocular Late Effects

The most common ocular effects are keratoconjunctivitis sicca (dry eye syndrome), cataracts, and retinopathy.

Dry eye syndrome is defined as the deficiency of tears or the evaporation of tears. About 50% of HSCT survivors develop dry eye syndrome by 6 months after HSCT. Forty percent of HSCT survivors with chronic GVHD experience dry eye syndrome, compared with 10% of HSCT survivors without GVHD. Risk factors for dry eye syndrome include TBI, use of methotrexate for GVHD prophylaxis, peripheral blood stem cell grafts, and chronic GVHD (Socie et al. 2003). Dry eye syndrome can occur in different stages. Symptoms are dry, gritty, sandy feeling or irritation in the eyes. A Schirmer test result of <5 mm is helpful in objectively identifying dry eye syndrome. Dry eye syndrome may contribute to damage to the ocular surface and increased risk for infection, which may lead to loss of vision. Survivors who are diagnosed with dry eye syndrome may further progress to a sicca syndrome that is characterized by dry mouth, dry skin, dry eyes, and vaginitis. Treatments for dry eye syndrome include preservative-free ocular lubricants, punctual occlusion, topical steroids, other topical immunosuppressive agents, and autologous serum tears (Leite et al. 2006). An ophthalmologist familiar with the ocular changes that HSCT survivors experience can also make recommendations for other products to improve symptom management.

A cataract is a clouding of the lens or the eye that becomes very dense and significantly impairs vision as it develops over time. Symptoms include blurry vision, double vision, sensitivity to light, and poor night vision. The most significant risk factors for cataract development in HSCT survivors are glucocorticoid use (longer than 3 months) and TBI. Patients who received 10-Gy single fractions of TBI are likely to develop cataracts by 4 years after treatment. About 80% of patients who received fractionated TBI were found to have cataracts by 6–10 years after HSCT (Socie et al. 2003). Early-stage cataracts are usually closely monitored and the patient is encouraged to use improved lighting, corrective lenses, glare-protection lenses, sunglasses, or magnifying lenses as appropriate for symptom management. As the cataract matures or ripens, surgical intervention to remove the affected lens and replace it with an artificial lens is generally required.

Retinal hemorrhage is described as the most frequent retinal complication of HSCT, with an incidence rate of 3.5–20% in survivors. Risk factors include GVHD-related vasculopathy, cytomegalovirus retinitis, and recurrence of leukemic diseases (Socie et al. 2003).

Ophthalmologic screening recommendations for ocular late effects include yearly review of ocular symptoms, dilated fundoscopic examination by an ophthalmologist, and visual acuity testing and tonimetry (ocular pressure testing). Survivors should be educated about the need for immediate evaluation by an ophthalmologist if sudden visual disturbance occurs. Frequently occurring or chronic visual disturbances should also prompt an ophthalmologic examination.

Oral Late Effects

The most common oral effects are dry mouth and increased prevalence of dental caries.

Dry mouth is decreased saliva production after HSCT. Dry mouth can be caused by damage to salivary glands as a result of chemotherapy, radiation therapy, and GVHD. This alters the oral environment, resulting in changes in oral tissues and an imbalance of chemicals and microbes, which often results in dental caries. Decreased saliva production may also be a side effect of common drugs used by the HSCT patients, such as antiemetics and antidepressants. As mucosal cells regenerate after HSCT and patients stop taking the offending medications, many report improvement in saliva production. Risk factors for ongoing dry mouth are TBI or radiation to the head and neck area and GVHD. In patients who have received radiation (either TBI or to the head and neck area), dry mouth may be a lifelong problem (Dobr et al. 2007). Review of oral symptomatology and assessment of the oral cavity should be performed at each follow-up visit. The finding of dry mouth can be important in the diagnosis of chronic GVHD and sicca syndrome, which may include dry skin, dry eyes, and vaginitis. Dry mouth may affect the patient's ability to taste, chew, and swallow. Counseling regarding use of beverages before and liberally during meals, addition of gravies and sauces on foods, and use of artificial saliva products may alleviate some of these issues. If dry mouth is associated with GVHD, systemic or topical treatment may also relieve dry mouth. Over-the-counter, alcohol-free oral moisturizers are readily available for dental and oral hygiene to soothe dry mouth and improve associated halitosis.

The incidence of dental caries is increased in patients who have extended symptoms of dry mouth and in patients with oral chronic GVHD. Prevention measures include good oral hygiene practices and daily use of fluoride rinses or gels, which improve the resistance of hard dental surfaces to bacterial acids and bacterial growth. Chlorhexidine mouthwashes can contribute to reduction in accumulation of plaque (Dobr et al. 2007).

Dental visits are recommended every 6–12 months for monitoring and restorative intervention of dental caries as well as thorough examination of the oral mucosa to check for suspicious lesions that may be early cancers.

Endocrine Late Effects

Thyroid and reproductive late effects are the most common endocrine-related late effects. Corticosteroid treatment for GVHD is commonly complicated by diabetes mellitus.

Thyroid dysfunction is one of the most common late sequelae of HSCT. Because development of thyroid disorder can predispose HSCT survivors to cardiac and metabolic disease, ongoing monitoring for thyroid dysfunction is important. The thyroid disorders most frequently seen are subclinical hypothyroidism, overt hypothyroidism, and, less commonly, autoimmune thyroid disease (Roziakova and Mladosievicova 2010).

About 30% of HSCT survivors develop subclinical compensated hypothyroidism and 15% develop overt primary hypothyroidism. The median time to diagnosis is reported to be about 50 months (Socie et al. 2003). Risk factors include treatment with 10-Gy single-dose TBI, which is associated with the highest incidence of hypothyroidism, as well as fractionated TBI and treatment with busulfan. Other chemotherapies, as well as prolonged chronic GVHD, are also risk factors.

Subclinical hypothyroidism is a compensated, benign, and most often a temporary finding in laboratory tests showing slightly increased thyroid-stimulating hormone (TSH) levels and normal T4 levels. Treatment of this condition is controversial because treatment can put patients at risk for problems such as osteoporosis or iatrogenic hyperthyroidism. Conversely, early treatment may decrease the risk of thyroid adenoma or carcinoma and prevent growth problems or delayed development in pediatric patients. Certainly if subclinical hypothyroidism persists or increases over many months, treatment should be considered.

Laboratory diagnosis of overt primary hypothyroidism shows high serum TSH levels and low concentrations of free T4. Many of the symptoms that are common with hypothyroidism are also commonly related to other effects of treatment, and thus laboratory testing should be used for confirmation. These symptoms include fatigue, weakness, weight gain, constipation, depression, memory loss, dry rough skin, coarse dry hair, irritability, decreased libido, muscle cramps or aches, abnormal menstrual cycles, and cold intolerance.

An uncommon but documented thyroid disorder, autoimmune thyroid disease, may occur as a late effect of HSCT. Autoimmune thyroid disease includes autoimmune thyroiditis and autoimmune-mediated hyperthyroidism. Autoimmune thyroiditis symptoms include the previously listed symptoms of hypothyroidism. Hyperthyroid symptoms include enlarged thyroid, nervousness, irritability, tremors, weight loss, sweating, palpitations, diarrhea, excessive tearing, double vision, pretibial myxedema, and exophthalmos.

Annual screening of laboratory TSH and free T4 levels is recommended. If subclinical hypothyroidism is noted, laboratory screening every 6 months should be considered until the decision is made to treat. A physical examination, including height and weight check and hair, skin, and thyroid examination, should be performed. More frequent screening and examination during periods of rapid growth should be considered in children. Treatment for hypothyroidism includes oral administration of L-thyroxine. Treatment for hyperthyroidism may require medication or radiation therapy to regulate or ablate the thyroid function.

Gonad and ovarian failure are known sequelae of treatment. Many HSCT survivors have undergone various modes and courses of treatment prior to HSCT, which contributes to poor fertility. The number of conceptions after autologous or allogeneic HSCT is low. However, if conception does occur, the likelihood of a live birth is favorable (Loren et al. 2011). Very few women who are conditioned with busulfan or TBI experience gonad recovery, and a low rate of gonad recovery has been observed in men conditioned with TBI. Among men who are conditioned with busulfan, about 17% show gonad recovery (Socie and Tichelli 2004).

Pretransplant strategies to preserve fertility (i.e., tissue/ova preservation or sperm banking) should be discussed with the patient and initiated if prior therapy, patient preference, and time before treatment allows. Posttreatment medical evaluation of hormone production and sperm analysis should be done to confirm infertility at 1 year or more after HSCT. Counseling should be provided regarding the use of birth control measures until confirmation of infertility can be made 1 or more years after HSCT. Fertility testing may be recommended at various time points after HSCT. Consultation with fertility specialists can be helpful for young adults, even after HSCT, to review all possible options.

The common use of corticosteroids to treat GVHD in allogeneic HSCT recipients frequently leads to hyperglycemia or diabetes mellitus. These conditions require close monitoring and treatment; they usually improve but may not resolve when corticosteroids are discontinued.

Skeletal Late Effects

Low bone mass as evidenced by osteopenia or osteoporosis, detected by bone mineral density testing, occurs in up to 50% of HSCT survivors by 12–18 months after HSCT. Osteopenia, with a t-score of −1 to −2.5, may occur in up to 30% of HSCT survivors, and osteoporosis, with a t-score of less than −2.5, occurs in about 10% of HSCT survivors. Nontraumatic fractures occur in 10% of HSCT survivors with low bone mass (Socie and Tichelli 2004). Risk factors for development of low bone mass include chemotherapy, radiation therapy, treatment with calcineurin inhibitors (tacrolimus, cyclosporine A), treatment with glucocorticoids (increasing with total dose and duration of therapy), hypogonadism, and nutritional and lifestyle factors (Socie et al. 2003). Preventive measures include sex hormone replacement therapy for those with hypogonadism or premature ovarian failure, oral supplementation of vitamin D, calcium supplementation using calcium-rich food sources and additional supplementation as needed, physical exercise that includes weight-bearing and resistance exercise, tobacco cessation, and moderation of alcohol intake. The use of bisphosphonate therapy for adults whose treatment with glucocorticoids is anticipated to last more than 3 months and for those with osteopenia is currently being studied.

Recommendations to avoid sun exposure and use sunscreens make vitamin D deficiency a common problem. This is a major issue for most allogeneic HSCT survivors. Vitamin D levels are checked using the 25-OH vitamin D test. If the vitamin D levels are lower than 20 ng/mL, vitamin D replacement using prescription oral ergocalciferol for 8–12 weeks followed by over-the-counter oral vitamin D supplementation of 800–1,000 international units per day is recommended. The baseline study of bone mass is obtained by bone mineral density study (dual photon densitometry) conducted at 6 months after HSCT. This study is repeated at 24 months after HSCT, unless the patient has a clinical reason to follow up earlier. HSCT survivors with osteopenia or osteoporosis, those receiving extended immunosuppressive therapy, or those with ovarian or gonad failure without hormone supplementation are instructed to undergo regular bone density studies.

Treatment is considered for HSCT survivors with a diagnosis of osteoporosis or high-risk osteopenia after evaluation of risk in regard to comorbid conditions, current clinical condition, and current drug therapy. Resumption of therapy for HSCT survivors for whom it was discontinued during the transplantation period should be directed by the primary HSCT physician.

Avascular necrosis (AVN) is the death of part of a bone because of an impaired blood supply. The incidence of AVN varies from 4% to >10% of HSCT survivors (Socie and Tichelli 2004). Timing is not well defined. Risk factors for AVN include TBI and cumulative exposure to corticosteroids. Incidence of AVN has been shown to be higher among HSCT survivors who received 10-Gy single-dose TBI than among those treated with fractionated TBI. AVN can lead to cracks in the affected bone and bone collapse. The femoral head is affected in 80% of cases of AVN (Socie et al. 2003). The wrist, shoulder, and knee are also frequently affected. Bones in the foot, ankle, spine, or jaw may be affected, but less frequently. The most common symptom is pain. If the hip is affected, pain is associated with standing and walking, and it is noted in the hip or groin and may radiate from thigh to knee. If the wrist is affected, pain in the wrist and weakness of the fingers may be noted. Shoulder pain and stiffness may be symptoms of shoulder involvement. Knee pain requires investigation.

Report of related symptoms should lead to further investigation. The diagnosis of AVN is best made by magnetic resonance imaging of the affected bone. A positive diagnosis warrants referral to an orthopedic specialist. Treatment in the early stage can include pain control and orthopedic measures to relieve pressure on the affected area. As AVN progresses, surgical replacement of the joint and affected bone is likely required.

Pulmonary Late Effects

Pulmonary effects in autologous HSCT survivors are generally related to chemotherapy and radiation lung toxicity and generally occur within 3 months after the end of treatment (Tichelli et al. 2008). Allogeneic HSCT survivors are more frequently affected by serious pulmonary late effects than are autologous HSCT survivors. Both infectious and noninfectious late effects can occur and have serious consequences. Air flow obstructive disorders are associated with the highest mortality rates. The most frequently occurring late-onset pulmonary complications are bronchiolitis obliterans syndrome (BOS), cryptogenic organizing pneumonia, sinopulmonary infections, and idiopathic pneumonia syndrome, also known as interstitial pneumonitis. These late-onset pulmonary effects are usually noted in the 6- to 12-month period after HSCT, but new onset has been reported 2–3 years after HSCT, and as many as 40% of allogeneic HSCT recipients may be affected.

BOS is the most common and lethal of air flow obstructive disorders. It is known to occur most frequently in HSCT recipients with GVHD, but cases of airflow obstruction disorders, specifically BOS, have also been reported in a small percentage of HSCT recipients who did not have other signs of GVHD (Pandya and Soubani 2010). Other risk factors include age >20 years at time of treatment, presence of pretransplant air flow obstruction (FEV1/FVC < .7), and viral respiratory infections within the first 100 days after HSCT (Dudek and Mahaseth 2006). The toxicity of chest irradiation, TBI, and chemotherapy, especially thiotepa and busulfan, is implicated in the development of pulmonary late effects. Because survivors who are diagnosed with serious pulmonary late effects have higher mortality rates than survivors who are not diagnosed with pulmonary late effects, close monitoring is recommended. Eighty percent of cases of BOS are noted between 6 and 12 months after HSCT. BOS that develops in the first 200 days after HSCT is associated with a worse prognosis than BOS that develops later (Patriarca et al. 2009). Progressive decline in FEV1 (≥20%) or FEV1/FVC < .7 with or without symptoms heightens the suspicion of BOS, and prompt pulmonary evaluation with a high-resolution computed tomographic scan and a transplantation center pulmonary service consultation should be considered. Often pulmonary function tests may not meet suggested criteria for BOS even though the patient presented with recent upper respiratory infection, wheezing, dry cough, and dyspnea. A chest x-ray may appear normal. In the absence of an infectious process, further evaluation for early airflow obstructive disorder should be initiated. An annual physical examination should include a review of pulmonary symptoms and a clinical chest examination (see Fig. 10.1 for screening recommendations).

Cardiovascular Late Effects

A broad range of cardiovascular late effects may occur, including coronary and peripheral arterial disease, cardiomyopathy, arrhythmia, autonomic neuropathy, and cerebrovascular events. Metabolic syndrome can also occur.

Survivors of HSCT are at increased risk for early cardiovascular events compared with the general United States population. Late cardiac effects occur more frequently in patients who have had allogeneic HSCT than in patients who have had autologous HSCT. Chemotherapy, radiation therapy, and GVHD can cause direct damage to the vascular or arterial endothelium, contributing to the development of atherosclerotic lesions. Anthracyclines and mediastinal radiation can cause direct cardiac damage. Other risk factors include arterial hypertension, dyslipidemia,

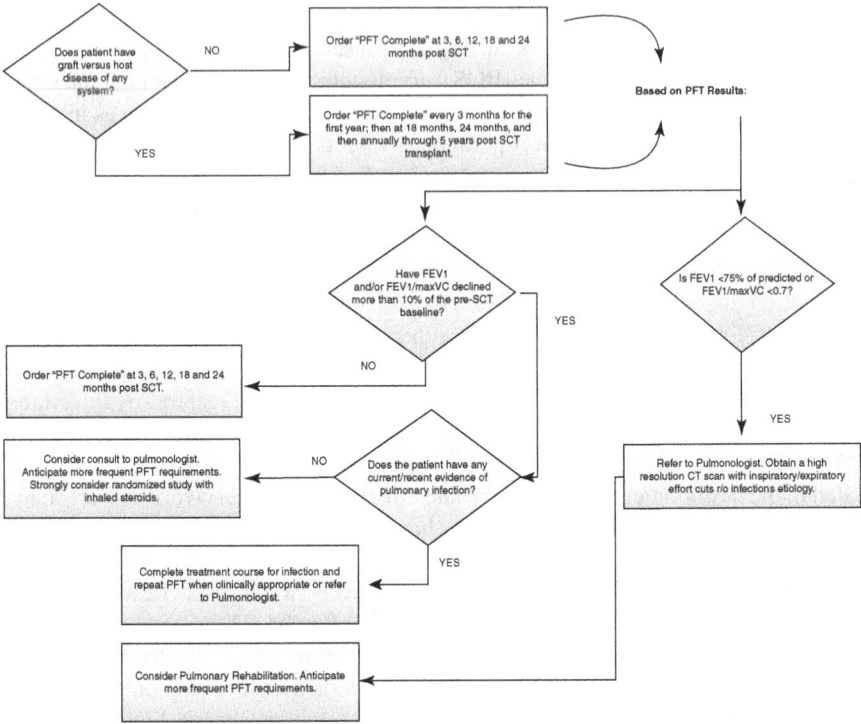

Fig. 10.1 Pulmonary screening recommendations for survivors of hematopoietic stem cell transplantation (*PFT* indicates pulmonary function test, *SCT* stem cell transplantation)

endocrine disorders, prolonged steroid use, and iron overload (Tichelli et al. 2007). Metabolic syndrome, which increases the absolute risk for cardiovascular disease in the general population, should be considered when developing a risk profile for the HSCT survivor (Grundy et al. 2005).

A diagnosis of metabolic syndrome can be made when the individual exhibits three of the following findings: elevated waist circumference, elevated triglyceride levels, reduced high-density lipid levels, hypertension, and elevated fasting glucose levels (Grundy et al. 2005). Smoking, obesity, and sedentary lifestyle are established risk factors for cardiovascular disease and are readily found in many HSCT survivors. Long-term follow-up recommendations include eliciting information regarding lifestyle and family history related to cardiovascular events and yearly physical examination and review of symptoms. A useful patient response inventory tool for heart failure symptoms is the MD Anderson Symptom Inventory-Heart Failure questionnaire (Fadol et al. 2008). Referral to cardiology services for further evaluation is strongly recommended for patients with preexisting cardiac disorders, for patients who exhibit early cardiac events during the transplantation process, or for patients who report heart failure symptoms.

Lifestyle and nutritional counseling should be initiated early in the survivorship recovery course. Body mass index measurement and hip-to-waist ratio are tools that can be explained to the patient to promote engagement in heart-healthy behaviors. Dietary recommendations should emphasize reducing trans-fatty acid intake, increasing nonsoluble fiber intake, and adhering to dietary measures to improve diabetes control. Lifestyle counseling includes tobacco cessation, alcohol abstinence or moderation, and increasing physical activity. A yearly fasting lipid profile should be initiated even when the survivor is demonstrating continuing robust recovery. Prior to pharmacologic intervention for dyslipidemia, current medication regimens should be considered for potential drug interactions. Ongoing renal or liver disorders may require a short delay of initiation or require more frequent monitoring of laboratory values and should be discussed with the transplantation team. When all immunosuppressant and prophylactic drugs have been discontinued, comprehensive management of hypertension, dyslipidemia, and diabetes can be managed by a primary care health care provider. Ferritin levels should be checked 1 year after HSCT, with more comprehensive iron overload evaluation and management if indicated, which may also benefit long-term cardiovascular health.

Renal Late Effects

The three most common renal pathologies with HSCT are thrombotic microangiopathy, nephrotic syndrome, and GVHD-related chronic kidney disease (Al-Hazzouri et al. 2008).

Chronic kidney disease is a well-described late effect in allogeneic HSCT survivors. The commonly used definition is a sustained decrease in the glomerular filtration rate below levels of 60 mL/minute per 1.73 m^2. The incidence is reported to be as high as 27% (Mohty and Apperley 2010). Chronic kidney disease generally occurs in the first 12 months after HSCT but new cases have been reported as long as 10 years after HSCT (Hingorani 2008). Risk factors include TBI (depending on the dose and amount of kidney shielding used), previous fludarabine exposure, GVHD, hypertension, preexisting renal dysfunction as noted by glomerular filtration rate, advanced age, and female sex (Kersting et al. 2007). Survivors with even mild chronic kidney disease may be at increased risk for further deterioration when the normal effects of aging on glomerular filtration rate are factored in over the years. Recommendations for long-term follow-up include testing for urine protein levels, blood urea nitrogen levels, and serum creatinine levels, as well as testing for glomerular filtration rate at 6 months and 1 year after HSCT. Continuing yearly urinalysis and testing for blood urea nitrogen levels and creatinine levels should be considered for survivors with even mild abnormalities. Hypertension should be aggressively managed.

Late Infections

Infections occurring after 100 days after HSCT are considered "late infections" and may be life-threatening. Allogeneic HSCT survivors are more frequently affected, especially those who have chronic GVHD or are receiving prolonged immunosuppressive therapy (Robin et al. 2007). The most common serious late infections are bacterial pneumonia, sepsis, central nervous system infections, disseminated varicella, and sinusitis. Fungal infections are less common after the first year. Prolonged cytomegalovirus surveillance and prophylaxis regimens have documented effectiveness in preventing serious late infections (Bjorklund et al. 2007). Updated guidelines for preventing infectious complications among HSCT survivors using prophylaxis and treatment are available (Tomblyn et al. 2009).

Thorough evaluation for infection when symptoms initially become apparent is indicated for all HSCT survivors, as is consideration of the current level of immunosuppression. HSCT survivors, particularly those with chronic GVHD, have defective splenic function and are at risk for late bacteremia from pneumococci or other organisms. Late infections can occur in survivors even years after HSCT (Bjorklund et al. 2007).

Immunocompromised HSCT survivors receive antibiotic prophylaxis to prevent bacterial, fungal, viral, and protozoal infections. Patient education regarding compliance with antibiotic prophylaxis is performed before the patient is discharged from the transplantation center and reinforced at each follow-up visit. Communication about the expected duration of these prophylaxis regimens with the referring oncologist or hematologist is critical. Patient education regarding frequent hand washing, meticulous cleanliness of food storage and preparation areas, sick child care, and crowd avoidance during respiratory illness season, as well as encouragement to immediately report fevers or other evidence of infection to their community physicians, is performed prior to discharge from the transplantation center.

Seasonal influenza vaccines with the inactivated vaccine should be offered to both autologous and allogeneic HSCT survivors who have no known contraindications starting at least 4 months after HSCT during influenza season (Tomblyn et al. 2009). A specific series of pneumococcal vaccines are given in the re-immunization plan series, which should be initiated for both autologous and allogeneic HSCT survivors at 6 months after HSCT. Guidelines are available for a recommended revaccination plan, including pneumococcal conjugate and polysaccharide vaccines; inactivated poliovirus; haemophilus influenza; hepatitis B; diphtheria, tetanus, and acellular pertussis; optional vaccines including meningococcal conjugate vaccine, hepatitis A, and human papilloma virus; and live vaccines including measles, mumps, and rubella and varicella vaccines.

Graft-Versus-Host Disease

GVHD represents one of the most common complications following allogeneic HSCT and has been the major barrier to wide-scale application of this therapy. Although advances in conditioning regimens, supportive care, and GVHD prophylaxis have improved the prognosis for HSCT recipients, the development of GVHD remains a significant source of morbidity and mortality and is the major cause of late nonrelapse death (Lee et al. 2002). GVHD results from the recognition of host tissues as foreign by immunocompetent donor cells. HLAs, the most immunogenic proteins in humans, are expressed by genes encoded by the major histocompatibility complex. The degree of disparity in HLA gene expression is the strongest predictor for GVHD; for this reason, the vast majority of HSCTs are performed from fully matched-HLA related or unrelated donors (Prasad et al. 1999; Flomenberg et al. 2004). Yet even in the setting of an HLA-matched donor, GVHD may still occur in up to 35–50% of HSCTs as a result of polymorphic genes outside of the major histocompatibility complex, referred to as minor histocompatibility antigens, which may be disparate between host and recipient (Gale et al. 1987; den Haan et al. 1995; Goulmy et al. 1996; Hahn et al. 2008). A fundamental problem for allogeneic HSCT is the close association between GVHD and the derived benefit resulting from a graft-versus-tumor effect. Both GVHD and graft-versus-tumor are mediated by mature donor T-cells contained within the infused graft; both effects are reduced when T-cells are depleted in so-called T-cell–depleted transplantations. Identifying and separating the target antigens resulting in GVHD and graft-versus-tumor is an active area of research that will hopefully result in maximizing the therapeutic potential of this modality while eliminating the frequent obstacle of GVHD (Molldrem et al. 2002).

Historically, GVHD has been divided into an acute and chronic form, using day 100 after HSCT to define these two entities. More recently, day 100 has come to be seen as an arbitrary distinction and an effort has been made to define GVHD as "acute" or "chronic" GVHD solely on the basis of disease manifestations (Filipovich et al. 2005). The skin (maculopapular rash), gastrointestinal tract (nausea, vomiting, or diarrhea), and liver (cholestatic jaundice or hepatitis) are the typical target organs for acute GVHD. Acute GVHD commonly manifests within the first 100 days following HSCT but may occur at a later time point in an entity referred to as "late acute GVHD." Chronic GVHD, on the other hand, has a median onset of 4–6 months following allogeneic HSCT, with disease manifestations resembling various autoimmune disorders such as sicca syndrome, systemic lupus erythema, and systemic sclerosis (Przepiorka et al. 2001; Remberger et al. 2002). The features of chronic GVHD are protean, with involvement of just about every organ having been described (Lee and Flowers 2008). The most common organ manifestations are detailed in Table 10.1, along with an associated review of symptoms that should be used for routine screening (Filipovich et al. 2005). Prior history of acute GVHD is one of the strongest risk factors for development of chronic GVHD; however, the chronic form may occur even in patients with no prior history of GVHD (referred to as "de novo" chronic GVHD; Lee and Flowers 2008). Typically, prophylactic immunosuppressants (such as tacrolimus or cyclosporine) are tapered within the first year following a matched related or unrelated donor HSCT in the absence of ongoing or prior history of significant GVHD. In this setting, the features of late acute or chronic GVHD may develop, requiring close monitoring by local practitioners and patients alike.

Corticosteroids (methylprednisone or prednisone, 1–2 mg/kg daily) are the standard first-line therapy for patients with suspected GVHD. Indications for the initiation of corticosteroids (or other therapies) vary, and for this reason GVHD treatment

Table 10.1 Common organ manifestations of chronic graft-versus-host disease and review of systems to be assessed

Organ system	Manifestation	Screening questions
Eyes	Keratoconjunctivitis	Do you have dry eyes, excessive tearing, foreign-object sensation, or morning crusting?
Mouth	Erythema, lichen-planus-like changes (striations), mucoceles, or ulcers	Do you have excessive oral dryness or oral pain or sensitivity to food or toothpaste?
Esophagus	Strictures, webs	Does food or liquid get stuck when you swallow?
Lungs	Bronchiolitis obliterans	Do you have shortness of breath or a persistent dry cough?
Gastrointestinal tract	Failure to thrive, diarrhea/malabsorption	Do you have weight loss or diarrhea, undigested material in stools, greasy stools, or diarrhea that improves with fasting?
Gynecologic organs	Lichen planus-like changes, vulvar erosions/fissures, vaginal scarring/stenosis	Do you have vaginal dryness or pain or dyspareunia?
Skin	Alopecia, angiomatous papules, bullae, erythema, hypo/hyperpigmentation, ichthyosis-like changes, keratosis-pilaris-like changes, lichen-planus-like changes, lichen-sclerosus-like changes, maculopapular changes, morphea-like changes, poikiloderma, scleroderma-like changes, sweat impairment, ulceration, changes to nails (brittleness, longitudinal ridging, onycholysis)	Do you have a rash, excessive dryness, new cellulitic skin changes, hair loss, or nail loss/brittleness?
Joints/fascial tissue	Fasciitis, panniculitis	Do you have any joint stiffness, impaired grip strength, or impaired "prayer sign"?
Blood	Eosinophilia, hypo/hypergammaglobulinemia, lymphopenia, thrombocytopenia	
Liver	Elevated total bilirubin, elevated alkaline phosphatase, elevated transaminases	

Information compiled from Filipovich et al. (2005)

decisions should be made in consultation with a patient's primary transplantation team. It is highly important for new symptoms suggestive of GVHD to be promptly discussed with the primary transplantation team so that therapy or workup are not delayed. Owing to the protean manifestations of GVHD, identification of local sub-specialists (such as ophthalmologic, pulmonary, gastrointestinal, dermatologic, and gynecologic practitioners) familiar with the organ-specific disease manifestation can be extremely helpful in treating patients with this complex illness. In addition, patients with GVHD are highly immunocompromised as a result of the immune dysregulation associated with the disorder and its treatment. In fact, infections are the leading cause of death in patients with GVHD (Witherspoon et al. 1984). For this reason, prophylactic antimicrobials are commonly used to prevent common bacterial (encapsulated organisms), fungal (pneumocystis, mold, candida), and viral (herpes simplex virus, cytomegalovirus) infections. Close monitoring and thorough evaluation and early (and often empiric) initiation of treatment for suspected infections is important to minimize morbidity in patients who suffer from GVHD.

The presence or absence of GVHD is the single best predictor for long-term quality of life in patients who have undergone HSCT (Fraser et al. 2006). The largest study evaluating quality of life in survivors of allogeneic HSCT has demonstrated that patients who do not develop GVHD have similar quality of life to that of age-matched controls. However, hope should not be lost for survivors who suffer from GVHD; the same study demonstrated that for patients who developed GVHD but were successfully treated, life experiences (quality of life) were similar to those of patients who had never suffered from the disorder. Therefore, a focused attention on the prevention and early treatment of GVHD is paramount to restoration of health in patients who have undergone allogeneic HSCT.

Neurologic and Psychosocial Late Effects

Cognitive Impairment

The cognitive impairments reported in both allogeneic and autologous HSCT survivors have been reported to follow a natural improvement over time, generally improving to population norms or better by about 1 year after HSCT (Jacobs et al. 2007). TBI, female sex, and prolonged immunosuppressive therapy are factors associated with the highest risk of cognitive deficit. We counsel survivors that cognitive impairment may occur during the first few months following treatment, but should continue to improve through the first year after HSCT. Neurocognitive testing and counseling can be offered to survivors who continue to have short-term memory problems, difficulty with concentration and focus, and trouble learning new things. These difficulties are most often noted when survivors return to work or school. Training in behavior modification and compensatory strategies may lessen the impact of the deficit (Poppelreuter et al. 2008).

Depression and Anxiety

Long-term assessment for symptoms of depression and anxiety are important not only in the first year after HSCT, but during all follow-up with health care providers throughout the survivorship continuum. Depression is associated with decreased survival (Loberiza et al. 2002), and quality of life can be adversely affected by moderate to severe depression (Syrjala et al. 2004). A structured evaluation of anxiety and depression may lead to earlier recognition so that treatment can be initiated. Twenty-six percent to 36% of survivors were found to have moderate to severe depressive symptoms in the first year after HSCT (Lee et al. 2005). Depressive disorders were noted most frequently in women and survivors coping with residual physical limitations and chronic GVHD at 3 and 5 years after HSCT and in both autologous and allogeneic HSCT survivors. Fifty-six percent of the survivors with depressive symptoms at 10 years after HSCT were found to not be receiving treatment for the depressive disorder (Syrjala et al. 2005).

Fatigue

Fatigue may be an issue for HSCT survivors for many years after the end of treatment. Fatigue can impact psychosocial functioning and can have an impact on the ability to return to work or school, resume participation in care of the family and household, participate in leisure time activities that were previously enjoyed, and engage in sexual activity. Fatigue and sleeping disorders have been reported to affect as many as 65% of long-term allogeneic HSCT survivors (Socie et al. 2003). Assessment of this physical symptom and its perceived impact on the HSCT survivor's daily life is an important and ongoing component in long-term follow-up. See Chap. 22 in this volume for more information about fatigue.

Sexuality and Sexual Functioning

Alterations in sexual functioning and sexuality are known late effects of treatment. Risk factors include radiation therapy, particularly TBI used in HSCT treatment regimens, and chemotherapy, particularly alkylating agents. A longitudinal study revealed clinically significant lower levels of sexual activity and functioning at 5 years after HSCT in survivors compared with case-matched controls. Forty-five percent of men and 80% of women reported problems in sexual functioning at 5 years after HSCT. Men most frequently reported problems with ejaculation, getting and maintaining an erection, and lack of desire. Women reported lack of desire, impaired orgasm ability, vaginal dryness, increased sensitivity to intimate touching, painful intercourse, vaginal tightness, and vaginal bleeding or irritation as the most commonly occurring problems (Syrjala et al. 2008).

Complex interactions of physical and psychosocial variables can contribute to varying levels of sexuality and sexual dysfunction. Laboratory studies of hormone levels, genital examination, erectile dysfunction testing, and open discussions with the patient and partner can reveal issues affecting sexuality and sexual function. When contributing factors are identified, interventions to improve the survivor's sexual health can be initiated. Strategies to improve sexual functioning should be employed early in recovery so that the cycle of avoidance behaviors and negative expectation does not continue to impact the problem (Syrjala et al. 2008).

Social Functioning

Resumption of roles and relationships with family and friends, as well as return to work or school, are global aspects of social functioning. Autologous HSCT survivors report good social functioning and start describing improvements at about 6 months after HSCT, which is earlier than for allogeneic HSCT survivors (Schulmeister et al. 2005). Long-term disease-free allogeneic and syngeneic HSCT survivors report high social functioning at 2–5 years after HSCT, with continued improvement after 5 years. One study noted a significantly lower social functioning score for patients who experienced chronic GVHD relative to those who did not (Worel et al. 2002).

Unemployment was another risk factor for decreased social functioning (Mosher et al. 2009). Most HSCT survivors return to work or school within 1–5 years after the end of treatment. Eighty-four percent of HSCT survivors who did not experience disease recurrence and who had a previous history of school or employment had returned to full-time work or school by 5 years after the end of treatment (Syrjala et al. 2004). At 10 years after HSCT, full-time employment rates for 74% of survivors did not differ from age-, sex-, and race-matched non-HSCT controls (Syrjala et al. 2005). Younger age and a higher education level were found to be associated with higher employment rates (Mosher et al. 2009). This evidence can help us encourage survivors who are anticipating their future. There have been reports of job discrimination with pressure to leave jobs and loss of job opportunities when a cancer diagnosis is revealed to a prospective employer. Eliciting work and school information as part of routine survivorship care can allow us to provide appropriate direction and resource information. Community resources can provide guidance regarding the Americans with Disability Act, which may provide survivors some protection against discrimination at work or require an employer to provide a reasonable accommodation for those who need a change in work conditions. Institutional, state, and community agencies also specialize in vocational counseling, aptitude testing, and assistance with re-enrollment in secondary education when a student leaves school abruptly because of a cancer diagnosis.

Life insurance denial is reported in 27% of 10-year HSCT survivors compared with 3.7% of controls. Ten-year HSCT survivors were denied health insurance at a reported rate of 24%, whereas no denials were reported in age-, sex-, and race-matched controls (Syrjala et al. 2005). HSCT survivors may be offered insurance with reduced coverage and higher premium rates because of their cancer history, which may leave them without coverage for late effects management or may simply be unaffordable. Uninsured individuals may be less likely to receive further preventive health care.

In summary, we have examined the potential late effects in the HSCT survivorship continuum and acknowledge that lifelong surveillance and preventive care can promote improved physiologic and psychosocial health for HSCT survivors.

Key Practice Points

- Patients who have received HSCT may have multiple overlapping complications from treatment for the primary disease and preparative regimens prior to HSCT.
- Late effects depend on cytotoxic agents used in the preparative regimen and the degree of myelosuppression and immunosuppression. Almost every organ system may be affected, and HSCT survivors are at increased risk for second malignancies.
- GVHD is a significant source of morbidity and is the major cause of late nonrelapse mortality.
- Chronic GVHD onset is usually 4–6 months after HSCT and symptoms resemble various autoimmune disorders.
- Infections, including opportunistic types, are a major complication after HSCT owing to the immunocompromised condition of survivors, and infections may be prolonged in the presence of GVHD. Prophylactic antimicrobials are commonly used to prevent common bacterial, fungal, and viral infections. HSCT survivors require revaccination starting at 6 months after HSCT.
- Psychosocial factors, including cognitive impairment, depression, fatigue, sexual dysfunction, and impaired social functioning, may affect quality of life for HSCT survivors.
- Lifelong surveillance and preventive care can promote improved health for HSCT survivors.

Suggested Readings

Al-Hazzouri A, Cao Q, Burns LJ, et al. Similar risks for chronic kidney disease in long-term survivors of myeloablative and reduced-intensity allogeneic hematopoietic cell transplantation. *Biol Blood Marrow Transplant* 2008;14:658–663.

Bjorklund A, Aschan J, Labopin M, et al. Risk factors for fatal infectious complications developing late after allogeneic stem cell transplantation. *Bone Marrow Transplant* 2007;40:1055–1062.

den Haan JM, Sherman NE, Blokland E, et al. Identification of a graft versus host disease-associated human minor histocompatibility antigen. *Science* 1995;268:1476–1480.

Dobr T, Passweg J, Weber C, et al. Oral health risks associated with HLA-types of patients undergoing hematopoietic stem cell transplantation. *Eur J Haematol* 2007;78:495–499.

Dudek AZ, Mahaseth H. Hematopoietic stem cell transplant-related airflow obstruction. *Curr Opin Oncol* 2006;18:115–119.

Fadol A, Mendoza T, Gning I, et al. Psychometric testing of the MDASI-HF: a symptom assessment instrument for patients with cancer and concurrent heart failure. *J Card Fail* 2008;14:497–507.

Filipovich AH, Weisdorf D, Pavletic S, et al. National Institutes of Health consensus development project on criteria for clinical trials in chronic graft-versus-host disease: I. Diagnosis and staging working group report. *Biol Blood Marrow Transplant* 2005;11:945–956.

Flomenberg N, Baxter-Lowe LA, Confer D, et al. Impact of HLA class I and class II high-resolution matching on outcomes of unrelated donor bone marrow transplantation: HLA-C mismatching is associated with a strong adverse effect on transplantation outcome. *Blood* 2004;104:1923–1930.

Fraser CJ, Bhatia S, Ness K, et al. Impact of chronic graft-versus-host disease on the health status of hematopoietic cell transplantation survivors: a report from the Bone Marrow Transplant Survivor Study. *Blood* 2006;108:2867–2873.

Gale RP, Bortin MM, van Bekkum DW, et al. Risk factors for acute graft-versus-host disease. *Br J Haematol* 1987;67:397–406.

Goulmy E, Schipper R, Pool J, et al. Mismatches of minor histocompatibility antigens between HLA-identical donors and recipients and the development of graft-versus-host disease after bone marrow transplantation. *N Engl J Med* 1996;334:281–285.

Grundy SM, Cleeman JI, Daniels SR, et al. Diagnosis and management of the metabolic syndrome. An American Heart Association/National Heart, Lung, and Blood Institute Scientific Statement. Executive summary. *Cardiol Rev* 2005;13:322–327.

Hahn T, McCarthy PL, Jr., Zhang MJ, et al. Risk factors for acute graft-versus-host disease after human leukocyte antigen-identical sibling transplants for adults with leukemia. *J Clin Oncol* 2008;26:5728–5734.

Hingorani S. Chronic kidney disease after liver, cardiac, lung, heart-lung, and hematopoietic stem cell transplant. *Pediatr Nephrol* 2008;23:879–888.

Jacobs SR, Small BJ, Booth-Jones M, et al. Changes in cognitive functioning in the year after hematopoietic stem cell transplantation. *Cancer* 2007;110:1560–1567.

Kersting S, Koomans HA, Hene RJ, et al. Acute renal failure after allogeneic myeloablative stem cell transplantation: retrospective analysis of incidence, risk factors and survival. *Bone Marrow Transplant* 2007;39:359–365.

Lee SJ, Flowers ME. Recognizing and managing chronic graft-versus-host disease. *Hematology Am Soc Hematol Educ Program* 2008:134–141.

Lee SJ, Klein JP, Barrett AJ, et al. Severity of chronic graft-versus-host disease: association with treatment-related mortality and relapse. *Blood* 2002;100:406–414.

Lee SJ, Loberiza FR, Antin JH, et al. Routine screening for psychosocial distress following hematopoietic stem cell transplantation. *Bone Marrow Transplant* 2005;35:77–83.

Leite SC, de Castro RS, Alves M, et al. Risk factors and characteristics of ocular complications, and efficacy of autologous serum tears after haematopoietic progenitor cell transplantation. *Bone Marrow Transplant* 2006;38:223–227.

Loberiza FR, Jr., Rizzo JD, Bredeson CN, et al. Association of depressive syndrome and early deaths among patients after stem-cell transplantation for malignant diseases. *J Clin Oncol* 2002;20:2118–2126.

Loren AW, Chow E, Jacobsohn DA, et al. Pregnancy after hematopoietic cell transplantation: a report from the late effects working committee of the Center for International Blood and Marrow Transplant Research (CIBMTR). *Biol Blood Marrow Transplant* 2011;17:157–166.

Majhail NS. Old and new cancers after hematopoietic-cell transplantation. *Hematology Am Soc Hematol Educ Program* 2008;2008:142–149.

Majhail NS, Brazauskas R, Rizzo JD, et al. Secondary solid cancers after allogeneic hematopoietic cell transplantation using busulfan-cyclophosphamide conditioning. *Blood* 2011;117:316–322.

Mohty M, Apperley JF. Long-term physiological side effects after allogeneic bone marrow transplantation. *Hematology Am Soc Hematol Educ Program* 2011;2010:229–236.

Molldrem JJ, Komanduri K, Wieder E. Overexpressed differentiation antigens as targets of graft-versus-leukemia reactions. *Curr Opin Hematol* 2002;9:503–508.

Mosher CE, Redd WH, Rini CM, et al. Physical, psychological, and social sequelae following hematopoietic stem cell transplantation: a review of the literature. *Psychooncology* 2009;18:113–127.

Pandya CM, Soubani AO. Bronchiolitis obliterans following hematopoietic stem cell transplantation: a clinical update. *Clin Transplant* 2010;24:291–306.

Patriarca F, Poletti V, Costabel U, et al. Clinical presentation, outcome and risk factors of late-onset non-infectious pulmonary complications after allogeneic stem cell transplantation. *Curr Stem Cell Res Ther* 2009;4:161–167.

Poppelreuter M, Weis J, Mumm A, et al. Rehabilitation of therapy-related cognitive deficits in patients after hematopoietic stem cell transplantation. *Bone Marrow Transplant* 2008;41:79–90.

Prasad VK, Kernan NA, Heller G, et al. DNA typing for HLA-A and HLA-B identifies disparities between patients and unrelated donors matched by HLA-A and HLA-B serology and HLA-DRB1. *Blood* 1999;93:399–409.

Przepiorka D, Anderlini P, Saliba R, et al. Chronic graft-versus-host disease after allogeneic blood stem cell transplantation. *Blood* 2001;98:1695–1700.

Remberger M, Kumlien G, Aschan J, et al. Risk factors for moderate-to-severe chronic graft-versus-host disease after allogeneic hematopoietic stem cell transplantation. *Biol Blood Marrow Transplant* 2002;8:674–682.

Rizzo JD, Curtis RE, Socie G, et al. Solid cancers after allogeneic hematopoietic cell transplantation. *Blood* 2009;113:1175–1183.

Robin M, Porcher R, De Castro Araujo R, et al. Risk factors for late infections after allogeneic hematopoietic stem cell transplantation from a matched related donor. *Biol Blood Marrow Transplant* 2007;13:1304–1312.

Roziakova L, Mladosievicova B. Endocrine late effects after hematopoietic stem cell transplantation. *Oncol Res* 2010;18:607–615.

Schulmeister L, Quiett K, Mayer K. Quality of life, quality of care, and patient satisfaction: perceptions of patients undergoing outpatient autologous stem cell transplantation. *Oncol Nurs Forum* 2005;32:57–67.

Schwartz JL, Kopecky KJ, Mathes RW, et al. Basal cell skin cancer after total-body irradiation and hematopoietic cell transplantation. *Radiat Res* 2009;171:155–163.

Socie G, Salooja N, Cohen A, et al. Nonmalignant late effects after allogeneic stem cell transplantation. *Blood* 2003;101:3373–3385.

Socie G, Tichelli A. Long-term care after stem-cell transplantation. *Hematol J* 2004;5 Suppl 3:S39–S43.

Syrjala KL, Kurland BF, Abrams JR, et al. Sexual function changes during the 5 years after high-dose treatment and hematopoietic cell transplantation for malignancy, with case-matched controls at 5 years. *Blood* 2008;111:989–996.

Syrjala KL, Langer SL, Abrams JR, et al. Recovery and long-term function after hematopoietic cell transplantation for leukemia or lymphoma. *JAMA* 2004;291:2335–2343.

Syrjala KL, Langer SL, Abrams JR, et al. Late effects of hematopoietic cell transplantation among 10-year adult survivors compared with case-matched controls. *J Clin Oncol* 2005;23:6596–6606.

Tichelli A, Bucher C, Rovo A, et al. Premature cardiovascular disease after allogeneic hematopoietic stem-cell transplantation. *Blood* 2007;110:3463–3471.

Tichelli A, Rovo A, Gratwohl A. Late pulmonary, cardiovascular, and renal complications after hematopoietic stem cell transplantation and recommended screening practices. *Hematology Am Soc Hematol Educ Program* 2008;2008:125–133.

Tichelli A, Rovo A, Passweg J, et al. Late complications after hematopoietic stem cell transplantation. *Expert Rev Hematol* 2009;2:583–601.

Tomblyn M, Chiller T, Einsele H, et al. Guidelines for preventing infectious complications among hematopoietic cell transplant recipients: a global perspective. Preface. *Bone Marrow Transplant* 2009;44:453–455.

Witherspoon RP, Deeg HJ, Lum LG, et al. Immunologic recovery in human marrow graft recipients given cyclosporine or methotrexate for the prevention of graft-versus-host disease. *Transplantation* 1984;37:456–461.

Worel N, Biener D, Kalhs P, et al. Long-term outcome and quality of life of patients who are alive and in complete remission more than two years after allogeneic and syngeneic stem cell transplantation. *Bone Marrow Transplant* 2002;30:619–626.

Chapter 11
Hematologic Cancer Survivorship Management: Leukemia

Etsuko Aoki

Contents

Chapter Overview The prognosis of patients with leukemia largely depends on the type of leukemia, clinical and pathologic prognostic factors of the leukemic cells, and patient characteristics. Over the past decade, long-term survival rates of patients with chronic myeloid leukemia (CML) have dramatically improved. On the other hand, these patients usually require life-long treatment, which may cause chronic physical, psychological, or socioeconomic complications that can affect patients' well-being. Chronic lymphocytic leukemia (CLL) is the most common

L.E. Foxhall, M.A. Rodriguez (eds.), *Advances in Cancer Survivorship Management*,
MD Anderson Cancer Care Series, DOI 10.1007/978-1-4939-0986-5_11,
© The University of Texas M.D. Anderson Cancer Center 2015

type of leukemia in the United States. The natural history of CLL is generally indolent, with median survival durations of 10 years. Patients with CLL are at risk for secondary malignancies and infectious complications with disease- and treatment-related pathogenesis. Patients with acute myeloid leukemia (AML) and acute lymphoblastic leukemia (ALL) are generally treated with intensive chemotherapy, which may result in chronic symptoms that interfere with patients' daily lives. Although some aspects of late or chronic toxic effects of treatment in patients with leukemia have been discussed, data concerning long-term effects remain limited. Further investigation is warranted to establish optimal monitoring schedules and effective interventions for survivors of adult-onset leukemia.

Introduction

The incidence of leukemia in the United States between 2005 and 2009 was 12.5 cases per 100,000 people, with a median age at diagnosis of 66 years (Surveillance Epidemiology and End Results data; http://www.seer.cancer.gov/statfacts/html/leuks.html). The natural history and prognosis of leukemia vary widely depending on the type of leukemia, clinical and pathologic prognostic factors, and the patient's health status. Improvements in therapy have substantially increased survival rates for some types of leukemia, especially chronic myeloid leukemia (CML).

In CML, patient outcomes have improved dramatically since the approval of imatinib, the first small-molecule tyrosine kinase inhibitor (TKI) against Bcr-Abl, as a frontline treatment for the chronic phase of CML in 2001. The 8-year overall survival rate for patients with CML is now 85% (Deininger et al. 2009). Second-generation TKIs, including dasatinib and nilotinib, have also been approved as frontline treatments for CML. In addition, newer TKIs, such as ponatinib and bosutinib, have recently been approved by the US Food and Drug Administration for CML that is resistant or intolerant to prior therapy.

The natural history of chronic lymphocytic leukemia (CLL) is variable but generally indolent, with survival times from initial diagnosis ranging from 2 to 20 years. The median survival duration is approximately 10 years. Many patients with CML and CLL enjoy long-term survival but often need continuous or intermittent treatments.

However, fewer patients with acute myeloid leukemia (AML) or acute lymphoblastic leukemia (ALL) survive for longer than 5 years without stem cell transplantation. According to Surveillance Epidemiology and End Results data, the 5-year relative survival rate for adult patients with AML was 23.4% between 2005 and 2009. Cure rates for ALL remain in the range of 30–50% in adults.

Historically, the main treatment for leukemia was cytotoxic chemotherapy. In some cases, radiation therapy has also been used in combination with chemotherapy for the treatment of extramedullary lesions. Some patients undergo high-dose chemotherapy or reduced-intensity chemotherapy with or without total body irradiation, followed by stem cell transplantation, with the intent of curing the disease. However, the sequelae of stem cell transplantation, such as chronic graft-versus-host disease, can profoundly affect survivors' long-term physical and psychological health.

More recently, targeted therapies have become available, as a result of improved understanding of the pathobiology of cancer. These treatments include monoclonal antibodies and small-molecule inhibitors against various molecular targets required for tumor development and proliferation. Immunotherapy using a monoclonal antibody against the cell surface markers on tumor cells, such as CD20, CD33, or CD52, was one of the earliest targeted therapies developed, and it is now widely used to treat leukemia. In contrast with monoclonal antibodies, small-molecule inhibitors can enter cells, thus interfering with the intracellular signaling pathway of tyrosine kinase. Small-molecule inhibitors are generally orally available. Several inhibitors against various molecular targets are now under preclinical and clinical development. Agents that can alter the epigenetic status (i.e., through methylation and acetylation) of tumor cell genes are also now available. Although these new agents are generally better tolerated than traditional cytotoxic chemotherapies, they are associated with their own toxic effects. As for late effects of these new agents, current knowledge remains limited, and further observation is needed.

Late Effects of Treatment

Numerous reports have discussed late effects of treatment in survivors of childhood leukemia, especially ALL. The late effects of childhood leukemia include secondary malignancies, adverse events involving the cardiovascular and neurologic systems, endocrine or metabolic abnormalities, infertility, and psychosocial effects. The best way to monitor for late effects and prevent their occurrence has also been discussed widely. In adult-onset leukemia, however, late effects of treatment have not been fully investigated, partly because of the relatively small number of survivors and lack of trials addressing the issue.

Adult-onset leukemia differs from childhood leukemia in various ways. CLL and AML are more common in adults, whereas ALL is the most prevalent childhood leukemia. The intensity of the therapy and the specific agents used differ between adult and pediatric patients. In addition, there are biological differences between adults and children. The most common long-term toxic effects observed in survivors of adult-onset leukemia treated with chemotherapy or targeted therapies are described in the following sections. We particularly focus on CML, for which the number of long-term survivors has greatly increased. The late effects of stem cell transplantation are discussed in a separate chapter.

Cardiovascular System

Anthracyclines

Anthracyclines are associated with an increased risk of cardiovascular adverse events. Anthracyclines may cause irreversible cardiomyopathy because of oxidative damage to myocytes, although other mechanisms have also been proposed. The cardiotoxicity of anthracyclines most commonly manifests as late congestive heart failure. Leukemia survivors treated with anthracyclines are also at increased risk for arrhythmia, pericarditis, myocarditis, and myocardial infarction. QT prolongation, which is detectable on an electrocardiograph, and increased risk of aortic stiffness have also been reported. Cardiotoxic effects may occur years after the treatment is completed, although one study reported that the median onset of left ventricular dysfunction was 4 months after completion of treatment with anthracyclines (Cardinale et al. 2010).

Cardiotoxicity in anthracyclines is strongly correlated with the cumulative dose. The cumulative dose of doxorubicin resulting in a 3–5% likelihood of congestive heart failure was reported to be 400 mg/m^2, and the dose resulting in a 7–26% likelihood of congestive heart failure was 550 mg/m^2 (Swain et al. 2003; Bird and Swain 2008). Also, patients receiving more than a 360–400 mg/m^2 cumulative dose of anthracyclines had the highest risk of cardiac mortality (Mertens et al. 2008; Tukenova et al. 2010). Thus, cumulative doses of doxorubicin are generally best limited to 450–500 mg/m^2. However, sensitivity to anthracyclines varies among patients, and no dose is considered to be safe. Several known risk factors predict cardiotoxic effects in patients treated with less than the recommended cumulative dose of anthracyclines. These include age older than 65 years; history of coronary artery disease, hypertension, or other heart disease; and cardiac irradiation (Steinherz et al. 1991; Swain et al. 2003; Hershman et al. 2008).

In addition to limiting cumulative doses of anthracyclines, several approaches have been investigated to reduce the risk of cardiotoxic effects. For example, in one study, fewer cardiotoxic effects were reported in patients receiving prolonged infusions of anthracyclines (6 hours or more) than in patients receiving bolus infusions of anthracyclines, with no differences between the patient groups in terms of response rates, remission rates, or survival durations (Smith et al. 2010). In the Department of Leukemia at MD Anderson, we currently employ 24-hour continuous infusion of doxorubicin in patients with ALL. More prolonged infusion protocol (48-hour continuous infusion) is used in patients with impaired cardiac function, as assessed by echocardiography.

The use of a liposomal formulation of doxorubicin or daunorubicin has been found to be associated with a significantly lower risk of cardiotoxic effects than the conventional formulation (Smith et al. 2010). Dexrazoxane, an EDTA-like chelator, was also reported to prevent anthracycline-induced damage in cardiac tissue. However, dexrazoxane may also interfere with the efficacy of anthracyclines, although the evidence is not concrete. At this point, dexrazoxane is not generally recommended for adult patients with leukemia who were treated with a doxorubicin-based regimen. Careful management of risk factors such as hypertension or hyper-lipidemia is also important for preventing cardiotoxic effects.

Cardiac function assessment is highly recommended before, during, and after potentially cardiotoxic chemotherapy, although the optimal monitoring method and schedule have not yet been determined. Most commonly, left ventricular function is assessed on an echocardiogram or ventriculogram (multiple-gated acquisition scan). In the Department of Leukemia at MD Anderson, we generally obtain an echocardiogram or ventriculogram prior to treatment and repeat assessment as necessary on the basis of the clinical picture and the patient's risk factors. Cardiac troponins and B-type natriuretic peptide have also been investigated as potential biomarkers for monitoring anthracycline-related cardiomyopathy. These biomarkers may help with early detection of cardiotoxic effects; however, the data remain limited, and further validation is needed.

Tyrosine Kinase Inhibitors

A small but worrisome risk of toxic effects in the cardiovascular system associated with some TKIs has also been reported. Cardiotoxic effects induced by TKIs are generally reversible when the suspected agent is discontinued. Hence, the cardiotoxicity of TKIs is most worrisome in patients who require chronic therapy for their disease, such as patients with CML.

The cardiotoxicity of imatinib has been debated. Severe congestive heart failure in patients treated with imatinib was first reported in 2006 (Kerkela et al. 2006). Reticulum stress and cell death in cardiomyocytes, likely induced by Abl inhibition, was suggested as the cause of the congestive heart failure in this study. However, in subsequent studies, congestive heart failure was observed in only 0.5–1.7% of patients, and most of them had comorbidities predisposing them to cardiac dysfunction (Atallah et al. 2007; Hatfield et al. 2007). Current available evidence suggests that cardiotoxic effects induced by imatinib are uncommon, occurring mostly in susceptible patients with predisposing factors. Close monitoring of patients with risk factors and symptoms suggestive of cardiac dysfunction is advisable.

Although data are limited, toxic effects in the cardiovascular system induced by other TKIs, including dasatinib, nilotinib, and ponatinib, have also been reported. Dasatinib is a TKI against Bcr-Abl, platelet-derived growth factor receptors a and b, c-Kit, and Src family kinases. Dasatinib is currently indicated for treatment of CML and Philadelphia chromosome–positive ALL. In one report, the incidence of congestive heart failure in patients treated with dasatinib was 2–4% (Yeh and Bickford 2009). Increased risks of QT prolongation, pericardial effusion, and pulmonary artery hypertension with dasatinib have also been reported. Nilotinib inhibits kinase activity of Bcr-Abl, c-Kit, and platelet-derived growth factor receptors a and b. In addition to QT prolongation, peripheral artery disease and other arteriopathy was observed in 6.15% of patients treated with nilotinib in one retrospective report (Le Coutre et al. 2011). Ponatinib was approved by the US Food and Drug Administration for the treatment of CML resistant or intolerant to first-line TKI therapy in 2012, with the inclusion of a boxed warning of potential arterial thrombosis and liver toxicity. Ponatinib is unique because of its potential activity in patients who harbor the T315I BCR-ABL mutation. Symptomatic bradyarrhythmia; supraventricular tachyarrhythmia, most predominantly atrial fibrillation; and serious heart failure were also observed in 1–5% of patients treated with ponatinib. Further observation is warranted to determine the cardiotoxicity of new kinase inhibitors.

Secondary Malignancies

Survivors of childhood or adolescent leukemia are known to be at increased risk for secondary malignancies. In survivors of childhood ALL, skin cancer and central nervous system neoplasms are the predominantly observed secondary malignancies, followed by solid tumors, including breast, soft tissue, and thyroid cancers. A study of the entire population of adults in Denmark focusing on thyroid cancer, brain cancer, and non-Hodgkin lymphoma revealed that the risk of developing these secondary malignancies was approximately 2–5 times higher in survivors of adult leukemia than in the general population (Nielsen et al. 2011).

Chemotherapy

Chemotherapy and radiation therapy can be associated with secondary myelodysplastic syndrome and leukemia, as well as solid tumors. Among chemotherapeutic agents, alkylating agents and topoisomerase II inhibitors are most frequently associated with secondary myelodysplastic syndrome or AML. Alkylating agents such as cyclophosphamide and chlorambucil, as well as radiation therapy, may cause secondary myelodysplastic syndrome or AML with a latency of 5–7 years. Typically the patient presents with myelodysplasia, and cytogenetic study often shows complex abnormalities, including deletion of chromosome 5 or 7. Secondary AML associated with topoisomerase II inhibitors generally has a latency of 1–3 years and presents as overt leukemia. The most common cytogenetic abnormalities observed with secondary AML involve 11q26 or 21q22 abnormalities.

Tyrosine Kinase Inhibitors in Patients with Chronic Myeloid Leukemia

TKIs have been found to potentially increase the risk of developing secondary malignancies. Multiple reports, including a few from MD Anderson, have demonstrated the development of chromosomal abnormalities in Philadelphia chromosome–negative metaphases, which may develop into myelodysplastic syndrome or AML, in patients with CML treated with imatinib or dasatinib (Kovitz et al. 2006; Jabbour et al. 2007). Because these chromosomal changes are not observed in patients treated with imatinib for diseases other than CML and the changes have also been observed in patients with CML treated with other agents, including interferon, the chromosomal changes are thought not to be solely caused by treatment with TKIs. The increased incidence of secondary malignancies other than myelo-dysplasia in patients with CML treated with imatinib was reported in a small cohort of patients, but subsequent studies have failed to confirm the association.

Chronic Lymphocytic Leukemia

Incidence of several malignancies, including melanoma, non-melanoma skin cancer, lung cancer, oropharyngeal cancer, prostate cancer, renal cancer, and lymphoma, is higher among patients with a history of CLL than in the general population (Wiernik 2004; Molica 2005; Tsimberidou et al. 2009). Previous reports have shown that the overall risk of malignancies (other than CLL) was almost twice as high in these patients than in the general population, especially the risk of skin cancers, and the risk remained elevated for at least 9 years after the diagnosis of CLL. Squamous cell skin cancer that is more aggressive than usual has also been reported in these patients. Treatment-related immunosuppression and shared risk factors are possible explanations for the increased risk of secondary malignancies in patients with CLL. Awareness of the risk could help increase early detection of secondary cancers. However, optimal cancer screening schedules for patients with CLL have not been established. At the very least, long-term monitoring with standard cancer screening should be performed. Protection from sun exposure using sunscreen or protective clothing to prevent skin cancers is also reasonable advice.

Reproductive Changes

Chemotherapy

Chemotherapeutic agents can be categorized into high, medium, and low risk according to their gonadotoxicity. Alkylating agents are considered high risk, resulting in oligospermia in men and follicular depletion, cortical fibrosis, and blood vessel damage to the ovaries in women. Agents considered medium risk include certain anthracyclines (e.g., doxorubicin) and platinum. Low-risk agents include vinca alkaloids and antimetabolites. Male patients with leukemia treated with chemotherapy may develop primary or secondary hypogonadism, which may or may not cause infertility. In female patients, premature ovarian failure and associated infertility may occur. Damage to the ovaries is usually irreversible because the number of germ cells is fixed during prenatal development. An increased risk of premature ovarian failure has been reported in adolescents and adults with leukemia compared with matched controls. Pregnancies that occur several years after completion of chemotherapy are not associated with an increased rate of fetal malformation or demise compared with pregnancies in the general population. However, it is recommended that female patients avoid conceiving during the first 2 years after the completion of chemotherapy to avoid fertilization of ova that might have been exposed to chemotherapy during the vulnerable period of folliculogenesis and growth.

Tyrosine Kinase Inhibitors

In preclinical studies, imatinib was found to cause teratogenic effects in mice. The findings of retrospective studies of female patients exposed to imatinib during pregnancy suggested a possible association between congenital abnormalities and imatinib exposure, although the number of patients was not large enough to draw definitive conclusions (Ault et al. 2006; Pye et al. 2008). On the basis of these findings, it is prudent to advise female patients to avoid conception while they are receiving treatment with imatinib. Current evidence does not suggest a risk of passing on congenital abnormalities in male patients, although oligospermia and reduced sperm motility have been observed. Women taking other TKIs are also advised not to become pregnant, although only a few anecdotal reports have described the effects of other TKIs on pregnancy.

Options to Preserve Fertility

For male patients, the simplest way to preserve fertility is to collect a semen sample for cryopreservation before starting the chemotherapy. However, this approach still has limitations; pretreatment semen quality may be poor in patients with acute leukemia, and most insurance companies will not cover the cost of maintaining the specimen. Another approach is hormonal manipulation during or after chemotherapy using testosterone or gonadotropin-releasing hormone agonists. However, current data indicate that the efficacy of this approach has been disappointing in humans.

The preservation of fertility in female patients is more challenging at this point. Possible options include cryopreservation of embryos and oocytes. Although embryo preservation is well established from a technical point of view, patients diagnosed with acute leukemia often do not have adequate time to undergo ovarian stimulation and oocyte retrieval, which takes 2–3 weeks, before they must start chemotherapy. In addition, this option is limited to patients who have a partner or are willing to use donor sperm. Oocyte preservation is still an investigational technology, and further advances in this area are needed. Administration of gonadotropin-releasing hormone agonist during chemotherapy has been attempted to decrease the gonadotoxic effects on ovaries; however, the efficacy and safety of this method remains controversial.

Quality of Life and Other Patient-Reported Outcomes

Quality of life (QOL) and other patient-reported outcome assessments are particularly important in patients with CML because these patients currently require life-long treatment, and adherence to medication is associated with increased survival durations. Data concerning QOL are needed to evaluate overall treatment effectiveness and clinical benefit because multiple TKIs are now available to treat CML. A study assessing QOL in patients with CML treated with imatinib revealed lower health-related QOL among young and female patients with CML, compared with their peers in the general population, because of physical and emotional problems (Efficace et al. 2011). The most frequently reported symptom was fatigue. Preliminary data on symptom burden gathered using the MD Anderson Symptom Inventory also suggested that fatigue and other symptoms were common among patients with CML treated with TKIs, affecting patients' ability to work and interact with others (Williams et al. 2008, 2011). In addition, different TKIs have been found to possibly produce different symptom burdens.

The diagnosis of CLL has a profound effect on QOL, even among patients with early-stage disease who do not have clinical symptoms or need treatment. One study demonstrated that overall QOL among patients with CLL was similar to population norms, but emotional well-being was significantly lower among patients with CLL compared with the general population and even compared with patients with other types of cancer (Shanafelt et al. 2007). Considering that the natural history of CLL is generally indolent and patients can be symptom-free for years, this emotional distress is unforeseen and should be noted by clinicians. The "watchful waiting" strategy currently recommended for patients with early-stage disease could leave patients with a feeling of uncertainty or a sense that they have been left alone with a serious, untreated disease.

In acute leukemia, most available data concerning long-term QOL are from studies conducted among patients who underwent stem cell transplantation, although some data are available concerning QOL in patients with AML who did not undergo stem cell transplantation. Among these patients, the most common and persistent symptom was fatigue, which greatly impairs QOL in affected individuals (Alibhai et al. 2007; Schumacher et al. 2002). Effective treatment measures have yet to be found.

Asking patients about the effects of the disease or treatment on their QOL, including physical, mental, and socioeconomic well-being, could unveil as-yet unknown issues and hence lead to further investigations to explore interventions to reduce symptom burden in patients. Validated tools for QOL assessment are available.

Neurologic Changes

Among adult survivors of childhood leukemia, even those who did not receive whole-brain irradiation, several long-term neurologic sequelae have been observed, including increased risks of headaches, seizures, focal neurologic deficits, late-onset auditory-vestibular-visual sensory deficits, and late-occurring stroke. However, data concerning long-term neurologic sequelae for adult-onset leukemia are limited.

Recently, problems with memory and concentration were reported by patients with CML who were being treated with TKIs (Pemmaraju et al. 2011). In addition, approximately one-third of patients with CML receiving treatment with TKIs reported ongoing problems with memory as one of the five most severe symptoms they experienced (Williams et al. 2011). Clinicians need to be aware of this issue, and further investigation is needed.

Bone Metabolism

High-dose steroids and antimetabolites used as a part of a chemotherapy regimen may cause late toxic effects on bone metabolism, such as osteoporosis or aseptic osteonecrosis of the femoral head. Currently, there is no well-established prevention or treatment for these problems, but lifestyle modification and bisphosphonates have been used. Careful follow-up of clinical symptoms and periodic bone density assessment may be advisable.

A study of the long-term effects of imatinib on bone remodeling in patients with CML showed increased total bone volume and decreased serum phosphorus and calcium concentrations. Although the clinical implications of these findings are largely unknown at this point, monitoring serum phosphorus and vitamin D levels may be a reasonable action. Further studies are warranted to determine the long-term effects of imatinib on bone metabolism in patients with CML.

Endocrine System

Imatinib may negatively affect patients who are receiving levothyroxine for hypothyroidism, although imatinib itself does not appear to cause hypothyroidism. Elevated thyrotropin levels and the need for increased doses of levothyroxine have been reported in patients with CML who are being treated with both imatinib and levothyroxine (de Groot et al. 2005). Another TKI against constitutive activation of the FLT3 receptor tyrosine kinase, sorafenib, which is currently in clinical trials as a treatment for FLT3-positive AML, may induce hypothyroidism.

Immune Function

Infections are a major complication in patients with CLL. Infections may be related to the disease itself or to the treatment. Disease-related pathogenesis is multifactorial, including hypogammaglobulinemia and perturbations in cell-mediated immunity, complement activity, or neutrophil function. Common bacterial organisms are the most common infectious pathogens observed in patients treated with alkylating agents or patients who are under observation. In patients treated with fludarabine-based regimens or alemtuzumab, a monoclonal antibody against CD52, infections may be caused by *Candida* spp, *Aspergillus* spp, *Pneumocystis jiroveci*, herpesvirus, or common bacterial organisms. Patients with frequent, recurrent infections should be evaluated for hypogammaglobulinemia. Intravenous replacement of immunoglobulin can reduce the risk of infection in patients with low immunoglobulin levels and frequent infections. Patients should be treated with appropriate antimicrobials, even for minor infections. Vaccination against influenza every year and against pneumococcus every 5 years is also recommended.

TKIs may also affect immune function. For example, imatinib may cause hypogammaglobulinemia and has been shown to suppress T-cell and natural killer cell activity in vitro. The clinical relevance of this phenomenon is unclear.

Conclusion

Possible late effects or chronic toxicity of treatments are becoming more evident, especially in patients with chronic leukemia. At this point, effective interventions have yet to be found. It is vital to establish optimal follow-up schedules to monitor physical, psychological, and socioeconomic health in leukemia survivors. This will allow potential issues in this population to be identified so that various interventions to improve survivor well-being can be tested.

Key Practice Points

- TKIs are a first-line treatment for CML. Patients with CML require life-long treatment with TKIs at this point, which can cause significant physical, emotional, or socioeconomic distress. Monitoring of clinical symptoms and QOL is recommended.
- Patients with CML who are receiving treatment with TKIs should be monitored for symptom burden, clinical symptoms suggestive of heart failure or cognitive dysfunction, serum phosphorus levels, serum gammaglobulin levels, and other cancers, as appropriate for their age. In patients who are also receiving thyroid hormone replacement therapy for hypothyroidism, more frequent monitoring of thyrotropin levels and dose adjustment of levothyroxine is warranted.
- Pregnancy should be avoided in female patients with CML while they are receiving treatment with TKIs.
- In patients with CLL, infections should be treated liberally with antimicrobial agents. Periodic vaccinations against influenza and pneumococcus are recommended.
- Patients with CLL and their physicians should be aware of the increased risk for second malignancies. Standard cancer screening, at the very least, is advised.
- For survivors of adult acute leukemia, long-term follow-up to assess physical, emotional, and socioeconomic well-being is vital. In particular, assessments for cardiovascular problems, infertility, osteoporosis, and symptom burden/QOL are necessary.

Suggested Readings

Alibhai SM, Leach M, Kowgier ME, et al. Fatigue in older adults with acute myeloid leukemia: predictors and associations with quality of life and functional status. *Leukemia* 2007;21: 845–848.

Atallah E, Durand JB, Kantarjian HM, et al. Congestive heart failure is a rare event in patients receiving imatinib therapy. *Blood* 2007;110:1233–1237.

Ault P, Kantarjian HM, O'Brien S, et al. Pregnancy among patients with chronic myeloid leukemia treated with imatinib. *J Clin Oncol* 2006;24:1204–1208.

Bird BR, Swain SM. Cardiac toxicity in breast cancer survivors: review of potential cardiac problems. *Clin Cancer Res* 2008;14:14–24.

Cardinale D, Colombo A, Lamantia G, et al. Anthracycline-induced cardiomyopathy: clinical relevance and response to pharmacologic therapy. *J Am Coll Cardiol* 2010;55:213–220.

de Groot JW, Zonnenberg BA, Plukker JT, et al. Imatinib induces hypothyroidism in patients receiving levothyroxine. *Clin Pharmacol Ther* 2005;78:433–438.

Deininger M, O'Brien SG, Guilhot F, et al. International randomized study of interferon vs STI571 (IRIS) 8-year follow up: sustained survival and low risk for progression or events in patients with newly diagnosed chronic myeloid leukemia in chronic phase (CML-CP) treated with imatinib. *Blood* 2009;114:1126a.

Efficace F, Baccarani M, Breccia M, et al. Health-related quality of life in chronic myeloid leukemia patients receiving long-term therapy with imatinib compared with the general population. *Blood* 2011;118:4554–4560.

Hatfield A, Owen S, Pilot PR. In reply to 'Cardiotoxicity of the cancer therapeutic agent imatinib mesylate'. *Nat Med* 2007;13:15–16.

Hershman DL, McBride RB, Eisenberger A, et al. Doxorubicin, cardiac risk factors, and cardiac toxicity in elderly patients with diffuse B-cell non-Hodgkin's lymphoma. *J Clin Oncol* 2008;26:3159–3165.

Jabbour E, Kantarjian HM, Abruzzo LV, et al. Chromosomal abnormalities in Philadelphia chromosome negative metaphases appearing during imatinib mesylate therapy in patients with newly diagnosed chronic myeloid leukemia in chronic phase. *Blood* 2007;110:2991–2995.

Kerkela R, Grazette L, Yacobi R, et al. Cardiotoxicity of the cancer therapeutic agent imatinib mesylate. *Nat Med* 2006;12:908–916.

Kovitz C, Kantarjian HM, Garcia-Manero G, et al. Myelodysplastic syndromes and acute leukemia developing after imatinib mesylate therapy for chronic myeloid leukemia. *Blood* 2006;108: 2811–2813.

Le Coutre P, Rea D, Abruzzese E, et al. Severe peripheral arterial disease during nilotinib therapy. *J Natl Cancer Inst* 2011;103:1347–1348.

Mertens AC, Liu Q, Neglia JP, et al. Cause-specific late mortality among 5-year survivors of childhood cancer: the Childhood Cancer Survivor Study. *J Natl Cancer Inst* 2008;100:1368–1379.

Molica S. Second neoplasms in chronic lymphocytic leukemia: incidence and pathogenesis with emphasis on the role of different therapies. *Leuk Lymphoma* 2005;46:49–54.

Nielsen SF, Bojesen SE, Birgens HS, et al. Risk of thyroid cancer, brain cancer, and non-Hodgkin lymphoma after adult leukemia: a nationwide study. *Blood* 2011;118:4062–4069.

Pemmaraju N, Kantarjian HM, Tanaka M, et al. Memory impairment in chronic phase (CP) chronic myeloid leukemia (CML) patients (pts) treated with dasatinib tyrosine kinase inhibitor (TKI) therapy. *Blood* 2011;118:3771a.

Pye SM, Cortes J, Ault P, et al. The effects of imatinib on pregnancy outcome. *Blood* 2008;111:5505–5508.

Schumacher A, Wewers D, Heinecke A, et al. Fatigue as an important aspect of quality of life in patients with acute myeloid leukemia. *Leuk Res* 2002;26:355–362.

Shanafelt TD, Bowen D, Venkat C, et al. Quality of life in chronic lymphocytic leukemia: an international survey of 1482 patients. *Br J Haematol* 2007;139:255–264.

Smith LA, Cornelius VR, Plummer CJ, et al. Cardiotoxicity of anthracycline agents for the treatment of cancer: systematic review and meta-analysis of randomised controlled trials. *BMC Cancer* 2010;10:337.

Steinherz LJ, Steinherz PG, Tan CT, et al. Cardiac toxicity 4 to 20 years after completing anthracycline therapy. *JAMA* 1991;266:1672–1677.

Swain SM, Whaley FS, Ewer MS. Congestive heart failure in patients treated with doxorubicin: a retrospective analysis of three trials. *Cancer* 2003;97:2869–2879.

Tsimberidou AM, Wen S, McLaughlin P, et al. Other malignancies in chronic lymphocytic leukemia/small lymphocytic lymphoma. *J Clin Oncol* 2009;27:904–910.

Tukenova M, Guibout C, Oberlin O, et al. Role of cancer treatment in long-term overall and cardiovascular mortality after childhood cancer. *J Clin Oncol* 2010;28:1308–1315.

Wiernik PH. Second neoplasms in patients with chronic lymphocytic leukemia. *Curr Treat Options Oncol* 2004;5:215–223.

Williams LA, Ault P, Garcia-Gonzalez A, et al. Identifying high symptom burden in patients with chronic myeloid leukemia on tyrosine kinase inhibitor therapy. *Blood* 2011;118:3138a.

Williams LA, Ault P, Wang XS, et al. The symptom burden of chronic myeloid leukemia. *Blood* 2008;112:2408a.

Yeh ET, Bickford CL. Cardiovascular complications of cancer therapy: incidence, pathogenesis, diagnosis, and management. *J Am Coll Cardiol* 2009;53:2231–2247.

Chapter 12
Hematologic Cancer Survivorship Management: Lymphoma

Maria Alma Rodriguez, Leslie Ballas, and Kristin Simar

Contents

L.E. Foxhall, M.A. Rodriguez (eds.), *Advances in Cancer Survivorship Management*,
MD Anderson Cancer Care Series, DOI 10.1007/978-1-4939-0986-5_12,
© The University of Texas M.D. Anderson Cancer Center 2015

Chapter Overview Lymphoid malignancies are a family of diverse cancers arising in the cells of the immune system. Lymphoid leukemia, lymphoma, and myeloma belong to this category of cancers. This chapter will focus on lymphomas and the late effects of treatment. Lymphomas are broadly categorized into Hodgkin lymphomas, which are uncommon, and non-Hodgkin lymphomas, which are the sixth most common malignancy in men and women. Incidence of non-Hodgkin lymphoma appears to be rising, although the reasons for this are unclear. Treatment for lymphoma has improved substantially over the past 50 years, resulting in a large population of long-term lymphoma survivors. Patients with lymphoma are treated principally with chemotherapy, immunotherapy, radiation, or stem cell transplantation. Surgery generally does not have a role in the treatment of these disorders except in rare cases. Different treatment modalities have different late side effects. In this chapter, we will summarize the most commonly known potential late effects of chemotherapeutic agents and radiation, the few situations in which surgery is used and its long-term effects, and recommended practice for surveillance of recurrence and late effects.

Introduction

Incidence of lymphoma has increased dramatically over the past 60 years, as reported by US and international registries. Approximately 66,000 new cases of non-Hodgkin lymphoma were diagnosed in the United States in 2011. It is the sixth most common cancer in both men and women, with a slight predominance in men compared with women (1.5:1). In the United States, the incidence is higher in whites compared with other racial or ethnic groups. The two most common subtypes of non-Hodgkin lymphoma are follicular lymphoma and diffuse large B-cell lymphoma. Hodgkin lymphoma constitutes less than 5% of all lymphomas. The overall 5-year survival rate for all lymphomas is 70% (Howlader et al. 2012). However, survival rates differ for each lymphoma subtype, depending on stage of the lymphoma, age of the patient, and inherent biologic risk factors of the lymphoma itself. In general, Hodgkin lymphoma is highly curable in early stages, as is diffuse large B-cell lymphoma, whereas other lymphoma subtypes, such as peripheral T-cell lymphoma, have a poor prognosis. Patients with other lymphomas, such as follicular lymphoma, may survive for many years but require intermittent treatment for repeated recurrences.

Treatment for most lymphomas has improved substantially over the past century. Radiation therapy was recognized early in the twentieth century as a potentially curative treatment for Hodgkin lymphoma, particularly for early-stage, localized disease. After World War I, nitrogen mustard, a neurotoxic agent used during the war as a chemical weapon, was also observed to be an active anticancer agent. This observation signaled the birth of a new therapeutic field: cancer chemotherapy. Lymphoid malignancies were the first type of cancer to be effectively treated with chemicals. Hodgkin lymphoma was the first type of cancer to be cured with a treatment regimen that combined four chemotherapy drugs, known as the MOPP regimen (nitrogen mustard, vincristine, procarbazine, and prednisone). Today many drugs can effectively treat lymphoma, and frontline treatment with some drugs may be curative for several subtypes of primary or relapsed lymphoma. The MOPP regimen is no longer used today; it has been superseded by the less toxic and equally efficacious ABVD drug combination (doxorubicin, bleomycin, vinblastine, and dacarbazine).

Over the past decade, several effective new immunotherapy agents have been introduced into the array of treatment options for patients with lymphoma (see Table 12.1). The population of lymphoma survivors today includes both patients who have been treated up front and those who have been treated in repeated episodes for recurrences, using a wide variety of approaches: chemotherapy, immunotherapy, combinations of chemotherapy and immunotherapy, radiation, and combinations of all of these modalities (The University of Texas MD Anderson Cancer Center 2012). In addition, patients who have experienced a relapse of the disease likely have also received intensive salvage chemotherapy and immunotherapy, often including stem cell transplantation. As treatments for lymphoma continue to improve and survival rates remain high, it is important to understand the potential late effects of the various therapies. The risk of secondary effects and complications of treatment depend on the type of treatment(s), as well as the age and health of the patient. The survivorship care plan must therefore be tailored to each patient's disease, treatment, and health history. We will review the late effects of the most commonly used chemotherapeutic and immunotherapeutic agents, as well as late effects of radiation. Survivorship concerns after stem cell transplantation are reviewed in a separate chapter.

Surgery

Laparotomy with lymph node sampling and splenectomy used to be an important procedure for staging Hodgkin lymphoma in the era preceding computed tomographic (CT) scanning technology. CT body imaging techniques, which became common in the late 1970s and early 1980s, now allow excellent visualization of internal nodal sites, including the spleen, for staging purposes. Hence, surgical staging procedures have become obsolete for lymphoma. Splenectomy is still considered appropriate, however, as a therapeutic and diagnostic modality for patients who present with splenic lesions or enlargement of the spleen indicating selectively localized disease, with no evidence of nodal or marrow disease. This is a classic presentation of a particular subtype of lymphoma called primary splenic marginal zone lymphoma. Splenectomy may also be indicated for patients with autoimmune thrombocytopenia or anemia syndromes that are related to the lymphoma but do not respond to medical therapy. The principal concern for long-term survivors after splenectomy is the risk of life-threatening infections by

Table 12.1 Chemotherapeutic agents commonly used to treat lymphoma

Regimen	Drugs included	Indication
Monoclonal antibodies targeted to specific cell surface antigens (given as single agents)	Rituximab; ofatumumab	Indolent B-cell lymphoma, frontline or relapse
	Brentuximab	Hodgkin lymphoma and CD30+ lymphoma, approved for relapsed disease (also effective when added to frontline chemotherapy; studies ongoing)
RCOP	R = rituximab, C = cyclophosphamide, O = vincristine, P = prednisone	Indolent B-cell lymphoma, frontline or relapse
BR, FR, FND, or FCR	B = bendamustine, R = rituximab, F = fludarabine, N = mitoxantrone, D = dexamethasone, C = cyclophosphamide	Indolent B-cell lymphoma, frontline or relapse
RCHOP, REPOCH, or RHCVAD/RMA	In RCHOP and REPOCH: R = rituximab, C = cyclophosphamide, H = doxorubicin, O = vincristine, P = prednisone, E = etoposide In RHCVAD/RMA: R = rituximab, H = "high-dose", C = cyclophosphamide, V = vincristine, A = doxorubicin (RHCVAD) or cytarabine (RMA), D = dexamethasone, M = methotrexate	Aggressive B-cell lymphomas, such as diffuse large B-cell lymphoma, mantle cell lymphoma, or Burkitt lymphoma; peripheral T-cell lymphoma, with rituximab excluded; usually frontline
ABVD	A = doxorubicin, B = bleomycin, V = vinblastine, D = dacarbazine	Hodgkin lymphoma, frontline (approval for addition of brentuximab pending)
ICE, RICE	I = ifosfamide, C = carboplatin, E = etoposide, R = rituximab	ICE: relapsed Hodgkin lymphoma or T-cell lymphoma; RICE: relapsed aggressive B-cell lymphoma; usually precedes autologous stem cell transplantation
DHAP (±R), ESHAP (±R)	D = dexamethasone, HA = high-dose cytarabine, P = platinum, E = etoposide, S = methylprednisolone, R = rituximab	−R: Relapsed Hodgkin lymphoma or T-cell lymphoma; +R: relapsed B-cell lymphoma; usually precedes autologous stem cell transplantation

encapsulated bacteria, such as meningococcus or pneumococcus. Vaccination is recommended prior to the splenectomy, with continual booster vaccines every other year for life, according to the Centers for Disease Control and Prevention (http://www.immunize.org/acip/).

Gastric surgery for resection of lymphoma is not generally indicated, unless the patient has a tumor-related ulcer that is actively bleeding, or if imminent perforation is a concern. Most gastric lymphomas will respond to medical management with chemotherapy or radiation, precluding resection. Preserving the gastrointestinal tract anatomy intact is the preferred option. In the event that a resection is required, long-term malabsorption of some nutrients may manifest as anemia. For example, patients with lesions in the terminal ileum and cecum may need to undergo resection of a portion of the distal bowel, which can lead to malabsorption of nutrients, such as vitamin B12, over the long term. Adhesions may also occur years later, presenting as bowel obstruction.

Late Effects of Chemotherapy

General Symptoms

Fatigue is the most common general complaint in lymphoma survivors, and it may persist for a long period of time after completion of treatment. The etiology of fatigue is complex, and many factors play into the equation. More information about fatigue is available in Chap. 22.

Patients also complain of a syndrome referred to as "chemobrain," which is described in various ways by the patients but in general indicates awareness that cognitive processes are slower than usual and short-term memory is somewhat impaired. This syndrome and its management are discussed in greater detail in Chap. 20.

Heart Problems

Cardiac adverse effects are the most common complication of the anthracycline family of chemotherapeutic agents. Doxorubicin is the most common anthracycline drug used in chemotherapeutic regimens for lymphoma (see Table 12.1). The classic injury caused by anthracyclines is myocardial muscle weakness, leading to congestive heart failure. Anthracyclines have a lifetime maximum dose threshold; therefore, if patients require additional treatment with anthracyclines for relapsing disease or secondary malignancies, cardiac evaluation and close monitoring for signs of congestive heart failure is imperative.

Lung Problems

Pulmonary adverse effects are not as common as cardiac adverse effects. Lung problems secondary to chemotherapy are most commonly caused by the drug bleomycin. This drug is one of the agents in the ABVD combination, which is the standard regimen used to treat Hodgkin lymphoma. Pulmonary adverse effects are also possible with fludarabine, cytarabine, and high-dose chemotherapy regimens used prior to stem cell transplantation. Patients most at risk for pulmonary adverse effects are those who smoke, are elderly, or have had other lung injury events, such as exposure to asbestos or other inhaled toxic chemicals.

Kidney Problems

A number of chemotherapy drugs, especially cis-platinum and ifosfamide, can cause renal adverse effects. Kidney damage caused by chemotherapy drugs may manifest as creatinine elevation or electrolyte disturbances, including profound loss of magnesium, which can persist for many years after treatment is completed. Susceptible patients are the elderly, those with diabetes, and those with hypertension or other renal disorders. Contrast material used for CT scans can worsen renal injury in patients with persistently elevated creatinine levels. Patients should also be counseled to avoid nonsteroidal anti-inflammatory drugs if they have renal damage.

Liver Problems

Many chemotherapeutic agents (e.g., methotrexate, cytarabine) can cause transient elevation of liver enzymes. High-dose regimens are also more likely to cause liver enzyme elevations than are low-dose regimens. However, lasting hepatic problems are rare unless they are associated with an underlying chronic infectious illness (e.g., hepatitis B or C) or toxic liver trauma (e.g., alcohol). Patients with chronic elevation of liver enzymes should be counseled to avoid acetaminophen-containing medications and to be aware of risks associated with medications that are known to cause liver enzyme abnormalities, such as statins. Patients should also avoid common substances that are toxic to the liver, such as alcohol. The monoclonal antibody rituximab may cause reactivation of a dormant hepatitis B virus in patients with a prior infection.

Neuropathy

Vinca alkaloids (i.e., vincristine and vinblastine) and proteasome inhibitors, such as bortezomib, can cause chronic neuropathy. Patients particularly at risk are the elderly and those with diabetes or peripheral vascular disease. Neuropathy may manifest in various ways, usually with sensory symptoms such as burning sensations or needle-like pains or with proprioceptive changes (e.g., loss of sensation of the location or position of one's feet on the floor). The most severe symptom of neuropathy, foot drop (loss of motor control of the ankle), is unusual.

Myelodysplasia

High-dose chemotherapy (as used prior to blood or marrow stem cell transplantation) or chronic doses of alkylators, such as cyclophosphamide, can cause myelodysplasia (pre-leukemia), with eventual transformation to leukemia. This complication may manifest as chronic unexplained anemia or slowly progressing pancytopenia, and it may occur years after treatment is completed.

Immunodeficiency

Antibodies directed at lymphoid cells (e.g., alemtuzumab, rituximab) and some other drugs, such as fludarabine, can cause lasting suppression of immunity that can lead to chronic infections. Another immune abnormality, graft-versus-host disease, is a potential chronic long-term effect of transplanted allogeneic stem cells. Late effects of allogeneic stem cell transplantation are discussed in Chap. 10.

Late Effects of Radiation Therapy

Late effects of radiation therapy are adverse effects that become apparent several years after the completion of treatment. Because many of these effects take years to manifest, most of the accumulated data are from patients treated with old technology and out-of-date radiation doses. Treatment-related adverse effects vary according to the area of the body treated. Here, we discuss effects related to radiation to the head and neck, pelvis, and mediastinum, as well as the increased risk of second malignancies that can accompany radiation therapy.

Xerostomia

The risk of long-term xerostomia associated with radiation has been well documented in patients with head and neck cancer. However, the risk of xerostomia associated with radiation therapy is unknown in patients with lymphoma, which is treated with lower doses than those used to treat head and neck cancers.

In the subacute setting (6 months after radiation therapy is completed), patients have a reduced risk of mouth dryness and sticky saliva if the mean dose to each of the parotid glands was less than 31 Gy and the mean dose to the minor salivary glands was less than 11 Gy (Rodrigues et al. 2009). This reduced risk is presumed to persist in the long term.

Thyroid Disorders

The most common late effect after radiation to the lower neck is hypothyroidism. The risk of thyroid disease 20 years after radiation therapy has been reported to be 52% (Hancock et al. 1991). In a childhood cancer survivorship study, survivors who had been treated with radiation had a 17 times higher risk of hypothyroidism than did siblings who did not receive radiation (Sklar et al. 2000). Thyroid disorders have also been closely linked to the doses of radiation received. In the pediatric population, 17% of children who received less than 26 Gy developed a thyroid disorder, whereas 78% of children who received more than 26 Gy developed thyroid problems (Constine et al. 1984). The median time to develop hypothyroidism after radiation therapy is approximately 6 years (Bhatia et al. 1989). Less common thyroid disorders that may develop after radiation therapy include Graves disease, thyroiditis, thyrotoxicosis, thyroid nodules, and thyroid malignancies.

Sterility

Radiation therapy alone is associated with sterility only if the patient receives pelvic radiation for disease below the diaphragm. Because radiation therapy is most commonly used in early-stage lymphomas, which rarely appear only in an infradiaphragmatic location, this is a rare side effect.

If the ovaries are exposed to radiation, they are at risk for DNA damage, atrophy, and decreased reserve. Sterility is not only related to the dose of radiation, but is also a function of age at the time of radiation therapy. A dose of 4 Gy is associated with a 30% risk of sterility in young women and a 100% risk of sterility in women older than 30 years (Ogilvy-Stuart and Shalet 1993). Displacing the ovaries to a different location within the pelvis, outside of the radiation field, can decrease the dose of radiation to the ovaries.

Male sex organs are even more sensitive to the effects of radiation. Men can have a decreased sperm count after a dose of 0.15 Gy and permanent sterility after a dose of 2 Gy. At MD Anderson, if possible, we use testicular shielding to decrease the dose of radiation to the testicles.

Cardiovascular Disease

Cardiovascular disease is the second leading cause of death in Hodgkin lymphoma survivors. Radiation-induced cardiac disease is caused by inflammation and fibrosis, and it usually manifests approximately 5–10 years after radiation therapy. Cardiac mortality secondary to radiation therapy has been shown to be related to both the dose of radiation and the age of the patient. The relative risk of cardiac death is 3.1 in patients treated with more than 30 Gy (Hancock et al. 1993), and the risk appears to be highest in patients treated with radiation before 20 years of age. Cardiac morbidity, such as valvular disorders, coronary artery disease, and congestive heart failure, is also of concern. The relative risks of myocardial infarction and congestive heart failure are 3.6 and 4.9, respectively, at 18 years after completion of radiation therapy. These relative risks become elevated 10 years after completion of treatment, and the increased risks persist for at least 25 years (Aleman et al. 2007). Chemotherapy has an independent effect on cardiovascular disease; the relative risk of cardiac death with ABVD without radiation is 7.8 (Swerdlow et al. 2007). The relative risk of cardiovascular disease associated with both chemotherapy and radiation therapy is elevated in those with known cardiac risk factors.

Smaller fields and lower doses used in modern techniques reduce the risk of cardiac morbidity and death. In addition, technological advances, such as respiratory gating, have decreased the dose of radiation to the heart. At MD Anderson, we have also started heavily screening patients for risk factors. We recommend echocardiograms starting 10 years after mediastinal radiation, and we recommend a lipid profile yearly.

Non-coronary vascular complications are also possible after radiation therapy. These include transient ischemic attack, stroke, carotid artery disease, and subclavian artery stenosis. The risk of such complications is approximately 2% at 5 years, 3% at 10 years, and 7% at 20 years after completion of radiation therapy (Hull et al. 2003). These risks are also dose-dependent. For example, subclavian artery stenosis is more likely to occur in those who received a dose of 44 Gy than in those who received 36 Gy; carotid artery stenosis is significantly more common in those who received 38 Gy than in those who received 36 Gy. Lastly, stroke is apparently more common in patients who receive mantle radiation, yet this same population does not have an increased risk of hypertension or diabetes mellitus.

Second Malignancies

When examining the role radiation therapy plays in the development of second malignancies, it is important to separate solid tumors from hematologic malignancies. In a study investigating the role of radiation therapy in the development of leukemia, patients who underwent both radiation therapy and chemotherapy did not have an increased risk of developing leukemia compared with those who underwent chemotherapy alone (van Leeuwen et al. 1994). However, patients who underwent chemotherapy combined with total nodal irradiation, a technique used infrequently today, had a 2.5 times higher risk of developing leukemia compared with those who underwent chemotherapy alone.

Solid tumors, which represent 75–80% of second malignancies induced by treatment for cancer, can be related to radiation therapy. Solid tumors induced by treatment most commonly appear in the breast, lung, and gastrointestinal tract. Second malignancies arise after a long latency period, and the risk for second tumors persists for many decades. Most of these tumors occur within or at the edge of the radiation field. As previously mentioned, because these tumors can take decades to appear, most of the available data concerning secondary malignancies are from studies of patients treated with larger treatment fields and higher radiation doses than are currently used. A meta-analysis examining the risk of breast cancer after radiation therapy showed that the risk of breast cancer was higher for those treated with extended fields (large treatment fields) than for those treated with the more modern involved-field radiation therapy (Franklin et al. 2006). Because few data have been accumulated since the transition to smaller fields, the risk for second malignancies has been modeled on the basis of known dose-related side effects. Models have predicted that the risk of secondary breast and lung cancers should be approximately 65% lower when smaller radiation fields are used.

Breast cancer is one of the most common second malignancies to appear after mediastinal radiation therapy in women. A dose of more than 4 Gy to the breast is associated with a 3.2 times higher risk of breast cancer, and a dose of more than 40 Gy to the breast is associated with an eight times higher risk (Travis et al. 2002). Risk of breast cancer is related to both the dose of radiation received and the age of the patient. For patients who receive treatment with mantle radiation (>40 Gy to the mediastinum and axilla) between the ages of 15 and 24 years, the relative risk of breast cancer is 19, whereas for those who receive treatment with radiation between the ages of 24 and 29 years, the relative risk is 7; those who are older than 30 years when they receive mantle radiation do not have an increased relative risk of breast cancer. The hormonal milieu also plays a role in risk of breast cancer. Women who experience premature menopause induced by either chemotherapy or pelvic radiation have been shown to have a decreased risk of breast cancer. Because of the known increased risk of breast cancer after chest radiation, and taking all of these factors into consideration, the American College of Radiology, as well as MD Anderson, recommends that breast magnetic resonance imaging and mammography start 8–10 years after chest radiation, with the aim of catching any potential cancers at an early stage.

Lung cancer is another concern in patients who receive radiation to the chest. The risk of lung cancer is increased after an exposure of more than 30 Gy (Travis et al. 2002). This risk is magnified if the patient smokes or used to smoke.

Although radiation therapy for lymphoma carries risks, it has also been shown to decrease local recurrence of disease, and the risks must be carefully weighed against the potential for disease recurrence. Moreover, not all of these potential risks apply to every patient and every radiation scenario. Radiation oncologists should provide each patient with an assessment of the patient's particular risks, considering the patient's characteristics and the treatment field that will be used.

Long-Term Survivorship Care

Increased risks for long-term and late sequelae exist years after treatment is finished. The transition from active treatment to posttreatment care is essential to maintain long-term health and well-being. To address the unique needs of long-term cancer survivors, MD Anderson clinical experts have synthesized the literature to develop evidence-based clinical practice algorithms as a guide for care of survivors of Hodgkin lymphoma and diffuse large B-cell lymphoma (see algorithms presented at the end of this chapter). The transition from oncologic care to survivorship occurs when the patient shows no evidence of disease and the posttreatment trajectory indicates that long-term survival is expected.

As illustrated in the algorithms, survivors of Hodgkin lymphoma or diffuse large B-cell lymphoma are eligible to transition to survivorship care at 5 years after diagnosis. The lymphoma survivorship algorithm contains four domains or components of care. These four domains guide the survivorship visit and the development of the treatment summary and follow-up care plan (referred to as a Passport Plan for Health; see below).

Surveillance

Every survivorship clinic visit includes an updated medical and family history. A full physical examination is performed. For all patients, complete blood count is evaluated and a chest x-ray is performed prior to the visit. The chest x-ray allows for evaluation of the mediastinal window and the lung fields for potentially problematic abnormalities. In addition, if new symptoms or changes are noted during the examination, appropriate imaging studies, such as CT scans, should be performed.

If a patient is found to have recurrent disease or a new lymphoma, the patient is referred back to the treating physician, and further anticancer therapy can be initiated. Patients who do not have any new findings return in 1 year.

Monitoring for Late Effects

Monitoring for second malignancies, late effects, and treatment-related comorbidities is an important component of survivorship care.

The MD Anderson Lymphoma Survivorship Algorithm recommends that the provider consider performing an annual low-dose, thin-slice, multidetector CT scan of the lungs to evaluate for an occult malignancy if the survivor received radiation to the thorax or if the patient is a smoker. According to the MD Anderson lung cancer screening algorithm, patients aged 50 years or older who have a 20+ pack-year history of smoking are eligible to undergo an annual low-dose, thin-slice, multidetector CT scan of the lungs. CT thorax screening in lymphoma survivors who are at high risk of developing a primary lung carcinoma, especially those who smoke and those who received radiation to the thorax, can potentially improve survival time if the lung carcinoma is detected at an early stage (Das et al. 2006). Additionally, if the survivor is an active smoker, smoking cessation should be discussed and offered.

Lymphoma survivors who received radiation to the chest are at increased risk of developing breast cancer. Breast screening with an examination and mammogram should begin 8 years after completion of chest radiation (if the radiation field overlapped the breast tissue) or at age 40 years, whichever comes first. The examination and mammogram should be repeated annually.

Thyroid screening (i.e., testing for levels of thyroid-stimulating hormone and free T4) is recommended annually if a survivor received radiation to the neck. An annual dermatologic examination is also recommended for all lymphoma survivors because of the increased risk of developing melanoma after radiation therapy (Abrahamsen et al. 2002). Infertility assessment or referral is offered if the patient is concerned about it.

For survivors treated with radiation to the thorax, an annual lipid panel is performed to screen for coronary artery disease. Cardiovascular screening is offered especially to survivors who received radiation to the neck or chest because of the long-term cardiovascular risk associated with radiation to these areas (Chen et al. 2009). For patients who received mantle or other extensive radiation modalities, a lipid screen is recommended, and survivors are strongly encouraged to see a cardiologist for a thorough cardiac evaluation and cardiovascular risk assessment (Heidenreich et al. 2007).

Psychosocial Functioning

Psychosocial health and functioning is assessed and evaluated at each survivorship visit. At the initial survivorship visit, the survivor speaks to a social worker. The survivor is assessed for body image concerns, relationship issues, distress, and employment or financial concerns. If these concerns extend beyond the expertise of an advanced practice nurse or physician assistant, appropriate referrals are made. Access to a primary care provider is evaluated. If the survivor does not have a primary care provider, the Case Management Department at MD Anderson can assist in locating a primary care provider near the survivor's home. Cancer survivors frequently report high rates of sexual dysfunction (Arden-Close et al. 2011). Survivors are referred to a sexuality counselor if desired.

Nutrition

All survivors also speak to a dietician at their initial visit. The dietician discusses with the patient any dietary-related concerns or questions. Basic nutrition information is given to the survivor, along with handouts discussing healthy eating practices.

Passport Plan for Health

The lymphoma survivorship Passport Plan for Health is a communication tool used to transmit cancer survivorship information to health care providers in the community. The MD Anderson provider assembles information about the patient's cancer history, therapy, actual or potential late effects of therapy, specific recommendations regarding cancer screening and surveillance, and general preventive and health maintenance strategies. The Passport enables the MD Anderson provider to individualize care and understand a specific patient's potential risks related to their cancer or treatment. The Passport is created by the health care provider (typically an advanced practice nurse or physician assistant) and a copy of the Passport is then given to the patient to keep as well as to pass along to their primary care provider or medical specialist (e.g., cardiologist). The Passport allows for the identification and evaluation of comorbid conditions that may complicate the patient's survivorship course.

Key Practice Points

- Patients with lymphoma can be treated with a variety of treatment modalities, which may lead to multiple overlapping complications after treatment is completed.
- Radiation toxicity depends on the site of radiation, but special attention should be given to thyroid, lung, and cardiac function in patients who received radiation to lymph node fields in the upper body. Smokers are at increased risk of pulmonary adverse effects and secondary lung malignancies, and thus smoking cessation is strongly recommended. Mammography or magnetic resonance imaging of the breast (if the patient was younger than 30 years during radiation treatment) should be performed as a baseline just after the completion of radiation therapy and then annually starting 8–10 years after completion of radiation therapy.
- Patients who have undergone splenectomy require life-long vaccination boosters every 2 years for encapsulated bacteria, as recommended by the Centers for Disease Control and Prevention.

- Cardiac disease is the most common long-term complication in long-term lymphoma survivors. Patients who received anthracyclines, especially combined with radiation to the thorax, must receive aggressive health management of other comorbid conditions, such as hyperlipidemia, hypertension, and obesity.
- Consistent screening examinations for secondary malignancies, including melanoma and other skin cancers, breast cancer, lung cancer, prostate cancer, colorectal cancer, and thyroid cancer, is very important because lymphoma survivors may be at increased risk of developing these malignancies compared with the general population.
- Unexplained anemia may be an early indicator of myelodysplasia, particularly in patients who received alkylators (e.g., cyclophosphamide) or fludarabine.
- The effects of the most recently developed immunologic treatment modalities on long-term outcomes have yet to be assessed, but preliminary data suggest that monitoring long-term survivors of lymphoma for manifestations of immune deficiency, such as recurrent infections, is recommended.

Suggested Readings

Abrahamsen AF, Andersen A, Nome O, et al. Long-term risk of second malignancy after treatment of Hodgkin's disease: the influence of treatment, age and follow-up time. *Ann Oncol* 2002;13:1786–1791.

Aleman BM, van den Belt-Dusebout AW, De Bruin ML, et al. Late cardiotoxicity after treatment for Hodgkin lymphoma. *Blood* 2007;109:1878–1886.

Alm El-Din MA, El-Badawy SA, Taghian AG. Breast cancer after treatment of Hodgkin's lymphoma: general review. *Int J Radiat Oncol Biol Phys* 2008;72:1291–1297.

Arden-Close E, Eiser C, Pacey A. Sexual functioning in male survivors of lymphoma: a systematic review. *J Sex Med* 2011;8:1833–1840.

Bhatia S, Ramsay NK, Bantle JP, Mertens A, Robison LL. Thyroid abnormalities after therapy for Hodgkin's disease in childhood. *J Nucl Med* 1989;30:255–257.

Centers for Disease Control and Prevention. Advisory committee on immunization practices vaccine recommendations, 2012. http://www.immunize.org/acip/. Updated October 12, 2012. Accessed November 19, 2012.

Chen AB, Punglia RS, Kuntz KM, Mauch PM, Ng AK. Cost effectiveness and screening interval of lipid screening in Hodgkin's lymphoma survivors. *J Clin Oncol* 2009;27:5383–5389.

Constine LS, Donaldson SS, McDougall IR, et al. Thyroid dysfunction after radiotherapy in children with Hodgkin's disease. *Cancer* 1984;53:878–883.

Das P, Ng AK, Earle CC, Mauch PM, Kuntz KM. Computed tomography screening for lung cancer in Hodgkin's lymphoma survivors: decision analysis and cost-effectiveness analysis. *Ann Oncol* 2006;17:785–793.

De Bruin ML, Burgers JA, Baas P, et al. Malignant mesothelioma after radiation treatment for Hodgkin lymphoma. *Blood* 2009;113:3679–81.

Diller L, Medeiros Nancarrow C, Shaffer K, et al. Breast cancer screening in women previously treated for Hodgkin's disease: a prospective cohort study. *J Clin Oncol* 2002;20:2085–2091.

Franklin J, Pluetschow A, Paus M, et al. Second malignancy risk associated with treatment of Hodgkin's lymphoma: meta-analysis of the randomised trials. *Ann Oncol* 2006;17:1749–1760.

Galper SL, Yu JB, Mauch PM, et al. Clinically significant cardiac disease in patients with Hodgkin lymphoma treated with mediastinal irradiation. *Blood* 2011;117:412–418.

Hancock SL, Cox RS, McDougall IR. Thyroid diseases after treatment of Hodgkin's disease. *N Engl J Med* 1991;325:599–605.

Hancock SL, Tucker MA, Hoppe RT. Factors affecting late mortality from heart-disease after treatment of Hodgkins-disease. *JAMA* 1993;270:1949–1955.

Heidenreich PA, Schnittger I, Strauss HW, et al. Screening for coronary artery disease after mediastinal irradiation for Hodgkin's disease. *J Clin Oncol* 2007;25:43–49.

Howlader N, Noone AM, Krapcho M, et al. SEER cancer statistics review, 1975–2009 (vintage 2009 populations). Bethesda, MD: National Cancer Institute. http://seer.cancer.gov. csr/1975_2009_pops09/. Published April 2012. Accessed November 21, 2012.

Hull MC, Morris CG, Pepine CJ, Mendenhall NP. Valvular dysfunction and carotid, subclavian, and coronary artery disease in survivors of Hodgkin lymphoma treated with radiation therapy. *JAMA* 2003;290:2831–2837.

Larsen RL, Jakacki RI, Vetter VL, Meadows AT, Silber JH, Barber G. Electrocardiographic changes and arrhythmias after cancer therapy in children and young adults. *Am J Cardiol* 1992;70:73–77.

Mauch PM, Kalish LA, Marcus KC, et al. Long-term survival in Hodgkin's disease relative impact of mortality, second tumors, infection, and cardiovascular disease. *Cancer J Sci Am* 1995;1:33–42.

Myrehaug S, Pintilie M, Tsang R, et al. Cardiac morbidity following modern treatment for Hodgkin lymphoma: supra-additive cardiotoxicity of doxorubicin and radiation therapy. *Leuk Lymphoma* 2008;49:1486–1493.

Ng AK, LaCasce A, Travis LB. Long-term complications of lymphoma and its treatment. *J Clin Oncol* 2011;29:1885–1892.

Ogilvy-Stuart AL, Shalet SM. Effect of radiation on the human reproductive system. *Environ Health Perspect* 1993;101(Suppl 2):109–116.

Orzan F, Brusca A, Gaita F, Giustetto C, Figliomeni MC, Libero L. Associated cardiac lesions in patients with radiation-induced complete heart block. *Int J Cardiol* 1993;39:151–156.

Rodrigues NA, Killion L, Hickey G, et al. A prospective study of salivary gland function in lymphoma patients receiving head and neck irradiation. *Int J Radiat Oncol Biol Phys* 2009;75:1079–1083.

Ron E, Lubin JH, Shore RE, et al. Thyroid cancer after exposure to external radiation: a pooled analysis of seven studies. *Radiat Res* 1995;141:259–277.

Saslow D, Boetes C, Burke W, et al. American cancer society guidelines for breast screening with MRI as an adjunct to mammography. *CA Cancer J Clin* 2007;57:75–89.

Sklar C, Whitton J, Mertens A, et al. Abnormalities of the thyroid in survivors of Hodgkin's disease: data from the childhood cancer survivor study. *J Clin Endocrinol* 2000;85:3227–3232.

Sung JS, Malak SF, Bajaj P, Alis R, Dershaw DD, Morris EA. Screening breast MR imaging in women with a history of lobular carcinoma in situ. *Radiology* 2011;261:414–420.

Swerdlow AJ, Higgins CD, Smith P, et al. Myocardial infarction mortality risk after treatment for Hodgkin disease: a collaborative British cohort study. *J Natl Cancer Inst* 2007;99:206–214.

Travis LB, Gospodarowicz M, Curtis RE, et al. Lung cancer following chemotherapy and radiotherapy for Hodgkin's disease. *J Natl Cancer Inst* 2002;94:182–192.

Tucker MA, D'Angio GJ, Boice JD Jr, et al. Bone sarcomas linked to radiotherapy and chemotherapy in children. *N Engl J Med* 1987;317:588–593.

The University of Texas MD Anderson Cancer Center. Clinical practice algorithms. http://www. mdanderson.org/education-and-research/resources-for-professionals/clinical-tools-and-resources/practice-algorithms/index.html. Published August 22, 2012. Accessed November 19, 2012.

van den Belt-Dusebout AW, Aleman BM, Besseling G, et al. Roles of radiation dose and chemotherapy in the etiology of stomach cancer as a second malignancy. *Int J Radiat Oncol Biol Phys* 2009;75:1420–1429.

van Leeuwen FE, Klokman WJ, Hagenbeek A, et al. Second cancer risk following Hodgkin's disease: a 20-year follow-up study. *J Clin Oncol* 1994;12:312–325.

Wethal T, Lund MB, Edvardsen T, et al. Valvular dysfunction and left ventricular changes in Hodgkin's lymphoma survivors. A longitudinal study. *Br J Cancer* 2009;101:575–581.

Yeh ET, Tong AT, Lenihan DJ, et al. Cardiovascular complications of cancer therapy: diagnosis, pathogenesis, and management. *Circulation* 2004;109:3122–3131.

Survivorship Algorithms

These cancer survivorship algorithms have been specifically developed for MD Anderson using a multidisciplinary approach and taking into consideration circumstances particular to MD Anderson, including the following: MD Anderson's specific patient population, MD Anderson's services and structure, and MD Anderson's clinical information. These algorithms are provided for informational purposes only and are not intended to replace the independent medical or professional judgment of physicians or other health care providers. Moreover, these algorithms should not be used to treat pregnant women.

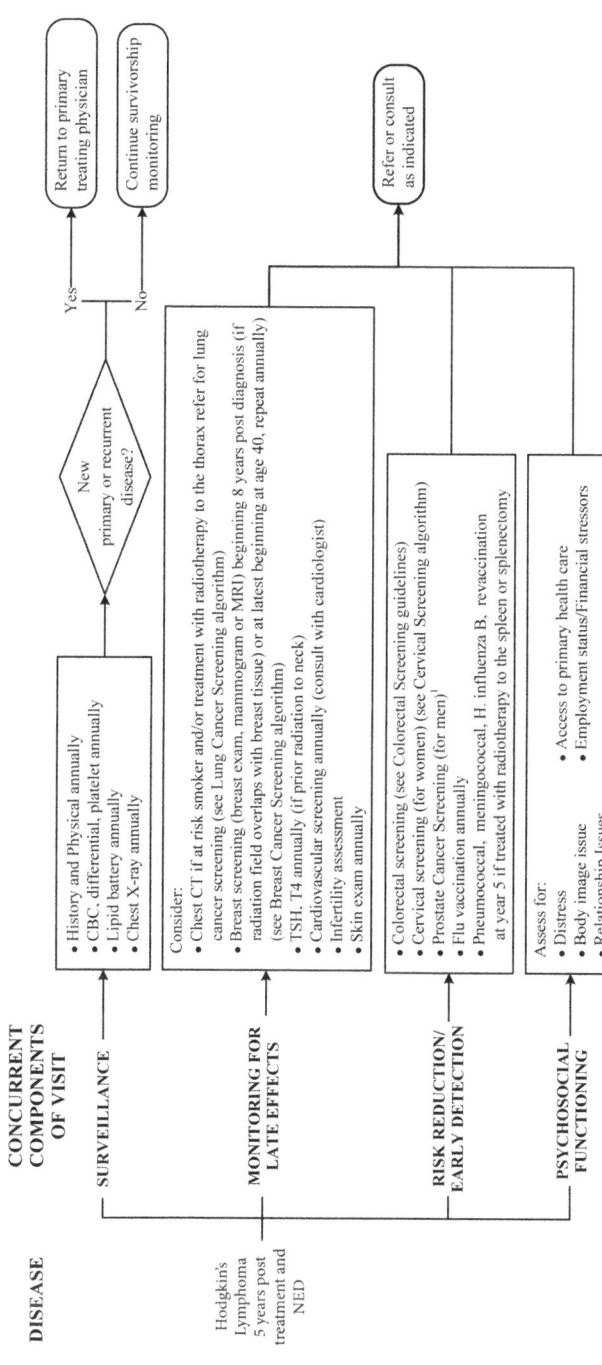

CONCURRENT COMPONENTS OF VISIT

DISEASE

Hodgkin's Lymphoma 5 years post treatment and NED

SURVEILLANCE
- History and Physical annually
- CBC, differential, platelet annually
- Lipid battery annually
- Chest X-ray annually

MONITORING FOR LATE EFFECTS
Consider:
- Chest CT if at risk smoker and/or treatment with radiotherapy to the thorax refer for lung cancer screening (see Lung Cancer Screening algorithm)
- Breast screening (breast exam, mammogram or MRI) beginning 8 years post diagnosis (if radiation field overlaps with breast tissue) or at latest beginning at age 40, repeat annually) (see Breast Cancer Screening algorithm)
- TSH, T4 annually (if prior radiation to neck)
- Cardiovascular screening annually (consult with cardiologist)
- Infertility assessment
- Skin exam annually

RISK REDUCTION/ EARLY DETECTION
- Colorectal screening (see Colorectal Screening guidelines)
- Cervical screening (for women) (see Cervical Screening algorithm)
- Prostate Cancer Screening (for men)[1]
- Flu vaccination annually
- Pneumococcal, meningococcal, H. influenza B, revaccination at year 5 if treated with radiotherapy to the spleen or splenectomy

PSYCHOSOCIAL FUNCTIONING
Assess for:
- Distress
- Body image issue
- Relationship Issues
- Access to primary health care
- Employment status/Financial stressors

New primary or recurrent disease?

Yes → Return to primary treating physician / Continue survivorship monitoring

No → Refer or consult as indicated

NED = No evidence of disease
[1] Based on American Cancer Society Prostate Cancer Screening Guidelines

Copyright 2012 The University of Texas M.D. Anderson Cancer Center

Department of Clinical Effectiveness V1
Approved by the Executive Committee of the Medical Staff on 02/28/2012

Algorithm 12.1 Survivorship—Hodgkin lymphoma

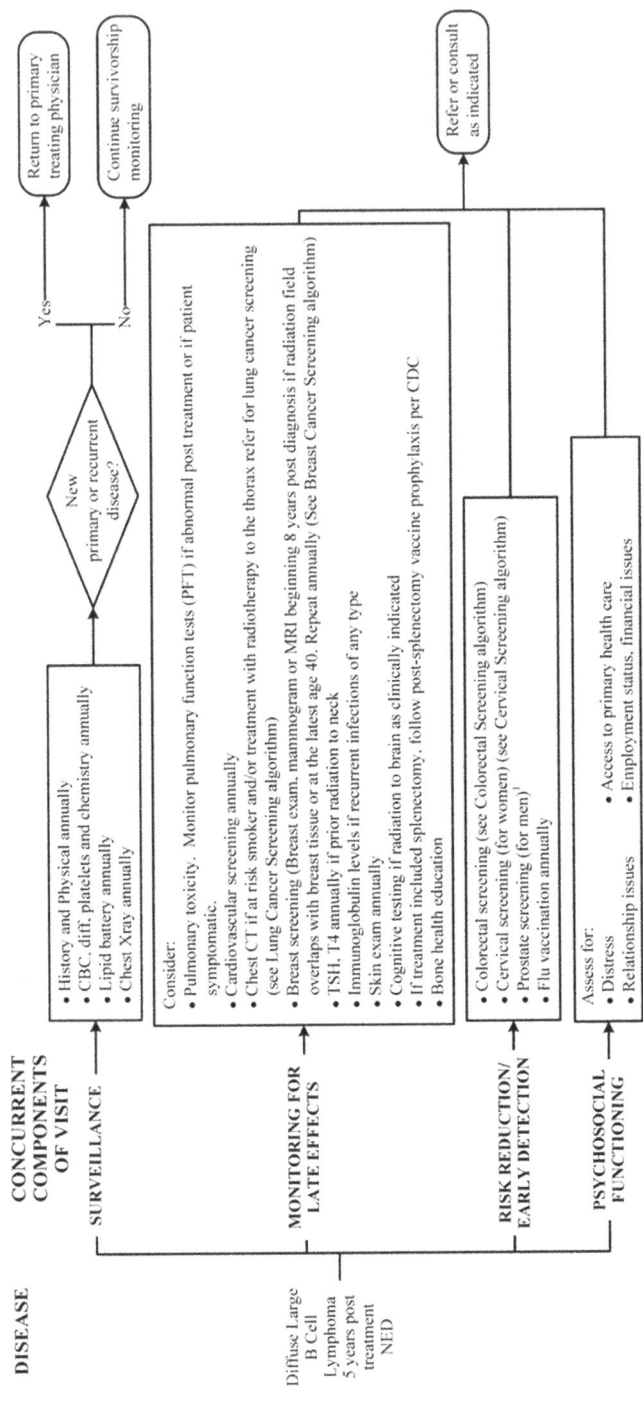

Algorithm 12.2 Survivorship—diffuse large B-cell lymphoma

Chapter 13
Melanoma Survivorship Management

Genevieve Marie Boland and Jeffrey E. Gershenwald

Contents

Chapter Overview Many important issues are relevant to melanoma survivors after initial melanoma diagnosis and treatment. A diagnosis of melanoma not only affects patients during the time of initial treatment, but also may play a significant role in their life for many years. These issues are broad and apply to many aspects of patients' lives. This chapter will discuss overall and stage-specific surveillance strategies and methods for risk reduction and prevention that are important to the melanoma survivor population. It is also important for patients and care providers alike to understand and learn to manage sequelae that may accompany various

L.E. Foxhall, M.A. Rodriguez (eds.), *Advances in Cancer Survivorship Management*,
MD Anderson Cancer Care Series, DOI 10.1007/978-1-4939-0986-5_13,
© The University of Texas M.D. Anderson Cancer Center 2015

melanoma treatments, from surgery to targeted therapies. Finally, this chapter will discuss issues relating to long-term survivorship such as psychosocial adjustment, reproductive issues, and health care costs.

Introduction

The goal of this chapter is to address topics relevant to melanoma survivors. A diagnosis of melanoma not only affects patients during the time of initial treatment, but also may play a significant role in their life for many years. Treatment sequelae may remain and factor into quality of life over time. The need for ongoing surveillance, the potential psychological and social effects of the diagnosis, and the need for associated treatments can have a substantial effect on an individual patient's life. Therefore, our goal is to establish a streamlined longitudinal plan for melanoma patients that addresses issues related to melanoma surveillance and monitoring, makes recommendations specific to melanoma treatments, and outlines approaches to optimize overall patient health, well-being, and quality of life.

Epidemiology

An estimated 76,100 people will be diagnosed with melanoma in 2014, and 9,710 patients will die of this disease (American Cancer Society 2014). Overall, the incidence of melanoma is increasing worldwide; in the United States specifically, the incidence has been rising by an average of 2.6% per year. Increasing awareness has led to both earlier detection and earlier treatment of melanoma. Given the increasing success of early identification and surgical treatment of melanoma, the overall number of melanoma survivors requiring surveillance has increased over time. It is estimated that almost one million melanoma survivors can be identified in the United States and an estimated 1.3 million melanoma survivors are expected to be living in the United States by 2022 (American Cancer Society 2013). A current challenge for both patients and providers is the fact that after the initial diagnosis and treatment of melanoma, surveillance and subsequent care for melanoma survivors may become fragmented between specialized cancer centers and primary care physicians. Efforts to create longitudinal guidelines for the delivery of evidence-based care to be followed during patient transition to survivorship are clearly needed; such guidelines must also continue to evolve. Overall, these guidelines should be simple and streamlined so that they can be applied to patients in a variety of clinical settings.

Melanoma survivors are generally aware of their stage-specific risk for recurrence. However, it is important to note that survivors also have an increased risk of developing a second or subsequent primary melanoma, compared with the risk of developing primary melanoma in the general population. Patient risk stratification can potentially guide recruitment of patients at high risk into more intensive screening regimens or even prevention trials. Although comprehensive integrated risk models are clearly warranted, it is well known that the risk factors of fair skin, increasing age, male sex, tanning bed use, sun exposure, and family or personal history of melanoma or nevi can also be used to stratify patients. Although more refinement is needed, this stratification can guide initial screening and inform posttreatment surveillance strategies for patients with a new primary melanoma.

Classification

Superficial spreading melanoma is the most common histologic subtype of melanoma (70% of cases); it usually occurs in the setting of a preexisting nevus. Nodular melanoma is the next most common type, accounting for 15–30% of all cases of melanoma. Lentigo maligna melanoma represents 4–10% of all cases of melanoma; it usually occurs in sun-exposed areas and is commonly found on the faces of elderly white women. Lentigo maligna melanoma is generally slow to become invasive, and a delay in initial diagnosis is not unusual. Acral lentiginous melanoma occurs more commonly in dark-skinned patients (35–60% of cases of melanoma occurring in dark-skinned individuals); it usually occurs on the palms, soles, and nail beds. Finally, in a small proportion of cases of melanoma, the lesion is amelanotic, lacks pigmentation, and is generally more difficult to diagnose.

In addition to the aforementioned histologic classifications, several molecular aberrations have been identified that can be used to classify and stratify patients with cutaneous melanoma. Molecular-based classifications of melanoma are now routinely used and are important in identifying tumors that, for example, may respond differently to specific treatment regimens than would other melanoma subtypes, or that may not respond to certain treatments at all. This is of particular relevance to patients with metastatic disease because these molecular criteria may ultimately help to determine the most appropriate treatment regimen for a specific tumor. In approximately 40% of cases of superficial spreading melanoma, a mutation in the *BRAF* gene is present, in most cases (>85%) a point mutation at V600E, which leads to a 400-fold increase in the activity of the BRAF protein, a serine/threonine protein kinase. However, approximately 80% of benign nevi also harbor *BRAF* mutations, suggesting that this mutation alone cannot account for the malignant potential of superficial spreading melanoma. Nonetheless, tremendous advances in the treatment of metastatic melanoma have been made by using therapies that target the *BRAF* mutation, contributing to the overall growing excitement about targeted therapies in melanoma. There is currently great interest in directing the growing knowledge of the molecular biology of melanoma toward new, more focused, and personalized therapeutic approaches.

Definition of Survivorship

A cancer survivor is anyone who has been diagnosed with cancer, from the time of initial diagnosis and treatment through the remaining years of life. The goal of survivorship care is to prevent, detect, and manage complications that arise from cancer or cancer treatments and to improve overall health and quality of life for survivors. The experience of living with a cancer diagnosis varies greatly from individual to individual. Some survivors may live with cancer as a chronic disease requiring periodic treatments, and others may enjoy long-term remission. Many survivors lead normal lives with minimal, if any, residual side effects.

It is important to note that the diagnosis of melanoma and associated initial treatments do not represent the end of the cancer experience. For most melanoma survivors, ongoing surveillance is critically important because of the increased risk for a second primary melanoma in addition to the stage-specific risk for recurrence. Additionally, the delayed sequelae of melanoma treatments may continue to affect the survivor's quality of life. Recovering from the social and emotional strain of cancer is an ongoing process that requires sensitivity on the part of health care providers to the stresses on both the patients and their families. Physicians and care teams now realize that many challenges remain to be addressed in helping survivors achieve good quality of life, even after the specific treatment(s) for melanoma have ended.

MD Anderson Mission

The survivorship mission at MD Anderson is three-fold: (1) to address the outcomes of cancer and cancer treatment; (2) to improve cancer survivors' health; and (3) to improve the quality of life of cancer survivors through integrated programs focusing on patient care, research, prevention, and education. Family, friends, and caregivers are also included in the process because they, too, are involved in the care of cancer survivors.

To facilitate the transition from initial cancer patient to survivor, a detailed survivorship care plan is very helpful. The goal of the survivorship plan is to effectively communicate information about the patient's diagnosis, treatment, and possible adverse effects associated with the treatment, including late adverse effects, to the patient and the patient's subsequent physicians to manage symptoms, optimize surveillance, and align expectations between the patients and the care team.

The components of the survivorship plan are cancer surveillance, risk-reduction strategies, management of late effects of therapy, and support for the psychosocial aspects of survivor treatment and long-term care. At MD Anderson, our goal is to establish guidelines that contribute to the continuity of care among the oncologic teams, consultants, and primary care physicians, as well as patients and their families, to allow individuals to successfully and smoothly transition to survivorship care.

Cancer Surveillance

Two essential elements of melanoma follow-up care are early detection of a new primary melanoma and detection of recurrent disease. Patients with a history of melanoma have an increased risk of developing a second primary melanoma, as well as a stage-specific risk of disease recurrence. The likelihood of recurrence depends on the stage and substage of the initial melanoma (Baughan et al. 1993); patients who present with early-stage disease have a lower likelihood of recurrence than those who present with advanced disease. A study of patients with melanoma at a large melanoma unit demonstrated recurrence rates of 5% for appropriately treated stage IA, 18% for stage IB, 29% for stage IIA, 40% for stage IIB, and 43% for stage IIC melanoma, after a median follow-up period of 6 years (Francken et al. 2008). In terms of survival, the 5-year disease-free survival rate for patients with stage I melanoma has been shown to be >90% (Kalady et al. 2003), and the 5-year recurrence-free survival rate for patients with stage III melanoma can vary substantially.

In both early-stage and late-stage disease, risk stratification is influenced by multiple factors, including the burden of disease in the regional lymph node basins. In patients with stage III melanoma, a distinction is made between those with micrometastatic disease and those with macrometastatic disease because the median 5-year overall survival rate of patients with micrometastases is approximately 70%, whereas among those with macrometastases, the median 5-year overall survival rate decreases to 43%. However, outcomes vary even within the overall cohort of patients with micrometastatic disease; 5-year overall survival rates range from 23% to 87% (Balch et al. 2010). Multivariate analyses have demonstrated that overall survival rates also vary with the thickness of the primary tumor, mitotic rate, patient age, tumor ulceration, anatomic site, and patient sex. Therefore, each patient must be individually assessed and stratified according to the patient's particular risk factors. It has also been noted that both primary and recurrent melanoma is often detected by patients rather than by medical practitioners (Moore Dalal et al. 2008; Romano et al. 2010). Therefore, patients should be active participants in their follow-up visits and should be encouraged to be involved in their own ongoing surveillance.

A 2003 study of the Surveillance, Epidemiology, and End Results database demonstrated that the risk of developing a second primary melanoma is high within this patient population; the risk of synchronous primary melanoma at the time of diagnosis was 0.5%, whereas the risk of metachronous primary melanoma was 1% at 1 year, 2% at 5 years, 3% at 10 years, and 5% at 20 years (Goggins and Tsao 2003); overall, these data highlight the importance of comprehensive skin examinations as part of overall surveillance.

Nieweg and Kroon (2006) demonstrated that approximately one-third of patients whose melanoma is treated locally for site-specific or regional lymph node recurrence can be treated until there is no evidence of disease with additional surgery or other therapies. The overall 5-year relapse-free survival rate for patients with stage III melanoma ranges from 63% for stage IIIA disease to 11% for stage IIIC disease (Romano et al. 2010). Although median 5-year overall survival rates for patients with stage IV disease have historically been only about 10%, a growing subset of patients with stage IV melanoma, particularly in the era of recently developed therapies such as immune modulators, achieve durable long-term survival. Overall, patients with early-stage disease have a low risk of recurrence but still have an increased risk of developing a second primary tumor. Patients whose primary disease is more advanced also have an increased risk of developing a second primary tumor, but they also have a higher risk of recurrence than patients with early-stage disease. In either case, close surveillance is warranted to evaluate any site of new disease or evidence of recurrence or metastasis.

In addition to having an increased risk of developing a second primary melanoma or recurrent disease, melanoma survivors may have an increased risk of developing other types of cancer, including breast cancer, prostate cancer, and non-Hodgkin lymphoma (Bradford et al. 2010). Therefore, survivorship programs should incorporate appropriate screening regimens for these patients and make efforts to optimize their overall health maintenance beyond single-organ or disease-specific care.

The melanoma surveillance plan proposed depends on the pathologic stage of the melanoma at the initial diagnosis and the interval of disease-free survival. Initial surveillance includes a clinical visit and physical examination of the skin and regional lymph node basins every 3–12 months, depending on the pathologic stage of the melanoma. At MD Anderson, patients have been broadly categorized into four groups for timing of transition into our survivorship program; each group has stage-specific surveillance strategies. Category 1 patients have stage 0 melanoma (i.e., melanoma in situ) and no evidence of disease after 6 months. Routine surveillance, which is initiated at 1 year after completion of treatment, includes an annual dermatologic examination and lymph node basin survey. Category 2 patients, who have stage IA melanoma and a disease-free interval of 3 years, are followed up with annual skin examinations and self-inspection. Category 3 patients have stage IB-II melanoma and no evidence of disease after 5 years, and category 4 patients have Stage III-IV disease and no evidence of disease after 5 years. Category 3 and 4 patients make annual visits to the clinic to undergo a skin examination and nodal basin survey. Category 4 patients may also receive interval radiologic imaging (e.g., chest x-ray, computed tomography scan, positron emission tomography/computed tomography scan) depending on their clinical history.

The use of imaging in surveillance has been studied, but results and recommendations of these studies have varied. For example, National Comprehensive Cancer Network guidelines recommend that a chest x-ray, computed tomography scan, or positron emission tomography/computed tomography scan be considered every 3–12 months to screen for recurrent or metastatic disease in patients with stage IIB-IV disease within the first 5 years of completion of treatment. After that time, if the patient is asymptomatic, routine radiologic imaging is not recommended. Additionally, annual brain magnetic resonance imaging may be considered in this group of high-risk patients (National Comprehensive Cancer Network 2013). The potential benefits of imaging must be balanced with the risk of false-positive results that may increase patient anxiety and necessitate unnecessary and potentially harmful interventions.

Several studies have examined the utility and cost-effectiveness of imaging for detection of pulmonary metastases in patients with melanoma (Pandalai et al. 2011). A cost-effectiveness analysis recommended against frequent use of chest x-rays given the low detection rate compared with the cost burden (Mooney et al. 1997), whereas other groups have recommended evaluation with a chest x-ray every

6–12 months for patients with melanoma (Morton et al. 2009). Additionally, ultrasound has increasingly been used for nodal basin surveillance, with reported sensitivities ranging from 24% to >80% (Machet et al. 2005; Uren et al. 2007; Boland and Gershenwald 2012); additional studies are needed to assess the role of ultrasound in surveillance.

Risk Reduction and Prevention

The risk of developing a subsequent primary melanoma or other new malignancy is increased in patients who have been diagnosed with and have previously been treated for melanoma, compared with the general population. Therefore, risk reduction and prevention strategies should focus on patient education, surveillance, and screening for skin malignancies. In addition, the toxicities of systemic and local melanoma treatments may increase the risk of other medical problems, such as cardiovascular disease or osteoporosis, which should be kept in mind during surveillance and follow-up. Given the possible increased risk for other cancers, routine cancer screening protocols should be considered for melanoma survivors.

Health maintenance strategies, such as routine gynecologic and breast or prostate screening, as well as weight loss counseling, tobacco cessation, and routine vaccines, are also important in preserving the overall health and well-being of survivors. The goal of a survivorship program is optimal health with the best possible quality of life for each individual survivor. At MD Anderson, survivors are enrolled in dermatologic screening programs, referred for gynecologic and breast or prostate screening as appropriate, offered counseling regarding diet or weight management and tobacco cessation programs as applicable, and provided with recommendations for routine vaccinations as needed.

Patient-guided, self-administered skin examinations are recommended and should focus on identification of new skin lesions or those changing in size, shape, or color. The ABCD rule can help distinguish an abnormal mole from a normal mole: A is for asymmetry, B is for border irregularity, C is for irregularity in color, and D is for diameter (particularly if larger than 0.25 in). However, not all cases of melanoma fit these guidelines, and skin lesions that do not heal, spread color from one area to the surrounding area, develop new redness beyond the border of the lesion, become itchy or tender, or develop surface changes should prompt dermatologic evaluation.

Risk-reduction strategies specific to melanoma, including avoiding sun exposure, should be emphasized to melanoma survivors (Table 13.1). A sampling of melanoma survivors suggests that they tend to use sunscreen and avoid exposure to ultraviolet light more than does the average person, but significantly less than expected in a population known to be at high risk. On the basis of these observations, there is clearly room for improvement in educating and counseling melanoma survivors about risk-reduction strategies, including avoiding sun exposure and tanning beds.

Table 13.1 Strategies for reducing your risk of melanoma

Avoid sunburn.

Limit sun exposure.

Do not use tanning beds or other artificial sunlight sources.

Wear a sunscreen rated at least SPF 30, a broad-brimmed hat, and a long-sleeved shirt when you are outside.

Wear sunglasses when you are outside.

Stay inside during the sun's peak hours between 10:00 am and 3:00 pm.

Protect children. Infants younger than 6 months should be completely shielded from direct sun exposure. Apply sunscreen to infants older than 6 months, and teach older children to make applying sunscreen a regular habit before they go outside.

Examine your skin monthly. Have any suspicious moles checked by a health care practitioner.

If you are at risk, have your skin examined at least once each year by a dermatologist.

For more information, see http://www.mdanderson.org/patient-and-cancer-information/cancer-information/cancer-topics/prevention-and-screening/sun-exposure/index.html

Melanoma Treatments and Their Sequelae

Surgery

Initial surgical management of early-stage primary melanoma in patients with clinically negative lymph nodes includes wide excision of the primary tumor with margins appropriate for tumor thickness (Ross and Gershenwald 2011). Evaluation of the regional nodal basins at risk may also be performed using the technique of lymphatic mapping and sentinel lymph node biopsy. The decision to perform sentinel lymph node biopsy is primarily based on the histologic characteristics of the primary tumor (Gershenwald and Ross 2011; Boland and Gershenwald 2012; Gershenwald et al. 2012). For patients with evidence of regional nodal disease, a completion lymph node dissection represents the current recommended standard practice, although trials are currently underway to assess whether this is required in all patients with sentinel lymph nodes positive for disease (Morton 2012).

Patients who undergo sentinel lymph node biopsy may experience some regional numbness or hyperesthesia owing to sensory nerve damage during surgery, although this is usually relatively minor and well tolerated by most patients. Of more concern is the potential for lymphedema, which can occur after sentinel lymph node biopsy but is more common after formal complete lymph node dissection. Interim analyses of the Multicenter Selective Lymphadenectomy Trial-I, an international randomized clinical trial comparing outcomes of patients who undergo wide excision of the primary site and observation of the regional nodes with the outcomes of patients who undergo wide excision of the primary site and sentinel lymph node biopsy, have thus far demonstrated a lower incidence of lymphedema in patients for whom lymphadenectomy was performed for early, clinically node-negative disease (i.e., those who underwent sentinel lymph node biopsy after a sentinel lymph node was found to be positive for disease) compared with those who underwent delayed lymphadenectomy for clinical regional node recurrence after wide excision alone (Faries et al. 2010). Thus, early detection and disease treatment are a primary goal for melanoma care for both oncologic and quality-of-life reasons.

For in-transit metastases (i.e., cutaneous or subcutaneous metastases generally located between the primary tumor site and the regional nodal basin) or more aggressive regional disease, regional approaches to treatment, including hyperthermic isolated limb perfusion or isolated limb infusion, are sometimes recommended. Hyperthermic isolated limb perfusion involves a formal lymph node dissection with isolation of the extremity vessels, placement of vascular cannulae, use of an extracorporeal bypass circuit, and tourniquet isolation of the limb for perfusion of chemotherapeutic agents, usually melphalan. In contrast, isolated limb infusion is a low-flow technique that uses percutaneously placed catheters and does not require oxygenation of the circuit. Given the relative technical simplicity of the infusion procedure compared with the perfusion protocol, the infusion procedure has become a more attractive option for many patients, particularly those with associated comorbidities. These treatment approaches may be accompanied by late sequelae such as lymphedema (see section on "Lymphedema" below) or tendon, nerve, or muscle injury secondary to melphalan, the chemotherapeutic agent most commonly employed for this approach. New regional perfusion or infusion agents are also being evaluated in clinical trials in an attempt to further improve response rates and decrease toxicity.

Lymphedema

Lymphedema is the condition resulting from interstitial edema that occurs when lymphatic drainage is blocked in a specific anatomic region. Lymphedema has many different causes, but secondary or acquired lymphedema accounts for most cases in the United States, and this can occur as a consequence of tumors, surgery, trauma, radiation, or any other mechanical insufficiency in the lymphatic system. A study examining the effects of lymphedema on almost 8,000 cancer survivors demonstrated a substantial effect of lymphedema on quality of life and functional outcomes (Cormier et al. 2010). Lymphedema in the postsurgical setting is often managed with compression garments and close surveillance for associated complications.

Given that no definitive cure for lymphedema exists, a major focus has been on prevention of lymphedema. Personal surveillance is important, and each patient should report any changes in size, sensation, color, or temperature of the limb to the health care provider to facilitate early identification of known lymphedema-associated complications. Obesity is also a known contributing factor for lymphedema; therefore, patients with lymphedema should be counseled in weight loss or weight maintenance. Additionally, stasis is a known contributing factor to symptomatic lymphedema, so counseling patients about increasing their levels of activity and avoiding stasis is also helpful.

Lymphedema awareness has increased in the health care professions. The National Lymphedema Network recommends that patients be managed by special teams or centers that have sufficient background in the pathophysiology of lymphedema as well as training in the techniques used for treatment. The website www. lymphnet.org has links to various lymphedema treatment centers, as well as health care professionals who specialize in the management of lymphedema and may serve as a useful resource. Early identification of lymphedema is important because early intervention generally affords a better chance for long-term control.

Patients with a confirmed diagnosis of lymphedema should optimally receive close follow-up from a team dedicated to lymphedema management and be fitted for a compression garment. Compression garments play a large role in the management of lymphedema by encouraging congested interstitial fluid to move into the vascular circulation rather than accumulating within the interstitial tissue of the affected region. The mechanism is dependent upon creating high working pressures in the area when the regional muscles contract; therefore, maintenance of the garments and interval replacement are essential for sustained function. Patients with lymphedema are more prone to infections of the involved extremity, so patient counseling regarding early signs of cellulitis and physician awareness of the need to aggressively treat infection are important. Patients should also be counseled regarding optimal skin care and avoidance of skin trauma. Assessment of patient range of motion should also be done routinely, either during clinical assessment or by the physical therapy service following up with the patient. Recommendations for lymphedema risk reduction by the National Lymphedema Network are summarized in Table 13.2.

The gold standard treatment for lymphedema is complete decongestive therapy, usually administered by a certified lymphedema therapist. The main components of the treatment phase include manual lymph drainage, multilayer compression bandaging, therapeutic exercises, skin care, and patient education in self-management. As lymphedema control is achieved, patients are eventually transitioned to lifelong self-care programs. Surgical treatments have been attempted, ranging from excisional operations to lymphatic reconstruction or tissue transfer procedures. Although some early surgical reports in patients with breast cancer were promising, most studies included very small patient cohorts or used inconsistent or nonstandardized measurement techniques. Therefore, at this time, the main focus of management and treatment is on the more traditional complete decongestive therapy (Cormier et al. 2012).

Late Effects of Surgery

Metastatic melanoma may occasionally be treated surgically with metastasectomy. Given the variance in location of recurrence and surgery required, patients may have delayed side effects relating to their surgical intervention and site. These can be managed on a case-by-case basis with knowledge of the surgical intervention required.

Table 13.2 Summary of the National Lymphedema Network lymphedema risk reduction practices[a]

I. Skin Care: avoid trauma or injury to reduce infection risk
Keep extremity clean and dry.

Apply moisturizer daily to prevent chapping or chafing of skin.

Practice good nail care; do not cut cuticles.

Protect exposed skin with sunscreen and insect repellent.

Use care with razors to avoid nicks and skin irritation.

If possible, avoid punctures such as injections and blood draws.

Wear gloves while doing activities that may cause skin injury (e.g., washing dishes, gardening, working with tools, using chemicals such as detergent).

If scratches or punctures to skin occur, wash with soap and water, apply antibiotics, and observe for signs of infection (e.g., redness).

If a rash, itching, redness, pain, increased skin temperature, increased swelling, fever, or flu-like symptoms occur, contact your physician immediately for early treatment of possible infection.

II. Activity/Lifestyle
Gradually build up the duration and intensity of any activity or exercise. Review the Exercise Position Paper.

Take frequent rest periods during activity to allow for limb recovery.

Monitor the extremity during and after activity for any change in size, shape, tissue, texture, soreness, heaviness, or firmness.

Maintain optimal weight. Obesity is known to be a major lymphedema risk factor.

III. Avoid Limb Constriction
If possible, avoid having blood pressure measured on the at-risk extremity, especially if the measurement involves repetitive pumping.

Wear nonconstrictive jewelry and clothing.

Avoid carrying a heavy bag or purse over the at-risk or lymphedematous extremity.

IV. Compression Garments
Garments should fit well.

Support the at-risk limb with a compression garment for strenuous activity (i.e., weight lifting, prolonged standing, and running) except in patients with open wounds or with poor circulation in the at-risk limb.

Patients with lymphedema should consider wearing a well-fitting compression garment for air travel. The National Lymphedema Network cannot specifically recommend compression garments for prophylaxis in at-risk patients.

V. Extremes of Temperature
Individuals should use common sense and proceed cautiously when using heat therapy such as a hot tub or sauna. If swelling in the at-risk limb or increased swelling in the lymphedematous limb occurs, cease use of heat therapy.

Avoid exposure to extreme cold, which can be associated with rebound swelling or chapping of skin.

Avoid prolonged (>15-minute) exposure to heat, particularly from hot tubs and saunas.

VI. Additional Practices Specific to Lower Extremity Lymphedema
Avoid prolonged standing, sitting, or crossing legs to reduce stagnation of fluid in the dependent extremity.

Wear proper, well-fitting footwear and hosiery.

Support the at-risk limb with a compression garment for strenuous activity, except in patients with open wounds or with poor circulation in the at-risk limb.

Note: Because there is little evidence-based literature regarding many of these practices, most recommendations must at this time be based on the pathophysiologic knowledge of experts in the field who have decades of clinical experience.

[a]Please refer to the Position Statement of the National Lymphedema Network (revised May 2012) for more details (Available at http://www.lymphnet.org/pdfDocs/nlnriskreduction.pdf)

Radiation

Radiation has been used selectively for adjuvant treatment of regional lymph node basins in patients deemed to have a high risk for recurrence, as defined by multiple positive lymph nodes, lymph nodes >3 cm, extracapsular extension, or recurrent regional disease. High-risk primary lesions, defined by satellitosis or close margins not amenable to re-resection, are also considered for adjuvant radiation therapy. A recent randomized clinical trial of >200 patients followed for 40 months demonstrated that risk of lymph node field relapse was reduced in the patients treated with adjuvant radiation compared with those not treated with adjuvant radiation, without an effect on overall survival. The most commonly reported adverse events associated with adjuvant radiation therapy were seroma, radiation dermatitis, and wound infection (Burmeister et al. 2012).

Desmoplastic melanoma, a subtype of melanoma characterized by associated collagen production, accounts for 1–4% of all melanomas, and many patients with desmoplastic melanoma have historically been offered radiation therapy in an attempt to improve local control. Focused radiation therapy has been employed for sinonasal and uveal melanoma; patients with mucosal melanomas not amenable to surgical resection, and those with unresectable metastases have also sometimes been offered radiation therapy. For patients with localized anorectal melanoma, a treatment approach that includes sphincter-sparing primary tumor excision followed by adjuvant radiation therapy, to avoid the significant morbidity and functional compromise associated with abdominoperineal resection, is currently recommended.

Radiation may also be used for palliation in patients with bone, brain, or visceral metastases. Stereotactic radiosurgery for brain metastases has been shown to be effective for local control of disease, particularly given the paucity of alternative treatment options for this site. Following both surgical resection and stereotactic radiosurgery, adjuvant whole brain radiation therapy may be employed. Clinicians should be aware of the potential sequelae of radiation, including acute reactions such as acute encephalopathy, cerebral edema, nausea or vomiting, radiation dermatitis or alopecia, hearing problems, myelosuppression, and mucositis or parotitis, or delayed reactions such as radiation necrosis, diffuse white matter injury, headaches, neurocognitive effects, cerebrovascular effects, effects on eyes and vision, ototoxicity, and endocrinopathies. Clinicians should also be familiar with potential risks of radiation therapy in the context of subsequent treatment. In this regard, focal brain necrosis has been reported in patients with a history of radiation therapy to the brain for metastatic melanoma who were later treated with ipilimumab.

Immunotherapy and Biological Therapy

Adjuvant Treatment

High-dose interferon alfa-2b was approved by the US Food and Drug Administration in 1996 and is considered a standard of care in the adjuvant setting for appropriately selected patients with melanoma who have a high risk of systemic recurrence.

The treatment regimen is time-intensive, requiring daily intravenous treatments 5 days per week for 1 month, followed by subcutaneous injections 3 days per week for an additional 48 weeks. More recently, pegylated interferon alfa-2b has been approved for the treatment of melanoma with microscopic or gross nodal disease. The dosing regimen of the pegylated form of interferon alfa-2b is a weekly injection. With both forms of interferon, substantial adverse effects make patient selection and adherence critical issues. Commonly reported adverse effects, many of which are flu-like symptoms, include fever, fatigue, headache, depression, anorexia, increased ALT/AST levels, myalgia, and nausea. During the induction phase, up to 58% of patients require dose reductions or delays in treatment owing to adverse effects.

Systemic Treatment

For patients with metastatic disease, many different treatment options are available, and selection of the appropriate treatment is based on the stage of disease, patient comorbidities, tumor susceptibilities, and anticipated patient tolerance of an individual treatment regimen. Interleukin-2 has been shown to have response rates ranging from 13% to 33%, and patients treated with interleukin-2 have been shown to have a greater durability of response than patients treated with chemotherapy. However, interleukin-2 may be associated with multiple adverse effects that make patient recruitment and compliance difficult. Interleukin-2 toxicity can manifest in many organ systems, including the heart, lungs, kidneys, and central nervous system. Most of the toxic effects are related to capillary leak syndrome, leading to decreased organ perfusion and accumulation of extravascular fluid.

Tremendous interest in harnessing the immune system in the setting of advanced melanoma has led to substantial advances in the understanding of immune checkpoint blockade. Treatments using antibodies targeting checkpoint blockade are generally well tolerated, with overall good results in the select group of patients who respond to treatment. Ipilimumab, a monoclonal antibody that clocks CTLA-4, a key immune regulator, has been approved as a treatment for metastatic melanoma (Hodi et al. 2010; Robert et al. 2011). Two fully human monoclonal CTLA-4 blocking antibodies, tremelimumab and ipilimumab, have been used clinically, with response rates ranging from 5% to 15%. A toxic effect relevant to the CTLA-4 antibodies is the development of autoimmune side effects, most commonly skin rashes and pruritus. More substantial potential adverse effects include colitis, hypophysitis (inflammation of pituitary gland), and hepatitis; if treated early with steroids or hormone replacement therapy, these adverse effects can usually be managed. Recently, exciting studies focused on the pathway involving programmed death ligand-1 (PDL-1), a negative regulator of T cell signaling, have suggested that this checkpoint is also a potential target for therapy; recently completed and ongoing trials of agents that target the programmed death 1 (PD-1) receptor on T cells have shown response rates of up to 28% in patients with metastatic melanoma (Topalian et al. 2012).

Substantial interest has also arisen in the development of tumor vaccines in the setting of advanced or metastatic melanoma, although no vaccines have yet been approved by the US Food and Drug Administration. Candidate vaccines range from DNA to dendritic cell to peptide to viral-based vaccines. Adoptive cell therapy, generally using a patient's own tumor-infiltrating lymphocytes for tumor targeting, has also garnered enthusiasm as a potential treatment for metastatic melanoma. In adoptive cell therapy, tumors are harvested from patients and the tumor-infiltrating lymphocytes or dendritic cells from the tumors are isolated and expanded ex vivo; these cells are then infused into the patient for adoptive immunotherapy, generally following a brief period of myeloablative therapy. Limitations of this approach, which remains experimental, include the highly personalized nature of the therapy and the need for substantial resources, time, and financial investment for each treatment.

Targeted Therapy

With the understanding that BRAF mutations (most commonly the V600E mutation) are present in up to 50% of patients with advanced melanoma, BRAF inhibitors have been developed and therapeutically employed for patients whose tumors contain the BRAF V600E mutation. Recently completed clinical trials have demonstrated improved overall survival and progression-free survival rates in patients treated with the BRAF inhibitor vemurafenib compared with those treated with dacarbazine (Chapman et al. 2011). Vemurafenib, the first BRAF inhibitor, was approved by the US Food and Drug Administration in late 2011 and is available as a treatment option for patients with advanced melanoma whose tumors have a BRAF V600 mutation. Despite this very substantial development, initial excitement over the remarkable initial patient responses to vemurafenib has been tempered by the observation that disease recurrence commonly occurs approximately 6–8 months after initiation of treatment with BRAF inhibitors, presumably as a result of the development of resistance to the treatment. Many investigators are actively exploring mechanisms of drug resistance and possible complementary targets in an effort to develop strategies to prolong or augment the effects of BRAF inhibitors.

In terms of melanoma survivorship, up to 25% of patients treated with BRAF inhibitors have been shown to develop squamous cell carcinoma (Flaherty et al. 2012a, b), which is important to keep in mind when developing a surveillance plan for these particular melanoma survivors. More recent studies have focused on downstream mediators of the BRAF pathway, including MEK signaling. A study by Flaherty et al. (2012a) demonstrated that MEK inhibition using trametinib in patients whose tumors have a BRAF mutation was associated with improved rates of progression-free and overall survival compared with BRAF inhibitor monotherapy; interestingly, the combination approach was also associated with a significantly decreased incidence of secondary skin neoplasms such as keratoacanthoma and squamous cell carcinoma (Flaherty et al. 2012a).

As our understanding of the molecular underpinnings of melanoma continues to rapidly expand, it is likely that an increasing proportion of patients with melanoma will be enrolled in clinical trials evaluating new agents for targeted treatment of melanoma. Therefore, appropriate communication with the patient and clinical trial team is important to optimize longitudinal care for the patient.

Chemotherapy

Single-agent chemotherapy has been used to treat metastatic melanoma, although the reported response rates have been poor. Treatment with dacarbazine has yielded response rates of approximately 16%. Other agents, including cisplatin, paclitaxel, docetaxel, and temozolomide, alone or as part of a combination therapy, have also been used with varying results. These therapies are associated with their own specific adverse effect profiles, and many of these adverse effects can be long-lasting. Therefore, individual patients should be counseled and followed up in light of their specific treatment history.

Long-Term Survivorship

Overall, it is clear that a diagnosis of cancer in general, and melanoma specifically, can substantially affect a patient's quality of life, even after initial treatment is completed. It should be noted that as surveillance and identification of early melanoma improve, most melanoma survivors will be those who had presented with early-stage disease. For these patients, treatment for melanoma may be predominantly surgical in nature and late effects may be minimal or relate principally to the surgical site(s) of treatment(s). However, patients undergoing systemic treatment for melanoma are generally more likely to believe that cancer has affected their overall health and are more likely to report lasting problems, most frequently arthritis or osteoporosis and circulatory problems. Adjuvant treatments such as interferon-alpha can be associated with substantial side effects that can reduce a patient's quality of life.

Psychological Adjustment

Variations in gender coping styles have been reported, but overall, men and women both demonstrate good long-term functioning and hardiness in regard to their diagnoses. However, women have consistently reported greater anxiety and psychological stress from the time of diagnosis than have men. It has also been noted that patients who report low quality-of-life scores prior to treatment are at a greater risk for poor tolerance of their treatment and increased emotional problems and overall poorer coping during treatments than other patients. This may be a group for whom early targeting and more aggressive psychosocial support approaches and interventions may be beneficial. Additionally, and not surprisingly, studies have found that patients with progressive disease have higher anxiety, more psychological and emotional strain, and poorer quality of life than their peers with stable disease.

At the time of clinical evaluation and surveillance, practitioners should assess survivors for distress, financial stressors, body image issues, or the need for improved social support. Multiple resources are available to melanoma survivors that can be recommended depending on the individual survivor's ongoing needs.

Reproductive Issues

Cancer survivors may face fertility issues after their cancer treatment(s), especially survivors who had chemotherapy as part of their treatment regimen(s). Many fertility-preserving initiatives are in place to address these issues in patients with cancer. Small studies in Europe have suggested that delayed reproductive difficulties are less of an issue in melanoma survivors than in survivors of cancers such as leukemia, cervical cancer, or breast cancer. However, reproductive health is a concern and remains an issue that should be addressed with melanoma survivors, particularly those diagnosed at young ages or during their reproductive years.

Health Care Costs

Similar to other malignancies, a diagnosis of melanoma incurs not only the initial costs of treatment, but also costs associated with surveillance and loss of patient productivity. A study examining the cost of melanoma in terms of projected loss of patient income estimated that annual productivity loss attributed to melanoma mortality in the United States was $3.5 billion, demonstrating the large financial burden this disease can create on a societal level. Other studies examining stage-specific costs have demonstrated that with stage I melanoma most of the cost incurred is from surveillance, whereas with later stages of melanoma, diagnosis and treatment-related costs are the main contributors. A diagnosis of stage IV disease has been estimated to be 2,200% more expensive than a diagnosis of stage I disease. This, too, highlights the importance of early diagnosis and treatment of melanoma to reduce the overall disease cost burden over time. Overall, prevention, early detection, and more streamlined surveillance programs may assist in cost containment in this growing patient population.

Key Practice Points

- Melanoma survivors have stage-specific risks for recurrence.
- Melanoma survivors have a higher risk of developing a new primary melanoma than the average population and should undergo routine dermatologic screening and surveillance.
- Given the high risk for new or recurrent skin cancers, patients with melanoma should be counseled regarding skin protection and sunscreen, sun avoidance, and directed self-skin examinations to identify suspicious lesions.
- Long-term follow-up of melanoma survivors should optimally be based on an understanding of the risks and sequelae of each patient's individual treatments, such as lymphedema in patients who have had surgery or squamous cell carcinomas in patients who received BRAF-targeted therapies.
- Patients with melanoma may have an increased risk of developing other types of cancer, such as breast cancer, prostate cancer, and non-Hodgkin lymphoma; health prevention strategies should be in place to address these other risks as well.
- Successful survivorship programs must not only address surveillance for at-risk lesions, but also assist in addressing psychosocial issues specific to cancer survivors.

Suggested Readings

American Cancer Society. Cancer treatment and survivorship: facts and figures, 2012–2013. http://www.cancer.org/acs/groups/content/@epidemiologysurveilance/documents/document/acspc-033876.pdf. Accessed September 27, 2013.

American Cancer Society. Cancer facts & figures 2014. http://www.cancer.org/acs/groups/content/@research/documents/webcontent/acspc-042151.pdf. Accessed June 23, 2014.

Balch CM, Gershenwald JE, Soong S-J, et al. Multivariate analysis of prognostic factors among 2,313 patients with stage III melanoma: comparison of nodal micrometastases versus macrometastases. *J Clin Oncol* 2010;28(14):2452–2459.

Baughan CA, Hall VL, Leppard BJ, Perkins PJ. Follow-up in stage I cutaneous malignant melanoma: an audit. *Clin Oncol (R Coll Radiol)* 1993;5(3):174–180.

Boland GM, Gershenwald JE. Sentinel lymph node biopsy in melanoma. *Cancer J* 2012;18(2):185–191.

Bradford PT, Freedman DM, Goldstein AM, Tucker MA. Increased risk of second primary cancers after a diagnosis of melanoma. *Arch Dermatol* 2010;146(3):265–272.

Burmeister BH, Henderson MA, Ainslie J, et al. Adjuvant radiotherapy versus observation alone for patients at risk of lymph-node field relapse after therapeutic lymphadenectomy for melanoma: a randomised trial. *Lancet Oncol* 2012;13(6):589–597.

Chapman PB, Hauschild A, Robert C, et al. Improved survival with vemurafenib in melanoma with BRAF V600E mutation. *New Engl J Med* 2011;364(26):2507–2516.

Cormier JN, Askew RL, Mungovan KS, Xing Y, Ross MI, Armer JM. Lymphedema beyond breast cancer: a systematic review and meta-analysis of cancer-related secondary lymphedema. *Cancer* 2010;116(22):5138–5149.

Cormier JN, Rourke L, Crosby M, Chang D, Armer J. The surgical treatment of lymphedema: a systematic review of the contemporary literature (2004–2010). *Ann Surg Oncol* 2012;19(2): 642–651.

Faries MB, Thompson JF, Cochran A, et al. The impact on morbidity and length of stay of early versus delayed complete lymphadenectomy in melanoma: results of the Multicenter Selective Lymphadenectomy Trial (I). *Ann Surg Oncol* 2010;17(12):3324–3329.

Flaherty KT, Infante JR, Daud A, et al. Combined BRAF and MEK inhibition in melanoma with BRAF V600 mutations. *New Engl J Med* 2012a;367(18):1694–1703.

Flaherty KT, Robert C, Hersey P, et al. Improved survival with MEK inhibition in BRAF-mutated melanoma. *New Engl J Med* 2012b;367(2):107–114.

Francken AB, Accortt NA, Shaw HM, et al. Follow-up schedules after treatment for malignant melanoma. *Br J Surg* 2008;95(11):1401–1407.

Gershenwald JE, Coit DG, Sondak VK, Thompson JF. The challenge of defining guidelines for sentinel lymph node biopsy in patients with thin primary cutaneous melanomas. *Ann Surg Oncol* 2012;19(11):3301–3303.

Gershenwald JE, Ross MI. Sentinel-lymph-node biopsy for cutaneous melanoma. *New Engl J Med* 2011;364(18):1738–1745.

Goggins WB, Tsao H. A population-based analysis of risk factors for a second primary cutaneous melanoma among melanoma survivors. *Cancer* 2003;97(3):639–643.

Hodi FS, O'Day SJ, McDermott DF, et al. Improved survival with ipilimumab in patients with metastatic melanoma. *New Engl J Med* 2010;363(8):711–723.

Kalady MF, White RR, Johnson JL, Tyler DS, Seigler HF. Thin melanomas: predictive lethal characteristics from a 30-year clinical experience. *Ann Surg* 2003;238(4):528–535.

Machet L, Nemeth-Normand F, Giraudeau B, et al. Is ultrasound lymph node examination superior to clinical examination in melanoma follow-up? A monocentre cohort study of 373 patients. *Br J Dermatol* 2005;152(1):66–70.

Mooney MM, Mettlin C, Michalek AM, Petrelli NJ, Kraybill WG. Life-long screening of patients with intermediate-thickness cutaneous melanoma for asymptomatic pulmonary recurrences: a cost-effectiveness analysis. *Cancer* 1997;80(6):1052–1064.

Moore Dalal K, Zhou Q, Panageas KS, Brady MS, Jaques DP, Coit DG. Methods of detection of first recurrence in patients with stage I/II primary cutaneous melanoma after sentinel lymph node biopsy. *Ann Surg Oncol* 2008;15(8):2206–2214.

Morton DL. Overview and update of the phase III Multicenter Selective Lymphadenectomy Trials (MSLT-I and MSLT-II) in melanoma. *Clin Exp Metastasis* 2012;29(7):699–706.

Morton RL, Howard K, Thompson JF. The cost-effectiveness of sentinel node biopsy in patients with intermediate thickness primary cutaneous melanoma. *Ann Surg Oncol* 2009;16(4):929–940.

National Comprehensive Cancer Network. NCCN clinical practice guidelines in oncology—melanoma, v2.2013. http://www.nccn.org/professionals/physician_gls/f_guidelines.asp#site. Accessed September 27, 2013.

Nieweg OE, Kroon BB. The conundrum of follow-up: should it be abandoned? *Surg Oncol Clin N Am* 2006;15(2):319–330.

Pandalai PK, Dominguez FJ, Michaelson J, Tanabe KK. Clinical value of radiographic staging in patients diagnosed with AJCC stage III melanoma. *Ann Surg Oncol* 2011;18(2):506–513.

Robert C, Thomas L, Bondarenko I, et al. Ipilimumab plus dacarbazine for previously untreated metastatic melanoma. *New Engl J Med* 2011;364(26):2517–2526.

Romano E, Scordo M, Dusza SW, Coit DG, Chapman PB. Site and timing of first relapse in stage III melanoma patients: implications for follow-up guidelines. *J Clin Oncol* 2010;28(18):3042–3047.

Ross MI, Gershenwald JE. Evidence-based treatment of early-stage melanoma. *J Surg Oncol* 2011;104(4):341–353.

Topalian SL, Hodi FS, Brahmer JR, et al. Safety, activity, and immune correlates of anti-PD-1 antibody in cancer. *New Engl J Med* 2012;366(26):2443–2454.

Uren RF, Sanki A, Thompson JF. The utility of ultrasound in patients with melanoma. *Expert Rev Anticancer Ther* 2007;7(11): 1633–1642.

Survivorship Algorithms

These cancer survivorship algorithms have been specifically developed for MD Anderson using a multidisciplinary approach and taking into consideration circumstances particular to MD Anderson, including the following: MD Anderson's specific patient population, MD Anderson's services and structure, and MD Anderson's clinical information. These algorithms are provided for informational purposes only and are not intended to replace the independent medical or professional judgment of physicians or other health care providers. Moreover, these algorithms should not be used to treat pregnant women.

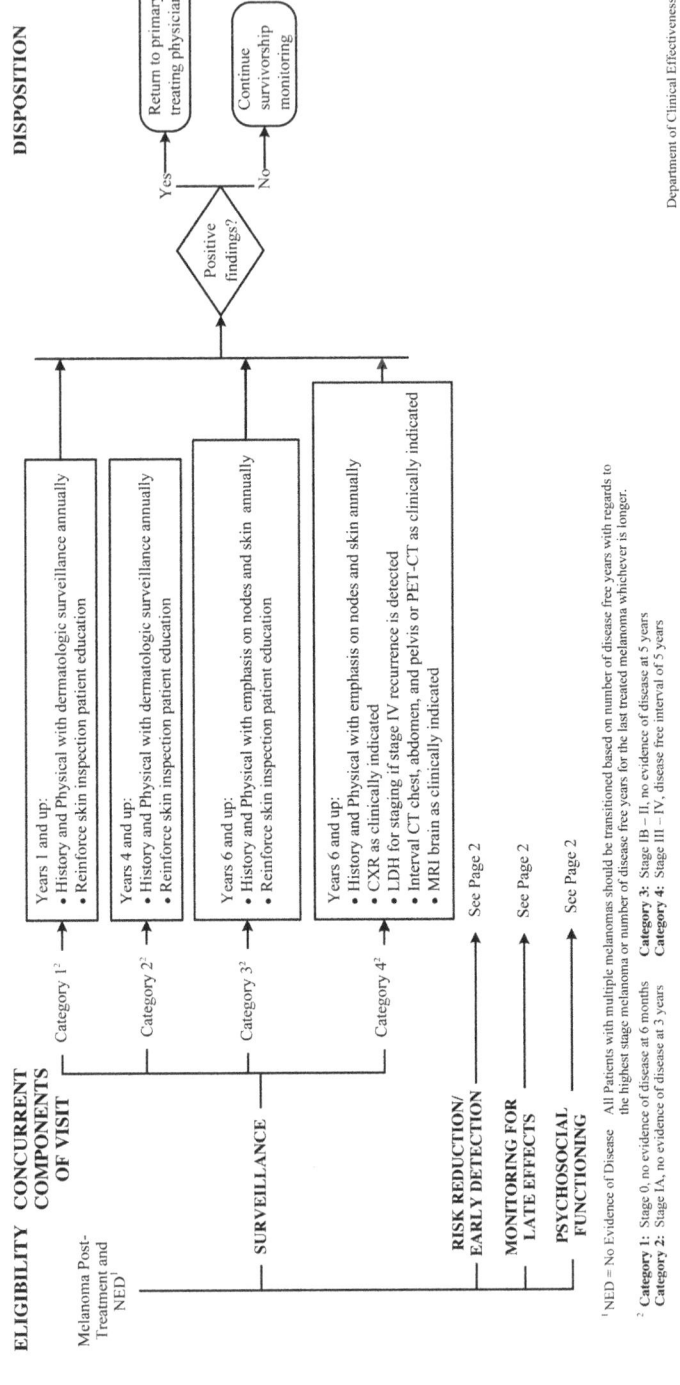

Algorithm 13.1a Survivorship—cutaneous melanoma (page 1)

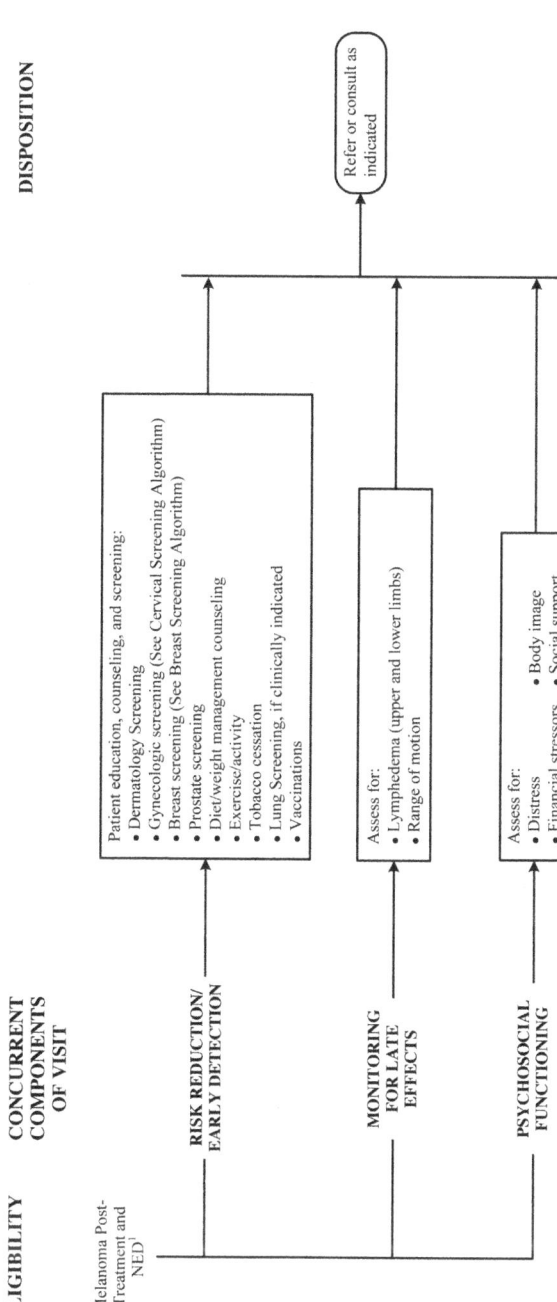

ELIGIBILITY

CONCURRENT
COMPONENTS
OF VISIT

DISPOSITION

Melanoma Post-
Treatment and
NED[1]

RISK REDUCTION/
EARLY DETECTION

Patient education, counseling, and screening:
• Dermatology Screening
• Gynecologic screening (See Cervical Screening Algorithm)
• Breast screening (See Breast Screening Algorithm)
• Prostate screening
• Diet/weight management counseling
• Exercise/activity
• Tobacco cessation
• Lung Screening, if clinically indicated
• Vaccinations

MONITORING
FOR LATE
EFFECTS

Assess for:
• Lymphedema (upper and lower limbs)
• Range of motion

PSYCHOSOCIAL
FUNCTIONING

Assess for:
• Distress
• Financial stressors
• Body image
• Social support

Refer or consult as
indicated

[1] NED = No Evidence of Disease

Department of Clinical Effectiveness V1
Approved by the Executive Committee of the Medical Staff on 12/18/2012

Algorithm 13.1b   Survivorship—cutaneous melanoma (page 2)

Chapter 14
Thyroid Cancer Survivorship Management

Sherrie L. Flores and Mouhammed Amir Habra

Contents

Chapter Overview Thyroid cancer survivors enjoy long life expectancy but may experience lifelong complications attributable to surgery, radioactive iodine therapy, or thyroid hormone suppression. The importance of these potential complications increases over time as the active initial cancer therapy is completed and the acute threat of the malignancy ebbs. Accordingly, a comprehensive examination of individuals treated for thyroid cancer should be undertaken as soon as possible to detect and correct problems and to improve quality of life in these patients. The Thyroid Cancer Survivorship Clinic at MD Anderson has been developed to provide an environment in which thyroid cancer survivors can be evaluated and potential future effects of cancer and cancer therapy can be addressed. In addition, providing this service can facilitate development of evidence-based guidelines for treatment goals and long-term surveillance.

L.E. Foxhall, M.A. Rodriguez (eds.), *Advances in Cancer Survivorship Management*,   241
MD Anderson Cancer Care Series, DOI 10.1007/978-1-4939-0986-5_14,
© The University of Texas M.D. Anderson Cancer Center 2015

Introduction

Awareness is growing that the life trajectory of individuals diagnosed with and treated for cancer can extend far beyond the often limited duration of active therapy. Thyroid cancer is the most common endocrine malignancy and is currently the fifth most common malignancy in women. Differentiated thyroid carcinoma, which includes papillary and follicular thyroid carcinoma, represents almost 95% of all cases of thyroid cancer. Medullary thyroid carcinoma, primary thyroid lymphoma, and anaplastic thyroid carcinoma represent about 5% of all cases of thyroid cancer. Recent projections estimate that 1,660,290 individuals will be newly diagnosed with cancer in the United States in 2013; of these, 60,220 individuals will be diagnosed with thyroid cancer but only 1,850 thyroid cancer-related deaths are expected to occur during the same period (Siegel et al. 2013). The number of patients with thyroid cancer is growing because of increasing incidence of the disease and improved survival durations of most patients with thyroid cancer. The overall 10-year survival rate for patients with differentiated thyroid carcinoma is about 90–95%, making this disease very attractive for the development of a survivorship model. Figure 14.1 illustrates the incidence of thyroid cancer between 1990 and 2011 in men and women as well as total mortality in both sexes. No guidelines have been formally established for thyroid cancer survivors and their health caregivers, and limited evidence-based information is available about thyroid cancer survivors' long-term management needs, goals, and targets.

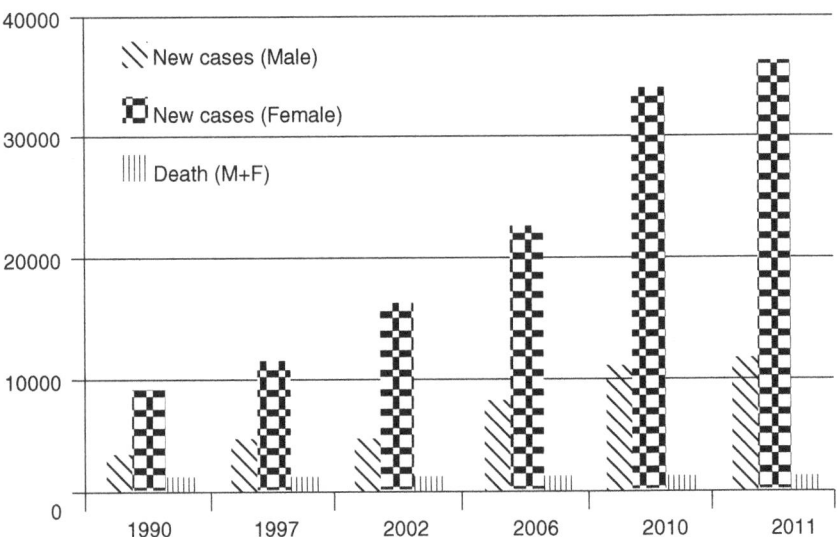

Fig. 14.1 New cases of thyroid cancer and thyroid cancer-related deaths that occurred each year in the United States between 1990 and 2011

Sequelae of Cancer Therapy in Thyroid Cancer Survivors

Thyroid cancer survivors are generally healthy individuals who lead a productive life after treatment. However, many survivors may face a wide range of long-lasting late effects of their disease in their near-normal lifespan. A report from MD Anderson showed that two-thirds of thyroid cancer survivors reported that their cancer or cancer treatment led to significant, lasting symptoms such as fatigue (Schultz et al. 2003). Similarly, reports from other institutions showed impaired quality of life in thyroid cancer survivors compared with control patients, independent of thyroid-stimulating hormone (TSH) levels (Tan et al. 2007; Hoftijzer et al. 2008).

Surgical Complications

Surgery is the most important initial treatment for thyroid carcinoma. Disease burden at the initial diagnosis and the presence of lymph node metastases determine the extent of initial surgical resection. Not surprisingly, more extensive surgery carries a higher risk for unwanted side effects, including vocal cord paralysis, regional pain, and hypocalcemia, among others. Fortunately, many of these complications tend to be transient, although some patients may experience long-lasting complications.

Hypoparathyroidism

Hypoparathyroidism is a known complication after total thyroidectomy. In most cases, patients develop transient hypocalcemia requiring short-term medical therapy. However, a small percentage of these patients may have permanent hypoparathyroidism, requiring frequent laboratory tests and medication adjustments as needed to maintain serum calcium levels in a narrow range to avoid problems from hypocalcemia, hypercalciuria, or hypercalcemia.

A growing number of surgical oncologists are performing central neck dissection with the initial total thyroidectomy in patients with differentiated thyroid carcinoma because of the high rate of lymph node metastasis in these patients. However, a higher incidence of transient and permanent hypoparathyroidism has been reported in patients who undergo central neck dissection than in patients who do not, and this should be considered when the patient is young and has a low risk of recurrence and a long life expectancy (Rosenbaum and McHenry 2009).

Implantation of parathyroid tissue can reduce both short-term hypocalcemia and permanent hypoparathyroidism after total thyroidectomy. The surgical expertise and extent of surgery are very important factors in determining the risk of surgical complications (hypoparathyroidism and vocal cord injury) in patients with thyroid cancer.

Vocal Cord Dysfunction

Preserving voice quality after thyroid surgery is an important goal for most patients. Transient recurrent laryngeal nerve dysfunction occurs in about 5–10% of all patients who undergo total thyroidectomy, and it usually improves spontaneously. Permanent recurrent laryngeal nerve injury is estimated to occur in about 1–2% of all patients who undergo total thyroidectomy. In some cases the injury may go unrecognized, but it can also lead to permanent hoarseness, coughing, and food aspiration. In a small number of patients with locally advanced thyroid cancer, those who underwent reconstruction of the recurrent laryngeal nerve at the time of thyroidectomy were found to have better vocal cord function than those who did not undergo this procedure (Hartl et al. 2005). In patients who develop unilateral recurrent laryngeal nerve damage, various procedures could be done to improve voice quality and reduce aspiration, including the medialization of the paralyzed vocal cord.

Limitation of Mobility

Limitation of neck-shoulder-arm mobility, local pain, and reduced sensation may occur after thyroid surgery, especially if wide neck dissection is also performed. In most cases, symptoms improve with conservative management and physical therapy. An estimated 5–15% of patients who undergo neck dissection are thought to be at risk for shoulder dysfunction, especially when the surgery is extended to the posterior neck triangle (level V). Upper extremity dysfunction can occur as a result of surgical injury, but it is usually mild; less than 10% of affected patients have reported severe impairment. Quality of life is also reduced in patients who develop neck pain and reduced shoulder mobility after surgery for head and neck malignancies (van Wilgen et al. 2004).

Radioactive Iodine Therapy Complications

Radioactive iodine (RAI) is often administered as an adjunct treatment in patients with differentiated thyroid carcinoma and is very well tolerated in most cases. However, concern is growing about unnecessary radiation exposure in patients with thyroid cancer who are at low risk for recurrence, who may not benefit from RAI therapy but could have a small risk for complications.

Oral and Ocular Complications

Because salivary and lacrimal glands have iodine uptake transporters, RAI uptake and accumulation occurs in these glands after RAI exposure, leading to problems such as salivary gland pain, xerostomia, altered taste, dental caries, salivary calculi, enlarged salivary glands, and excessive tearing secondary to lacrimal duct obstruction. A significant reduction in lacrimal gland secretion was observed in patients who had undergone RAI therapy, but similar reductions were also observed in patients who had not undergone the therapy (Fard-Esfahani et al. 2007). Furthermore, no correlation was found between RAI dose and tear production based on results of the Schirmer test. RAI therapy can also exacerbate coexisting Graves ophthalmopathy. Because some patients with differentiated thyroid carcinoma have Graves disease at the time of initial diagnosis, careful assessment is needed in these patients to avoid progression of exophthalmos.

Reduced salivary function in the first year after RAI therapy has been reported in 26–58% of patients with thyroid cancer who received the treatment, but only 5% had long-term side effects (Hyer et al. 2007; Grewal et al. 2009). The long-term adverse effects of RAI therapy on the salivary glands are most noticeable in the parotid glands, leading to a sense of dysphagia. Although conclusive evidence of benefit is lacking, sour candies are widely used to increase salivary flow at the time of RAI therapy with the hope of reducing salivary gland damage. However, emerging literature has suggested that this practice is potentially harmful, increasing salivary gland exposure to radiation by stimulating the salivary gland cells (Nakada et al. 2005).

Amifostine was proposed as a cytoprotective agent to reduce salivary gland damage after RAI therapy; however, a recent review article did not find conclusive evidence to support this claim (Ma et al. 2010), and the use of amifostine to protect salivary glands after RAI treatment remains questionable. The use of pilocarpine along with dexamethasone and intensive oral hygiene also was not found to reduce oral complications after RAI therapy (Silberstein 2008). Sialendoscopy has recently been used to treat selected patients who developed sialadenitis after RAI therapy. A retrospective review in 12 women with RAI-induced sialadenitis showed that mucous plugs and ductal stenosis were the most common abnormalities in these patients and that sialendoscopy use resulted in symptomatic improvement in 75% of patients (Bomeli et al. 2009).

Gonadal Effects

In male patients, testosterone levels have been shown to remain stable after RAI therapy. However, dose-dependent increases in follicle-stimulating hormone and luteinizing hormone levels have been observed in male patients during the first 6 months after RAI exposure, followed by spontaneous normalization after about 18 months, suggestive of RAI-related damage to the germinal epithelium. The radiation dose to the testicles has been found to depend on the RAI dose used, with an estimated median radiation dose of 6.4 cGy to each testicle in patients receiving 3 GBq (81 mCi) of RAI and 21.2 cGy to each testicle in patients receiving 9.2 GBq (249 mCi) of RAI (Hyer et al. 2002). Children born to men treated with RAI have not been found to have an increased risk for congenital malformations. Although the testicular exposure to radiation that occurs with RAI therapy is not enough to cause permanent damage to the testicles, one-third of male patients who underwent RAI therapy were found to experience reduced sperm count during follow-up (Esfahani et al. 2004). Patients concerned about fertility issues can request semen analysis and possibly opt for semen banking prior to RAI therapy.

In women treated with RAI, menopause was shown to occur at an earlier age compared with women with goiters who did not receive RAI (Ceccarelli et al. 2001). A minority of young women (younger than 40 years) who underwent RAI therapy were found to experience transient irregular menses without obvious harmful effects on fertility or pregnancy outcomes (Vini et al. 2002).

Secondary Malignancies

The risk of secondary malignancies after RAI therapy is less well established. However, in a review of a large cohort of patients with thyroid cancer, the risk of second primary malignancies in patients treated with RAI increased in a dose-dependent manner compared with the risk of second primary malignancies in the general population; an estimated extra three cases of leukemia were observed in every 10,000 patients receiving 100 mCi of RAI during 10 years of follow-up (Rubino et al. 2003). The risk of developing leukemia after RAI therapy is significantly increased, although the risk of developing solid tumors is less clear. Other studies have also shown an increased risk of developing leukemia and salivary gland malignancies after exposure to RAI but disputed the increased risk of developing other solid tumors (Sawka et al. 2009; Iyer et al. 2011). However, patients with thyroid cancer are subject to close clinical monitoring and surveillance, and this could lead to detection bias (i.e., more malignancies are found in this group compared with the general population).

Most new cases of differentiated thyroid carcinoma involve low-volume disease. Reports of the potential toxicity of RAI therapy are creating the need to critically reexamine the clinical application of this very targeted and effective modality to optimize its use in patients with more extensive disease, who are more likely to derive clinical benefit from RAI therapy, while limiting exposure to RAI in patients at low risk for recurrence. Despite these recent reports, no specific recommendations have been made to screen thyroid cancer survivors differently from the general population. We have formulated our thyroid cancer survivorship algorithm (presented at the end of the chapter) on the basis of consensus of experts and available evidence.

Thyroid Hormone Suppression Complications

Thyroid hormone replacement therapy aims to replace thyroid hormone after thyroid ablation and to suppress TSH levels to reduce the risk of cancer recurrence. Although most patients do well with thyroid hormone replacement therapy, some patients have a poorly explained sense of chronic fatigue despite seemingly appropriate thyroid hormone dosing; some of these patients continue to complain of fatigue well after the acute cancer treatment. It is possible that patients have a selective defect in thyroid hormone replacement at a tissue level that is not reflected in laboratory test results. Treatment with the combination of levothyroxine (T4) and liothyronine (T3) has anecdotally helped alleviate fatigue in some patients, but recently conducted clinical trials have been unable to document an objective clinical benefit of this treatment (Joffe et al. 2007). In addition, some patients who undergo TSH-suppressive therapy may develop hyperthyroid symptoms that could exacerbate other coexisting disorders such as postmenopausal hot flashes and anxiety disorders.

Patients with differentiated thyroid carcinoma, compared with patients with other types of thyroid cancer, often receive higher doses of thyroid hormone replacement agents to suppress TSH production. Although TSH suppression improves long-term outcomes in patients with advanced differentiated thyroid carcinoma, the benefit of this practice is less clear in patients with more limited disease. Long-term thyroid hormone suppression can be an additional source of comorbidity.

The incidence of atrial fibrillation is three times higher in patients older than 60 years who have TSH levels of less than 0.1 mU/L, compared with other patient groups (Sawin et al. 1994). Similarly, subclinical hyperthyroidism is associated with left ventricular dysfunction, increased heart rate, and potentially increased risk for ischemic events. Short-term studies in a small number of patients with endogenous subclinical hyperthyroidism showed that normal sinus rhythm, normal heart rate, and left ventricular mass were restored after TSH was normalized with medical therapy or RAI (Biondi et al. 2002; Sgarbi et al. 2003). Still, no large, randomized studies with long-term follow-up have been conducted to verify these findings.

Echocardiographic evidence has shown increased left ventricular dimensions with impaired myocardial systolic and diastolic functions in patients with differentiated thyroid carcinoma. However, these changes are reversible after restoration of euthyroid state.

The prevalence of premature atrial and ventricular beats is higher in patients with subclinical hyperthyroidism than in euthyroid controls. Although transitioning to a euthyroid state has not been shown to have any effect on atrial premature beats in these patients, it has been shown to significantly reduce the frequency of ventricular premature beats. Patients with differentiated thyroid carcinoma who have undergone long-term TSH suppression have also been shown to have reduced arterial elasticity, increased left ventricular mass index, and increased interventricular septum thickness compared with age- and sex-matched healthy controls.

A meta-analysis did not find an association between subclinical hyperthyroidism and risk of coronary heart disease or cardiovascular mortality (Singh et al. 2008). However, a population-based study of 5,860 patients aged 65 years or older found that the prevalence of atrial fibrillation was twice as high in patients with subclinical hyperthyroidism (9.5%) than in euthyroid controls (4.7%; Gammage et al. 2007).

Studies examining the effects of subclinical hyperthyroidism on bone health have shown conflicting results. Reduced bone density in cortical bones was reported in some studies of women with subclinical hyperthyroidism (Paul et al. 1988). In a cross-sectional study, men with thyroid carcinoma who underwent TSH-suppressive therapy did not differ from healthy controls in terms of bone turnover markers, bone density scores, or asymptomatic vertebral fractures (Reverter et al. 2010). In a prospective cohort study of patients aged 65 years or older, men with subclinical hyperthyroidism had a three times higher risk of developing hip fractures compared with euthyroid men (hazard ratio = 3.27, 95% confidence interval = 0.99–11.30), but subclinical dysfunction in women in the same study did not affect hip fracture risk (Lee et al. 2010). A meta-analysis found reduced cortical bone density in postmenopausal women with exogenous subclinical hyperthyroidism compared with controls, whereas men and premenopausal women with subclinical hyperthyroidism did not have significant declines in bone density (Uzzan et al. 1996). Some literature suggests that estrogen and calcium supplementation could ameliorate the effect of TSH suppression on bone loss. Long-term TSH suppression (>6 years) in women with differentiated thyroid carcinoma has been shown to reduce the efficacy of bisphosphonate therapy compared with no TSH suppression or TSH suppression for a shorter period (3 years).

Second Primary Cancer in Thyroid Cancer Survivors

Thyroid cancer survivors carry a higher risk of developing future second primary malignancies compared with the general population. This could in part be a consequence of previous cancer treatments such as RAI therapy or external beam radiation therapy in the early years after initial diagnosis. Differentiated thyroid carcinoma can also occur as part of certain cancer genetic predisposition syndromes. Differentiated thyroid carcinoma may occur in about 10% of patients with Cowden syndrome, which is associated with *PTEN* gene mutations (10q23.31) and also carries a high risk of developing breast carcinoma and uterine carcinoma. Differentiated thyroid carcinoma can also occur in about 2% of individuals with familial adenomatous polyposis, which is an autosomal dominant disorder associated with *APC* gene mutations (5q22.2). Affected individuals develop multiple adenomatous colon polyps, leading to the development of colon cancer at an early age.

Risk factors for second primary malignancies include age (50 years or older at the time of thyroid cancer diagnosis), RAI dose of at least 3 GBq (81 mCi), and external beam radiation therapy. Risk factors for death associated with second primary malignancies include age (50 years or older) and development of a second primary malignancy other than breast cancer.

Key Practice Points

- Incidence of thyroid cancer is rapidly increasing, and thyroid cancer is currently the fifth most common cancer in women.
- Because of the relatively low mortality rate associated with thyroid cancer, an increasing number of patients are added yearly to the existing pool of thyroid cancer survivors.
- Substantial morbidity could result from the initial treatments offered to thyroid cancer survivors, and the treatments may lead to long-term complications.
- Although TSH suppression is a standard treatment, especially in the first few years after a thyroid cancer diagnosis, complications could erupt from prolonged and unnecessary TSH suppression.
- Patients with thyroid cancer may have a higher risk of developing other malignancies compared with the general population and should undergo cancer screening as appropriate for their age and medical history.

Suggested Readings

Biondi B, Palmieri EA, Lombardi G, et al. Effects of subclinical thyroid dysfunction on the heart. *Ann Intern Med* 2002;137(11):904–914.

Bomeli SR, Schaitkin B, Carrau RL, et al. Interventional sialendoscopy for treatment of radioiodine-induced sialadenitis. *Laryngoscope* 2009;119(5):864–867.

Ceccarelli C, Bencivelli W, Morciano D, et al. 131I therapy for differentiated thyroid cancer leads to an earlier onset of menopause: results of a retrospective study. *J Clin Endocrinol Metab* 2001;86(8):3512–3515.

Esfahani AF, Eftekhari M, Zenooz N, Saghari M. Gonadal function in patients with differentiated thyroid cancer treated with (131)I. *Hell J Nucl Med* 2004;7(1):52–55.

Fard-Esfahani A, Mirshekarpour H, Saghari M, et al. The effect of high-dose radioiodine treatment on lacrimal gland function in patients with differentiated thyroid carcinoma. *Clin Nucl Med* 2007;32(9):696–699.

Gammage MD, Parle JV, Holder RL, et al. Association between serum free thyroxine concentration and atrial fibrillation. *Arch Intern Med* 2007;167(9):928–934.

Grewal RK, Larson SM, Pentlow CE, et al. Salivary gland side effects commonly develop several weeks after initial radioactive iodine ablation. *J Nucl Med* 2009;50(10):1605–1610.

Hartl DM, Travagli JP, Leboulleux S, et al. Clinical review: current concepts in the management of unilateral recurrent laryngeal nerve paralysis after thyroid surgery. *J Clin Endocrinol Metab* 2005;90(5):3084–3088.

Hoftijzer HC, Heemstra KA, Corssmit EP, van der Klaauw AA, Romijn JA, Smit JW. Quality of life in cured patients with differentiated thyroid carcinoma. *J Clin Endocrinol Metab* 2008;93(1):200–203.

Hyer S, Kong A, Pratt B, et al. Salivary gland toxicity after radioiodine therapy for thyroid cancer. *Clin Oncol* 2007;19(1):83–86.

Hyer S, Vini L, O'Connell M, et al. Testicular dose and fertility in men following I(131) therapy for thyroid cancer. *Clin Endocrinol* 2002;56(6):755–758.

Iyer NG, Morris LG, Tuttle RM, Shaha AR, Ganly I. Rising incidence of second cancers in patients with low-risk (T1N0) thyroid cancer who receive radioactive iodine therapy. *Cancer* 2011;117(19):4439–4446.

Joffe RT, Brimacombe M, Levitt AJ, et al. Treatment of clinical hypothyroidism with thyroxine and triiodothyronine: a literature review and metaanalysis. *Psychosomatics* 2007;48(5):379–384.

Lee JS, Buzkova P, Fink HA, et al. Subclinical thyroid dysfunction and incident hip fracture in older adults. *Arch Intern Med* 2010;170(21):1876–1883.

Ma C, Xie J, Jiang Z, et al. Does amifostine have radioprotective effects on salivary glands in high-dose radioactive iodine-treated differentiated thyroid cancer. *Eur J Nucl Med Mol Imaging* 2010;37(9):1778–1785.

Nakada K, Ishibashi T, Takei T, et al. Does lemon candy decrease salivary gland damage after radioiodine therapy for thyroid cancer? *J Nucl Med* 2005;46(2):261–266.

Paul TL, Kerrigan J, Kelly AM, Braverman LE, Baran DT. Long-term L-thyroxine therapy is associated with decreased hip bone density in premenopausal women. *JAMA* 1988;259(21):3137–3141.

Reverter JL, Colome E, Holgado S, et al. Bone mineral density and bone fracture in male patients receiving long-term suppressive levothyroxine treatment for differentiated thyroid carcinoma. *Endocrine* 2010;37(3):467–472.

Rosenbaum MA, McHenry CR. Central neck dissection for papillary thyroid cancer. *Arch Otolaryngol Head Neck Surg* 2009;135(11):1092–1097.

Rubino C, de Vathaire F, Dottorini ME, et al. Second primary malignancies in thyroid cancer patients. *Brit J Cancer* 2003;89(9):1638–1644.

Sawin CT, Geller A, Wolf PA, et al. Low serum thyrotropin concentrations as a risk factor for atrial fibrillation in older persons. *New Engl J Med* 1994;331(19):1249–1252.

Sawka AM, Thabane L, Parlea L, et al. Second primary malignancy risk after radioactive iodine treatment for thyroid cancer: a systematic review and meta-analysis. *Thyroid* 2009;19(5):451–457.

Schultz PN, Stava C, Vassilopoulou-Sellin R. Health profiles and quality of life of 518 survivors of thyroid cancer. *Head & Neck* 2003;25(5):349–356.

Sgarbi JA, Villaca FG, Garbeline B, et al. The effects of early antithyroid therapy for endogenous subclinical hyperthyroidism in clinical and heart abnormalities. *J Clin Endocrinol Metab* 2003;88(4):1672–1677.

Siegel R, Naishadham D, Jemal A. Cancer statistics, 2013. *CA Cancer J Clin* 2013;63(1):11–30.

Silberstein EB. Reducing the incidence of 131I-induced sialadenitis: the role of pilocarpine. *J Nucl Med* 2008;49(4):546–549.

Singh S, Duggal J, Molnar J, et al. Impact of subclinical thyroid disorders on coronary heart disease, cardiovascular and all-cause mortality: a meta-analysis. *International J Cardiol* 2008;125(1):41–48.

Tan LG, Nan L, Thumboo J, Sundram F, Tan LK. Health-related quality of life in thyroid cancer survivors. *Laryngoscope* 2007;117(3):507–510.

Uzzan B, Campos J, Cucherat M, et al. Effects on bone mass of long term treatment with thyroid hormones: a meta-analysis. *J Clin Endocrinol Metab* 1996;81(12):4278–4289.

van Wilgen CP, Dijkstra PU, van der Laan BF, et al. Shoulder and neck morbidity in quality of life after surgery for head and neck cancer. *Head & Neck* 2004;26(10):839–844.

Vini L, Hyer S, Al-Saadi A, Pratt B, Harmer C. Prognosis for fertility and ovarian function after treatment with radioiodine for thyroid cancer. *Postgraduate Medical Journal* 2002;78(916):92–93.

Survivorship Algorithms

These cancer survivorship algorithms have been specifically developed for MD Anderson using a multidisciplinary approach and taking into consideration circumstances particular to MD Anderson, including the following: MD Anderson's specific patient population, MD Anderson's services and structure, and MD Anderson's clinical information. These algorithms are provided for informational purposes only and are not intended to replace the independent medical or professional judgment of physicians or other health care providers. Moreover, these algorithms should not be used to treat pregnant women.

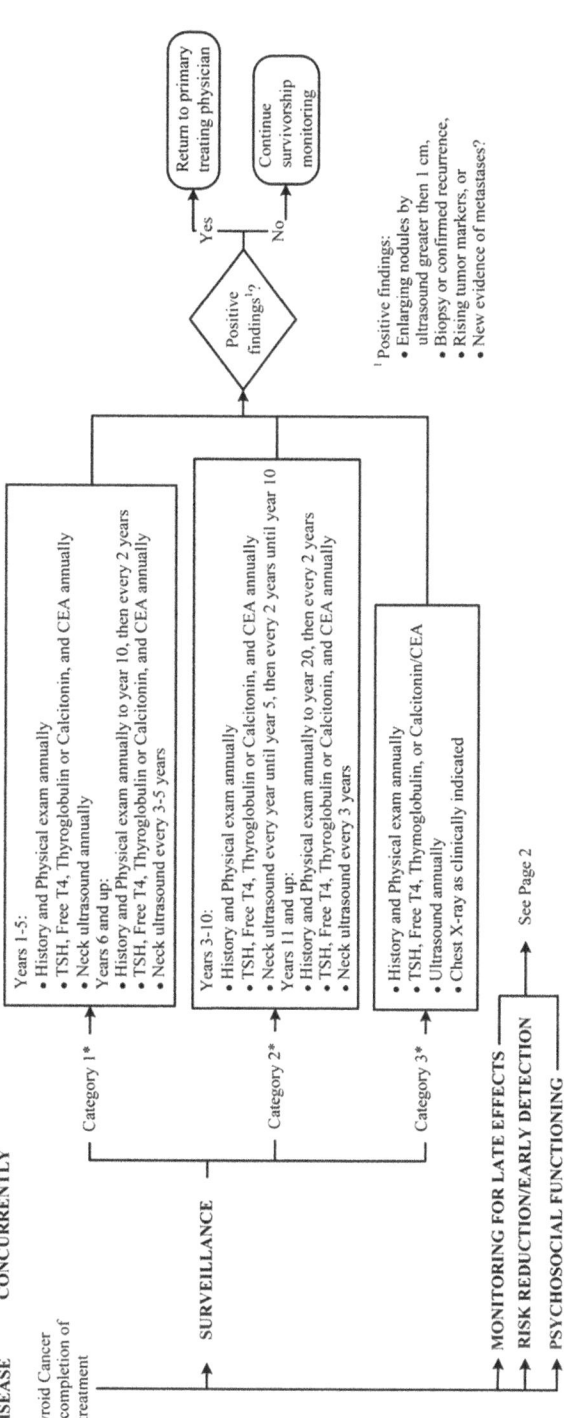

DISEASE   CONCURRENTLY

Thyroid Cancer
after completion of
treatment

SURVEILLANCE

Category 1*

Years 1-5:
• History and Physical exam annually
• TSH, Free T4, Thyroglobulin or Calcitonin, and CEA annually
• Neck ultrasound annually
Years 6 and up:
• History and Physical exam annually to year 10, then every 2 years
• TSH, Free T4, Thyroglobulin or Calcitonin, and CEA annually
• Neck ultrasound every 3-5 years

Category 2*

Years 3-10:
• History and Physical exam annually
• TSH, Free T4, Thyroglobulin or Calcitonin, and CEA annually
• Neck ultrasound every year until year 5, then every 2 years until year 10
Years 11 and up:
• History and Physical exam annually to year 20, then every 2 years
• TSH, Free T4, Thyroglobulin or Calcitonin, and CEA annually
• Neck ultrasound every 3 years

Category 3*

• History and Physical exam annually
• TSH, Free T4, Thymoglobulin, or Calcitonin/CEA
• Ultrasound annually
• Chest X-ray as clinically indicated

Positive findings[1,2]?

Yes → Return to primary treating physician

No → Continue survivorship monitoring

[1] Positive findings:
• Enlarging nodules by ultrasound greater then 1 cm,
• Biopsy or confirmed recurrence,
• Rising tumor markers, or
• New evidence of metastases?

MONITORING FOR LATE EFFECTS
RISK REDUCTION/EARLY DETECTION → See Page 2
PSYCHOSOCIAL FUNCTIONING

* Category 1: T1 N0 M0, no evidence of disease (thyroglobulin less than or equal to 1 or calcitonin less than or equal to 5; no suspicious lymph nodes or thyroid bed lesions by ultrasound) at 1 year.
Category 2: T2-4 N0-1 M0, no evidence of disease (thyroglobulin less than or equal to 1 or calcitonin less than or equal to 5; no suspicious lymph nodes or thyroid bed lesions by ultrasound) at 3 years.
Category 3: T2-4 N0-1 M0, stable minimal evidence of disease (thyroglobulin less than or equal to 5 or or calcitonin less than or equal to 50; no suspicious lymph nodes or thyroid bed lesions or stable subcentimeter lesions by ultrasound) at 5 years.

Department of Clinical Effectiveness V2
Approved by the Executive Committee of the Medical Staff 05/31/2011

Algorithm 14.1a Survivorship—thyroid cancer, including papillary, follicular, and medullary carcinoma (page 1)

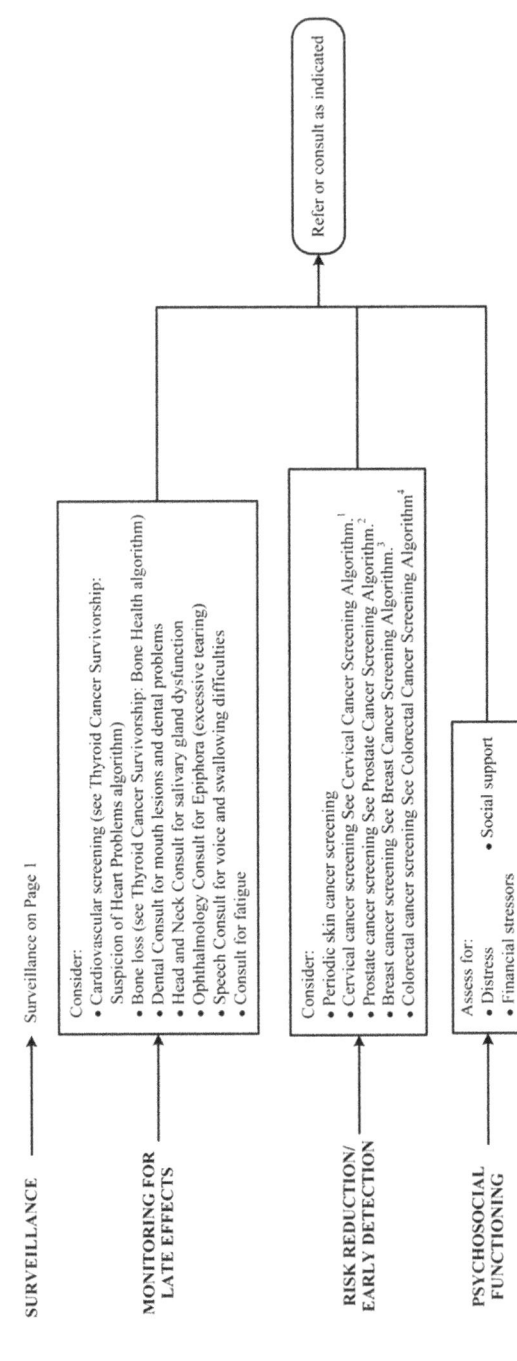

CONCURRENTLY

SURVEILLANCE → Surveillance on Page 1

MONITORING FOR LATE EFFECTS

Consider:
- Cardiovascular screening (see Thyroid Cancer Survivorship: Suspicion of Heart Problems algorithm)
- Bone loss (see Thyroid Cancer Survivorship: Bone Health algorithm)
- Dental Consult for mouth lesions and dental problems
- Head and Neck Consult for salivary gland dysfunction
- Ophthalmology Consult for Epiphora (excessive tearing)
- Speech Consult for voice and swallowing difficulties
- Consult for fatigue

RISK REDUCTION/ EARLY DETECTION

Consider:
- Periodic skin cancer screening
- Cervical cancer screening See Cervical Cancer Screening Algorithm.[1]
- Prostate cancer screening See Prostate Cancer Screening Algorithm.[2]
- Breast cancer screening See Breast Cancer Screening Algorithm.[3]
- Colorectal cancer screening See Colorectal Cancer Screening Algorithm[4]

PSYCHOSOCIAL FUNCTIONING

Assess for:
- Distress
- Financial stressors
- Social support

Refer or consult as indicated

[1] Cervical screening - begin 3 years after sexual intercourse, but no later than 21 years old. Screening annually with conventional PAP test or every 2 years using liquid based Paptest. If greater than 30 years old with 3 normal PAP smears, may get screened every 3 years.
[2] Prostate screening - begin at age 50 (age 45 for family history and/or African American) until age 75 annually.
[3] Breast screening - begin at age 40.
[4] Colorectal screening - begin at age 50; colonoscopy every 10 years.

Department of Clinical Effectiveness V2
Approved by the Executive Committee of the Medical Staff 05/31/2011

Algorithm 14.1b Survivorship—thyroid cancer, including papillary, follicular, and medullary carcinoma (page 2)

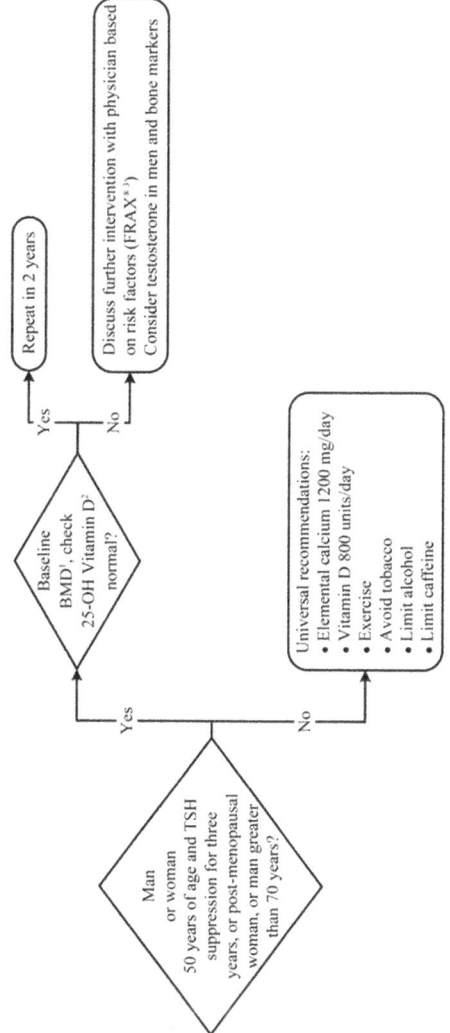

[1] BMD – Bone Mineral Density
[2] 25-hydroxyvitamin D, also know as 25-hydroxycholecalciferol, caldiciol or abbreviated as 25-OH VitD, the main vitamin D metabolite circulating in plasma.
[3] FRAX - WHO Fracture Risk Assessment Tool at www.shef.ac.uk/frax

Department of Clinical Effectiveness V1
Approved by the Executive Committee of the Medical Staff 05/31/2011

Algorithm 14.2 Thyroid cancer survivorship: bone health

Part III
Cancer Prevention and Screening

Chapter 15
Tobacco Cessation

Maher Karam-Hage and Paul M. Cinciripini

Contents

Chapter Overview Tobacco use is behind most preventable diseases with disabling consequences and death. These diseases are among the most serious, including cancer, cardiovascular diseases (brain strokes, cardiac infarcts, peripheral artery disease), and respiratory system diseases (emphysema, chronic infections). It is estimated that one-third of cancers are attributable to tobacco use and in theory can be prevented. Therefore, a comprehensive tobacco cessation program is a crucial element of successful survivorship and cancer prevention programs. Smoking cigarettes is the most common and deadliest method of consuming tobacco, and nicotine is the reinforcing substance in any tobacco use that with long-term exposure leads to dependence (addiction). Nicotine dependence involves biological, behavioral, and cognitive elements; an optimal approach to treatment

L.E. Foxhall, M.A. Rodriguez (eds.), *Advances in Cancer Survivorship Management*,   257
MD Anderson Cancer Care Series, DOI 10.1007/978-1-4939-0986-5_15,
© The University of Texas M.D. Anderson Cancer Center 2015

for nicotine dependence should address each of these three dimensions. A comprehensive tobacco/smoking cessation program should include cognitive behavioral techniques, motivational interviewing approaches, and appropriate medications. Currently the medications approved by the US Food and Drug Administration for the treatment of nicotine dependence include nicotine replacement therapies, bupropion-SR (sustained release), and varenicline; these treatments can be used individually or in combination. Combining medications capitalizes on the synergy resulting from differing mechanisms of action.

Introduction

Cigarette smoking is the principal cause of preventable morbidity and mortality in the United States (US Centers for Disease Control and Prevention [CDC] 2010) and around the globe. In the United States alone, 443,000 deaths per year are attributable to cigarette smoking, according to the CDC; around the world, that number is estimated to be about six million deaths per year. Although tobacco use in general correlates with many cancers, cigarette smoking in particular is reported to be causally linked to at least 18 types of cancer. Smoking-related health care expenditures in the United States are estimated to be around $96 billion, and costs related to the accompanying loss in productivity are about $97 billion, resulting in an economic burden from smoking of about $193 billion per year (CDC 2012).

Approximately 12 million people are living with cancer in the United States (CDC 2012); lung cancer, ischemic heart disease, and chronic obstructive pulmonary disease constitute the three leading causes of smoking-attributable mortality. Smoking cigarettes accounts for the vast majority of tobacco use and addiction, as well as for the vast majority of nicotine dependence (for the purpose of this chapter we will use the term "tobacco addiction" interchangeably with "smoking cigarettes" or "nicotine dependence"). Therefore, treating tobacco addiction must be an essential component of any campaign to eradicate cancer, in particular because of the staggering statistics pointing to smoking as the cause of one out of every three deaths from cancer and as the cause of four out of five deaths from chronic obstructive pulmonary disease. Because the consequences of smoking take many years or decades to become apparent, declining smoking rates and increasing public health campaigns against tobacco will take years or even decades to make a dent in the current death toll.

Unfortunately, smoking cigarettes remains the leading cause of death in the United States even though cigarette use has declined substantially in United States and other industrialized nations. However, there is reason for hope, as evidenced by outcomes of public health programs in the state of California, where aggressive campaigns with provisions for treatment did ultimately decrease cigarette use, which is currently at around 15% in the state (CDC 2011). This is the second lowest smoking rate in the nation, after Utah (13%). Interestingly, this decrease in smoking in California was followed by a substantial reduction in lung cancer incidence within 5 years and thereafter. For 2009 the incidence of new lung cancer cases/year was at 60 and 78 per 100,000 for California versus the US respectively, while in 1999 that incidence was at 75 and 93 cases per 100,000 for California versus the US respectively. This provides concrete evidence at the population level of the causal relationship between smoking and lung cancer and between quitting smoking and decreased lung cancer incidence.

Overall, despite several public health campaigns, one-fifth of the US population (<20%) currently smokes cigarettes. Unfortunately, smoking rates are substantially higher among certain groups; rates increase gradually with lower education levels and lower income levels. Yet 70% of smokers, when asked, say they would like to quit, and 40% of current smokers have made at least one quit attempt of at least 24 hours in the previous year, although only 6% manage to maintain abstinence from cigarettes when they quit without assistance (US Department of Health and Human Services 2000). Evidence shows that the difficulty in maintaining abstinence after quitting, whether assisted or not, is strongly related to affective and cognitive dysfunction, which may persist for some time after the initial cessation. In addition, cravings for cigarettes after cessation can result in a slip to smoking (less than 24 hours of smoking), and those slips often lead to full relapse to regular smoking.

Biological and Behavioral Determinants of Nicotine Dependence

The Reward Pathway

Cigarettes contain nicotine, a highly addicting substance. Like most drugs that are used for prolonged periods, nicotine can lead to dependence (traditionally referred to as addiction) because it acts on and stimulates specific receptors. Because nicotine receptors are spread in most areas of the brain, the administration of nicotine leads to a rapid increase in dopamine release within the nucleus accumbens and the ventral tegmental area (the two main areas of the reward pathway). This stimulation typically starts within 10 seconds of smoking a cigarette. It has been established that natural rewards such as food consumption, social affiliation, and sexual activity, which are linked to survival of the individual or species, also activate these two central areas of the reward pathway within the brain. The reward pathway has projections to many areas of the brain; of particular importance are the projections from the nucleus accumbens and ventral tegmental area to the prefrontal cortex, the amygdala, and the olfactory tubercle (Fig. 15.1). Several other brain systems (neurotransmitters and pathways) are thought to be involved in the process of developing

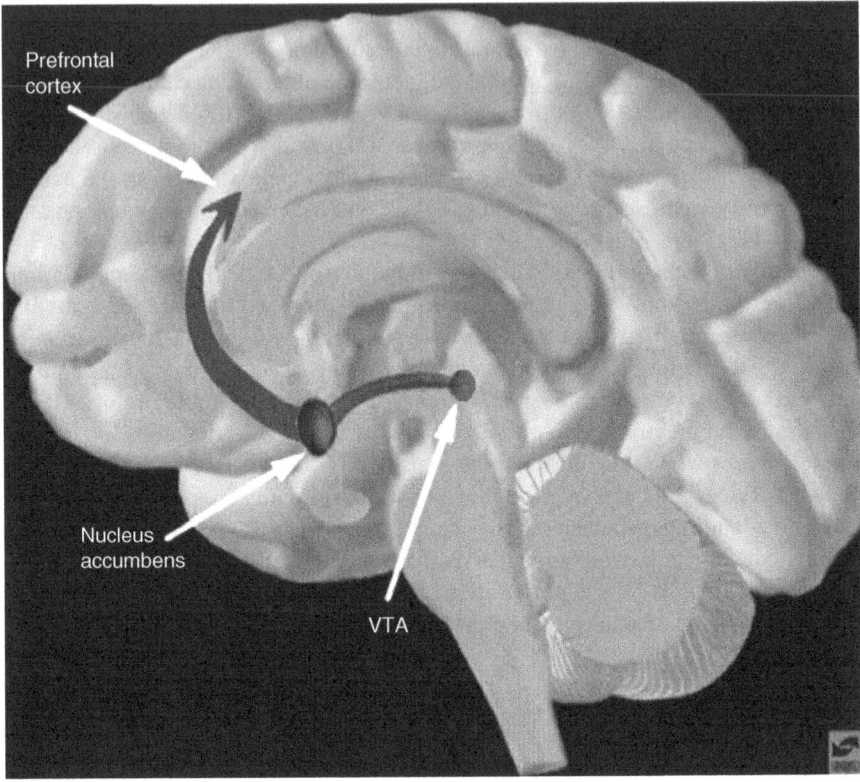

Fig. 15.1 The nucleus accumbens and ventral tegmental area (VTA) project to the prefrontal cortex as part of the reward pathway

dependence to a substance, although dopamine is referred to as the final or common neurotransmitter in the reward pathway.

Neuronal Adaptation

A pleasurable sensation from the activation of the reward pathway is associated with the acute use of a substance of abuse such as nicotine. However, repeated administration of a substance such as nicotine over months or years is likely to lead to increased tolerance, which in turn produces a state of withdrawal in the absence of the substance. Tolerance and withdrawal are the physiologic hallmarks of dependence and are thought to be the result of neuroadaptive effects occurring within the brain (Benowitz 2008). Interestingly, the chronic use of drugs of abuse and dependence (including nicotine) appears to result in a generalized decrease in dopaminergic neurotransmission. This decrease is likely to be a homeostatic response to the intermittent yet repetitive increases in dopamine induced by the frequent and sustained use of such drugs (Volkow et al. 2002).

Diagnosis of Nicotine Dependence

Because specific biological markers are absent, nicotine dependence is a clinical diagnosis. The Diagnostic and Statistical Manual of Mental Disorders, fifth edition (DSM-5; American Psychiatric Association 2013), employs universal criteria for all substance dependence, including nicotine use disorder (formerly nicotine dependence). According to DSM-5, a substance use disorder is diagnosed when the patient meets two or more of the 11 total criteria within a 12-month period. The DSM-5 criteria offer ease of use for the clinician because of the universality of the criteria to all substances of dependence. However, because of their universality, the DSM-5 criteria are not specific to tobacco and therefore do not capture many of the particular aspects of tobacco use and nicotine dependence. This nonspecific categorization has led to the development of specific scales to quantify nicotine dependence. Traditionally, the Fagerström Test of Nicotine Dependence has been used, although recently the Wisconsin Inventory of Smoking Dependence Motives has become more accepted as a more comprehensive scale.

Smoking and Psychiatric Comorbidities

Smoking rates among individuals with no mental illness, past-month mental illness, and lifetime mental illness have been reported to be 22%, 34%, and 41%, respectively. These rates indicate that having a current mental disorder effectively doubles the chances of being a smoker. Furthermore, in a nationally representative sample, smokers who had a mental disorder in the past month were reported to consume 44% of all cigarettes smoked (Lasser et al. 2000). Smoking seems to be closely linked with several psychiatric comorbidities, including dependence on other substances, suggesting a shared biological pathway between nicotine dependence and these other psychiatric conditions. Evidence of co-occurrence of mental illness with smoking also highlights the importance of screening and treating mental health disorders among smokers, whether the co-occurrence is causal or a simple correlation. Treating these comorbid mental disorders would at least reduce the impact of the disorders on patients' ability to quit smoking, and treating such disorders may increase patients' resilience against relapsing to cigarette use. This is of particular importance among patients who are in remission from cancer (survivors) who relapse to or continue to smoke and are unable to quit because they may still be recovering from the emotional toll of cancer, which often leads to clinical depression or anxiety disorders.

Treatment for Tobacco Use

To achieve maximum benefits, the treatment approach for tobacco use disorder (nicotine dependence) must be comprehensive, because the disease itself has multiple components. Similarly, the approach must be ongoing or longitudinal because dependence is a chronic relapsing disorder. The essential components of a treatment program are psychosocial therapies and medications. Therapies such as cognitive behavioral therapy, motivational interviewing, skills building, and problem solving have been shown empirically to be effective.

First-line medications approved by the US Food and Drug administration (FDA) comprise three major categories: (1) nicotine replacement therapies (NRTs); (2) sustained-release bupropion (bupropion-SR), a nicotine receptor antagonist; and (3) varenicline (Chantix), a nicotine receptor partial agonist. The US Department of Health and Human Services updated the Clinical Practice Guideline for Treating Tobacco Use and Dependence (CPG-TTUD) in 2008 (Fiore et al. 2008). This guideline is evidence-based and is considered the standard of practice in providing treatment for tobacco and smoking cessation; it can be summarized in ten key recommendations (Table 15.1). Medications have a big impact on smoking cessation, reduction of cravings, and mitigation of nicotine withdrawal symptoms. NRTs, bupropion-SR, and varenicline are first-line therapies for nicotine dependence (Table 15.2), whereas nortriptyline (Pamelor) and clonidine (Catapres) are not approved by the FDA for this particular use and are considered second-line therapies owing to their side effect profiles.

Nicotine Replacement Therapies

NRTs were the first pharmacologic treatments to be offered for smoking cessation. In general, the quit rate among smokers who use an NRT is double that of smokers who do not use an NRT (Karam-Hage and Cinciripini 2007). The FDA has approved the following NRTs for smoking cessation: 16- or 24-hour prescription or over-the-counter patch, prescription nasal spray or buccal inhaler, and over-the-counter polacrilex gum, flavored gum, and flavored lozenges and mini-lozenges (Table 15.2).

In a review of 103 trials of NRTs, the overall odds ratio for maintaining abstinence from cigarette smoking when using a single NRT, compared with placebo, was 1.77 (95% confidence interval, 1.66–1.88; Silagy et al. 2004). However, combinations of NRTs, in particular combining the patch with an episodic NRT (gum, lozenge, inhaler, or nasal spray), seemed to be more effective than any single NRT and may be more effective than any other pharmacologic treatment available today. Silagy et al. (2004) concluded that (1) 8 weeks of patch therapy is as effective as longer courses of patch therapy, and there is no evidence that tapering off patch therapy is better than ending patch therapy abruptly; (2) wearing a patch only during waking hours (for 16 hours per day) is as effective as wearing a patch for 24 hours per day; (3) gum may be offered on a fixed-dose or as-needed basis; (4) highly dependent smokers (e.g., those who need to smoke within 30 minutes of waking) and those who have been unable to quit with the 2-mg dose gum need the 4-mg dose gum; and (5) the effectiveness of NRTs appears to be largely independent of the intensity of psychosocial therapeutic support provided to the smoker.

Table 15.1 Ten key recommendations for tobacco and smoking cessation treatment programs

The overarching goal of these recommendations is that clinicians strongly recommend the use of effective tobacco dependence counseling and medication treatments to their patients who use tobacco, and that health systems, insurers, and purchasers assist clinicians in making such effective treatments available.

1. Tobacco dependence is a chronic disease that often requires repeated intervention and multiple attempts to quit. Effective treatments exist, however, that can significantly increase rates of long-term abstinence.

2. It is essential that clinicians and health care delivery systems consistently identify and document tobacco use status and treat every tobacco user seen in a health care setting.

3. Tobacco dependence treatments are effective across a broad range of populations. Clinicians should encourage every patient willing to make a quit attempt to use the counseling treatments and medications in this Guideline.

4. Brief tobacco dependence treatment is effective. Clinicians should offer every patient who uses tobacco at least the brief treatments shown to be effective in this Guideline.

5. Individual, group, and telephone counseling are effective, and their effectiveness increases with treatment intensity. Two components of counseling are especially effective, and clinicians should use these when counseling patients making a quit attempt:
   Practical counseling (problem solving/skills training)
   Social support delivered as part of treatment

6. Numerous effective medications are available for tobacco dependence, and clinicians should encourage their use by all patients attempting to quit smoking—except when medically contraindicated or with specific populations for which there is insufficient evidence of effectiveness (i.e., pregnant women, smokeless tobacco users, light smokers, and adolescents).
   Seven first-line medications (five nicotine and two non-nicotine) reliably increase long-term abstinence: bupropion-SR, nicotine gum, nicotine inhaler, nicotine lozenge, nicotine nasal spray, nicotine patch, and varenicline.
   Clinicians also should consider the use of certain effective combinations of medications in this Guideline.

7. Counseling and medication are effective when used individually for treating tobacco dependence. The combination of counseling and medication, however, is more effective than either treatment alone. Thus, clinicians should encourage all individuals making a quit attempt to use both counseling and medication.

8. Telephone quitline counseling is effective with diverse populations and has broad reach. Therefore, both clinicians and health care delivery systems should ensure patient access to quitlines and promote quitline use.

9. If a tobacco user currently is unwilling to make a quit attempt, clinicians should use the motivational treatments shown in this Guideline to be effective in increasing future quit attempts.

10. Tobacco dependence treatments are both clinically effective and highly cost-effective relative to interventions for other clinical disorders. Providing coverage for these treatments increases quit rates. Insurers and purchasers should ensure that all insurance plans include the effective counseling and medication in this Guideline as covered benefits.

From the US Department of Health and Human Services Clinical Practice Guideline for Treating Tobacco Use and Dependence (Fiore et al. 2008)

Table 15.2 Dosage and availability of US Food and Drug Administration–approved pharmacologic agents for smoking cessation

Cessation agent	Dosage	Label indication and use	Availability in the United States	OR of efficacy (95% CI)
Nicotine gum	2 and 4 mg	2 mg for ≤25 cigarettes per day and 4 mg for >25 cigarettes per day; minimum 8 pieces per day, maximum 20 pieces per day	OTC; traditional, mint, and orange flavors; generic available	1.66 (1.52–1.81)[a]
Nicotine patch	21, 14, and 7 mg	≥10 cigarettes per day: 21 mg for 6 weeks, then 14 mg for 2 weeks, then 7 mg for 2 weeks	OTC; clear and skin color; generic available	1.81 (1.63–2.02)[a]
Nicotine nasal spray	10 mg/mL, 0.5 mg per squirt	2 squirts (1 dose) per hour, minimum 8 doses per day, maximum 40 doses per day	Prescription only, 100 mg per bottle; no generic	2.35 (1.63–3.38)[a]
Nicotine oral inhaler	10 mg per cartridge, 4 mg delivered	6–16 cartridges per day up to 12 weeks, then gradual reduction for 12 weeks	Prescription only, 168 cartridges per box; no generic	2.14 (1.44–3.18)[a]
Nicotine lozenges	2 and 4 mg	If first cigarette is ≤30 minutes after waking, use 4-mg lozenge; if >30 minutes, use 2-mg lozenge; minimum 8 lozenges per day, maximum 20 lozenges per day	OTC; mint and cherry flavors; no generic	2.05 (1.62–2.59)[a]
Bupropion-SR	100 and 150 mg	150 mg every morning for 3 days, then 150 mg twice daily for 3 months	Prescription only; generic available	1.94 (1.72–2.19)[b]
Varenicline	0.5 and 1 mg	0.5 mg every morning for 3 days, then 0.5 mg twice daily for 4 days, then 1 mg twice daily up to 3 months; if quit, another 3 months	Prescription only; no generic	High dose 3.09 (1.95–4.91)[c]; low dose 2.66 (1.72–4.11)[d]

Adapted from Karam-Hage and Cinciripini (2007)

OR indicates odds ratio, *CI* confidence interval, *OTC* over the counter

[a]OR for comparative efficacy of nicotine replacement therapies and control (placebo), as reviewed by Silagy et al. (2004)

[b]OR for overall bupropion-SR efficacy, as reviewed by Hughes et al. (2007)

[c]OR for varenicline efficacy compared with placebo; Gonzales et al. (2006)

[d]OR for varenicline efficacy compared with placebo; Jorenby et al. (2006)

Patient education and management of expectations are key aspects of the clinical visit before treatment begins. This is especially true for combination approaches, such as the simultaneous use of two NRTs, use of bupropion-SR plus an NRT, or use of bupropion-SR plus varenicline. Although NRTs carry a warning that patients should not use them while continuing to smoke, the use of any NRT, such as gums, inhalers, and patches, has been deemed safe even in patients who continue to smoke. In fact, studies have shown that the use of NRTs while continuing to smoke helped reduce the number of cigarettes smoked per day by as much as 50% among participants who were not motivated to quit, without any significant nicotine toxicity or major adverse events. NRTs have a minor side effect profile: the patch can cause local skin irritation, nausea, or headaches in some patients; oral NRTs may cause nausea, sore throat, or mouth sores in those receiving chemotherapy; and the nasal spray may cause nasal irritation (Physicians' Desk Reference 2013).

A trend in smoking cessation pharmacotherapy is the combination of NRTs or the combination of NRTs with bupropion-SR, which has a different mechanism of action. A recent large and well-designed placebo-controlled trial was conducted among volunteers recruited from the community (Piper et al. 2009). In that trial, three monotherapies (bupropion-SR, patch, and lozenge) and two combination therapies (bupropion-SR plus lozenge and patch plus lozenge) were compared; the patch and lozenge combination produced the greatest benefit relative to placebo for smoking cessation, and bupropion-SR plus lozenge came in as a close second best (Piper et al. 2009). An effectiveness trial by the same research group using the same monotherapies and combinations was conducted in a primary care patient population (Smith et al. 2009). The combination of bupropion-SR plus lozenge was superior to each monotherapy tested and resulted in a smoking abstinence rate of 30% at 6-month follow-up. In addition, the combination of the patch and lozenge was the second-best therapy tested and was superior to any of the monotherapies (Smith et al. 2009).

Bupropion-SR

In 1991 the FDA approved bupropion-SR, under the name Zyban, for the treatment of nicotine dependence, although it was originally approved as an antidepressant. Bupropion is considered an atypical antidepressant because it does not have a clearly known mechanism of action. However, its pharmacodynamic properties include inhibition of norepinephrine reuptake and, to some extent, dopamine reuptake. These inhibitory properties are thought to play a role in its mechanisms of action as an antidepressant and possibly as a treatment for nicotine dependence. In addition, bupropion was found to have some activity as a noncompetitive antagonist on high-affinity $\alpha 4\beta 2$ subnicotinic acetylcholinergic receptors. One of the drug's metabolites, (2S,3S)-hydroxybupropion, could have more powerful antagonist activity against $\alpha 4\beta 2$ receptors than bupropion itself. This metabolite may also reduce nicotine reward, withdrawal symptoms, and cravings. Bupropion-SR therapy is typically started 1–2 weeks before the planned quit date at a dosage of 150 mg per day for 3–7 days; then it is increased to 150 mg twice per day.

Unfortunately, use of bupropion-SR is limited by its contraindication for patients with a family or personal history of seizure, a personal history of head trauma, or a history of bulimia and anorexia nervosa. The most commonly reported adverse events with use of bupropion-SR are anxiety, insomnia, dry mouth, and tremors; therefore, bupropion-SR should be used cautiously in patients who may already have these symptoms. Bupropion-SR is also relatively contraindicated in patients who have elevated liver enzyme levels (>3× the upper limit of normal) because it is metabolized extensively in the liver and its metabolites may accumulate and lead to toxic effects.

A recent meta-analysis based on 44 clinical trials that included more than 13,000 smokers showed that bupropion-SR was more effective than placebo in helping patients achieve long-term (6–12 months) abstinence from smoking (risk ratio, 1.62; 95% confidence interval, 1.49–1.76; Hughes et al. 2014). Bupropion-SR also has been shown to be effective in primary care settings and in several special clinical populations, such as patients with schizophrenia, patients with depression, veterans (Beckham 1999), and patients who have posttraumatic stress disorder (Hertzberg et al. 2001).

Bupropion-SR offers unique advantages for cancer survivors, especially those who have depression or attention deficit hyperactivity disorder, because it may alleviate the comorbid symptoms in addition to helping with smoking cessation. Another advantage of bupropion-SR is its potential attenuation of the weight gain associated with smoking cessation, an important issue for smokers who are obese, overweight, or afraid of gaining weight after quitting. Bupropion-SR also has a subtle positive effect on sexual dysfunction (through an unknown mechanism); this is an important advantage because smoking and cancer treatment are known to cause impotence and other sexual dysfunction.

Bupropion-SR has some side effects, most commonly dry mouth, insomnia, and hand tremors, and rarely seizures, depression, or suicidal ideation (Physicians' Desk Reference 2013).

Varenicline

Varenicline (Chantix in the United States, Champix in other countries) is the first pharmaceutically designed compound with partial agonist effects on nicotinic receptors to become available on the market. Varenicline is a selective partial agonist that occupies and stimulates $\alpha 4\beta 2$ nicotinic cholinergic receptors; consequently, it stimulates dopamine release in the nucleus accumbens, although to a lesser extent (40–60% less) than nicotine itself. By binding competitively to nicotinic receptors throughout its relatively long half-life of 24 hours, varenicline also displays antagonistic properties, in that it prevents the full stimulation of the nicotinic receptors that ensues when nicotine is co-administered. Because of these mixed properties, varenicline may provide relief from withdrawal symptoms, via its agonist effect, while blocking the rewarding effects of nicotine, via its antagonist effect (Gonzales et al. 2006).

Two initial randomized, double-blind clinical trials showed that varenicline (2 mg per day) is more effective for smoking cessation than placebo (odds ratio ≈ 3) and bupropion-SR (300 mg per day; odds ratio ≈ 2). The overall continuous smoking abstinence rates from the end of the 12-week treatment through 1-year follow-up were 21% for varenicline, 16% for bupropion-SR, and 8% for placebo in one study (Gonzales et al. 2006) and 23%, 14%, and 10%, respectively, in the other study (Jorenby et al. 2006). In a combined analysis of the two trials, treatment with varenicline resulted in significantly higher continuous smoking abstinence rates at 1 year than did treatment with placebo alone or bupropion-SR alone ($p < 0.05$ for both comparisons). In this pooled analysis, compared with placebo, varenicline nearly tripled the odds of a smoker quitting, even when a conservative definition (continued abstinence during the last 4 weeks of treatment with the medication) was used as the outcome measure (odds ratio, 3.09; 95% confidence interval, 1.95–4.91; $p < 0.001$).

In a randomized, double-blind continuation study of the same treatments, an additional 12 weeks of treatment with varenicline or placebo (for a total of 24 weeks of treatment) was administered to patients who had abstained from smoking at some point during the first 3 months of treatment with varenicline. In that trial, patients who received varenicline during the 12-week extension period reported significantly fewer cravings and diminished withdrawal symptoms throughout the trial, and 70% of them remained abstinent at the end of the 12-week extension period. In contrast, only 50% of patients who were randomized to receive a placebo during the 12-week extension period remained abstinent at the end of the study. Furthermore, the 1-year follow-up abstinence rate (i.e., 1 year after treatment was completed) in patients who had received 24 weeks of treatment with varenicline was twice that of patients who had received only 12 weeks of treatment with varenicline (25 and 12%, respectively; Tonstad et al. 2006).

The most commonly observed adverse effect of varenicline was nausea, which occurred in up to 30% of patients receiving the medication (approximately twice the rate of nausea observed in patients receiving a placebo); fortunately, the nausea was mild to moderate in most cases. Other commonly reported adverse events were flatulence and abnormal dreams. Recently, the FDA has received a large amount of MedWatch voluntary reports indicating an increased risk for neuropsychiatric events among people taking varenicline. Most of these events consisted of depressive symptoms, irritability, aggression, or suicidal ideation, as well as difficulty with motor coordination. As a result, the FDA mandated the inclusion of specific warnings about the possibility of occurrence of these symptoms on the medication label; it also recommended that patients stop the medication immediately and report to their health care providers if they develop such symptoms. The FDA has commissioned further analysis of existing data and mandated that the manufacturer conduct postmarket prospective studies to clarify the relationship between these adverse effects and varenicline and the magnitude of such occurrences (FDA 2008).

For many patients, the prospect of trying a new treatment option (i.e., varenicline) could motivate them to try to quit smoking again, especially among those who have not succeeded in quitting with prior established smoking cessation medications. In addition, a combination strategy such as adding bupropion-SR to varenicline or vice versa may increase the efficacy of smoking cessation (Ebbert et al. 2009). The combination may also mitigate the emergence of depression and other neuropsychiatric symptoms (Karam-Hage et al. 2010); bupropion-SR is expected to counterbalance the neuropsychiatric side effects that may occur with varenicline.

A recent Cochrane review concluded that, at 6-month follow-up, treatment with varenicline at the standard dose (2 mg per day) more than doubled the chances of abstaining from smoking compared with treatment with placebo. Low-dose varenicline (1 mg per day) roughly doubled the chances of quitting compared with placebo and reduced the number and severity of side effects compared with the standard dose of varenicline. The number of patients who quit smoking after treatment with varenicline was higher than the number of patients who quit smoking after treatment with bupropion-SR. Interestingly, the Cochrane review also reported that two trials of nicotine patches did not show that varenicline had a clear benefit over the nicotine patch at 6-month follow-up (Cahill et al. 2011). Another important factor in an era of cost containment is the cost-effectiveness of a new treatment; the review indicated that varenicline seemed to be more cost-effective than bupropion-SR in most cost-effectiveness models studied.

Nonpharmacologic Treatments

Behavioral therapy delivered by physicians, psychologists, nurses, pharmacists, dentists, and other clinicians increases patients' smoking abstinence rates; this is especially true when "the 5 A's" are applied: Ask patients if they smoke, Advise them to quit, Assess motivation for change, Assist if they are willing to change, and Arrange for follow-up.

Sixty-four behavioral therapy studies met selection criteria for meta-analyses performed for the CPG-TTUD in 2000; these meta-analyses were needed to examine the effectiveness of interventions using various types of counseling and behavioral therapies. In these meta-analyses, four specific categories of counseling and behavioral therapy yielded statistically significant increases in smoking abstinence rates relative to no contact (i.e., untreated control conditions). These categories were (1) providing practical counseling such as problem solving, skills training, or stress management; (2) providing support during a smoker's direct contact with a clinician (intratreatment social support); (3) intervening to increase social support in the smoker's environment (extratreatment social support); and (4) using aversive smoking procedures (rapid smoking, rapid puffing, other smoking exposure). These recommendations remained the same for the updated CPG-TTUD in 2008 because no newer studies or therapies were available to warrant additional analysis.

Of interest is the finding that even minimal interventions lasting less than 3 minutes increased overall cigarette abstinence rates. Every smoker should be offered at least a minimal intervention, whether or not he or she is eventually referred to an intensive intervention. In addition, a strong dose-response relationship has been observed between the session length of person-to-person contact and successful treatment outcomes. Intensive interventions are more effective than less intensive interventions and should be used whenever possible. Person-to-person treatment delivered for four or more sessions appears especially effective in increasing cigarette abstinence rates. Therefore, if feasible, clinicians should strive to meet four or more times with individuals trying to quit smoking. In a meta-analysis for the CPG-TTUD of 2000 and 2008, incremental improvements in abstinence rates were observed with an increasing number of sessions and total duration of treatment. These incremental improvements were categorized into intervals: abstinence rate of 22% (odds ratio, 1) with one session, abstinence rate of 28% (odds ratio, 1.4) with 2–3 sessions, abstinence rate of 27% (odds ratio, 1.3) with 4–8 sessions, and abstinence rate of 33% (odds ratio, 1.7) with >8 sessions. Unfortunately, the vast majority of pharmacologic trials provide only minimal behavioral therapy of around 10 minutes' duration as the minimal standard to show efficacy of a medication, which seems to carry on to clinical practice by necessity owing to the pressures on clinical providers to deliver more services in less time.

Strategies to Treat Cancer Survivors Who Are Hard-Core Smokers

Despite exposure to the best treatments, about 60–65% of smokers do not manage to quit smoking after a single quit attempt, and less than a quarter of the 35–40% who do succeed are able to stay abstinent 1 year later (Fiore et al. 2008). This is probably due to a multitude of factors, including genetic predisposition to nicotine dependence, psychiatric comorbidities, and readiness to quit. These resilient smokers are often called "hard-core" smokers, because they did not respond to treatment and remain smoking even after major health events related to smoking, such as cancer. Among this group of hard-core smokers are many cancer survivors, some of whom may have quit temporarily out of fear and the shock of "having cancer" or in response to pressure from their doctors and family, only to return to smoking once they started to feel healthier. Therefore, it is not sufficient to provide cancer survivors with basic smoking cessation therapy and expect them to have the same response as the average smoker in the community. Despite lack of controlled trials, cancer survivors need intensive interventions, including both behavioral and pharmacologic approaches.

As mentioned above, the CPG-TTUD of 2008 shows clear evidence of a dose-response relationship in exposure to psychosocial interventions, in terms of both duration and frequency. A variety of techniques have been suggested and other novel approaches can be used to help hard-core smokers. Two types of combination pharmacotherapy have been used successfully: (1) combinations of different forms of NRT with different pharmacokinetic profiles (e.g., nicotine patch+nicotine gum), and (2) combinations of treatments with different therapeutic targets, such as NRT+non-nicotine medications or two non-nicotine medications (e.g., bupropion-SR+NRT or bupropion-SR+varenicline; Ebbert et al. 2010).

The Tobacco Treatment Program at MD Anderson

The Tobacco Treatment Program (TTP) at MD Anderson is a fully integrated multidisciplinary program because it provides an integrated mental health and substance use treatment model. The TTP model consists of providing psychosocial treatment from counselors with master's degrees or PhDs and providing medical and psychiatric treatment from a physician assistant, nurse, and psychiatrist specializing in addiction treatment. The addiction psychiatrist provides the specialized expertise on treatment plans and treats mental health and other substance use disorders (in addition to nicotine dependence).

A common clinical dilemma faced by the TTP team is whether it is best to treat co-occurring disorders simultaneously, sequentially, or in any particular order. Unfortunately, the literature is scant, and some of it is conflicting with regard to this issue. Our treatment philosophy at the TTP is to provide individualized treatment for each patient. For patients who are interested and feel that they are able to initiate treatment for both disorders simultaneously, we help them to do so, whereas for others who are reluctant or not ready to quit smoking, we try to treat the comorbid conditions first, in hope of building therapeutic alliances and stabilizing patients' mood and affect. This approach almost always improves patients' self-esteem and self-efficacy while it builds a therapeutic alliance that prepares them to then tackle smoking cessation. Of note, self-efficacy has been found to be correlated at various levels with the ability to initiate and succeed at quitting smoking.

The MD Anderson TTP, which was launched in 2006, was modeled on the CPG-TTUD for 2000. Through the end of August 2013, the TTP had served 4,111 new patients and conducted about 35,000 follow-up appointments since its inception in January 2006. The TTP has served patients from more than 50 MD Anderson clinical departments.

The demographics and other common measures of our patient population have remained somewhat constant, as illustrated in Table 15.3 (showing both demographics over time and for the 2013 fiscal year specifically) and Table 15.4. It is noteworthy that a substantial number of our patients also present with one or more psychiatric diagnoses (Fig. 15.2). In 2011, we analyzed our 6-month follow-up data, on the basis of cohorts treated from the start of the program in 2006 until the end of 2010. The 6-month abstinence rate (7-day point prevalence at 6 months after the end of treatment) among those who were able to reach abstinence (respondent-only) was 46% (n=1,291; response rate, 74%); however, when an intention-to-treat model is used (including all patients treated at baseline and assuming all those lost to follow-up have relapsed to smoking), the 6-month abstinent rate (7-day point prevalence at 6 months after the end of treatment) dropped to 34% (n=1,670). Also of interest is

Table 15.3 MD Anderson Tobacco Treatment Program patient demographics for 2006–2013 and for fiscal year 2013 (FY13)

Characteristic	FY13 (%)	2006–2013 (%)
Ethnicity		
Black	10.7	10.3
Hispanic	5.2	5.2
Other	6.5	7.1
White	77.7	77.4
Sex		
Female	49.5	50.4
Male	50.5	49.6
Location		
Houston metro	61.0	57.7
Texas	25.2	26.3
Other state	12.4	15.0
Outside United States	1.3	1.0

Table 15.4 MD Anderson Tobacco Treatment Program patient clinical characteristics for fiscal year 2013

Characteristic	Mean	SD
Age (years)	56.1	11.6
Cigarettes per day	15.8	10.5
Drinks per day	1.9	3.5
Years smoked	33.3	13.9
Fagerström Test for Nicotine Dependence score	4.3	2.2
Center for Epidemiologic Studies-Depression score	14.0	11.5
Positive and Negative Affect Schedule scores		
Negative affect	20.7	8.4
Positive affect	30.3	7.6

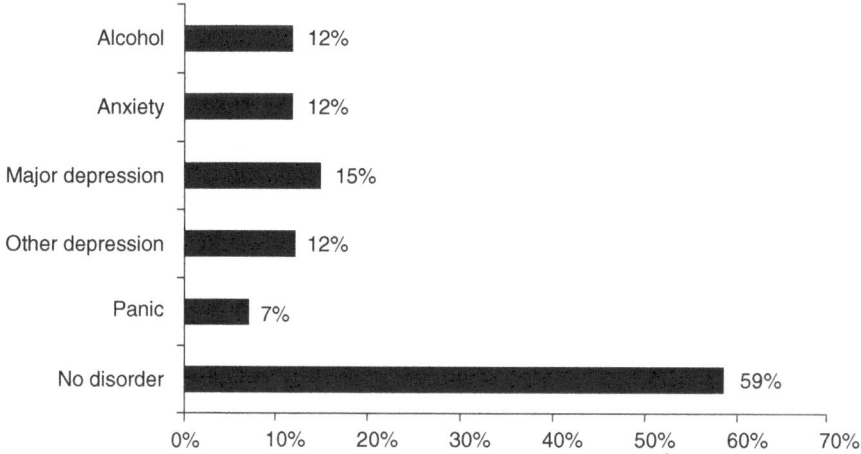

Fig. 15.2 Frequency of co-occurring psychiatric disorders among patients who visited the MD Anderson Tobacco Treatment Program in fiscal year 2013

our finding that non-quitters reduced their daily cigarette consumption by ~44% from baseline to the end of treatment (from 16 [standard deviation, 12.2] to nine [standard deviation, 9.1] cigarettes per day; n=1,034) and by ~38% from baseline to 6 months after the end of treatment (from 16 to 10 cigarettes per day; n=663). This reduction represents a significant change in behavior.

We pride ourselves with our program's success, measured by the 34–46% of patients who were abstinent from cigarettes at the 6-month follow-up point (7-day point prevalence of smoking abstinence rates). By comparison, the 4-week point prevalence smoking abstinence rates in a highly motivated population of healthy smokers were shown to range from 24% in patients treated with bupropion-SR to 35% in patients treated with varenicline, after 12 weeks of treatment (Gonzales et al. 2006; Jorenby et al. 2006).

Key Practice Points

- Tobacco use is responsible for more than 30% of cancer-related mortality and is the top cause of death in the United States. About 450,000 people in the United States and about five million globally die every year from tobacco-related illnesses.
- Nicotine is the addictive substance in tobacco; it stimulates nicotine receptors and consequently the reward areas of the brain.
- Behavioral and pharmacologic therapies successfully treat tobacco use; however, they work best when used together.
- Seven medications have been approved by the FDA for use as monotherapy for tobacco cessation.
- When used in certain combinations, medications can be a useful tool for tobacco cessation, especially among cancer survivors who are "hard-core" smokers.
- Minimal counseling can make a difference in smoking cessation rates; however, there is a dose-response rate in frequency and total amount of time dedicated to counseling smokers.
- Comprehensive cancer treatment needs to include tobacco cessation treatment, in particular to avoid treatment complications and disease recurrence among survivors.

Suggested Readings

American Psychiatric Association. *Diagnostic and Statistical Manual of Mental Disorders*. 5th ed. Washington, DC: American Psychiatric Association; 2013.

Beckham JC. Smoking and anxiety in combat veterans with chronic posttraumatic stress disorder: a review. *J Psychoactive Drugs* 1999;31:103–110.

Benowitz NL. Neurobiology of nicotine addiction: implications for smoking cessation treatment. *Am J Med* 2008;121:S3–S10.

Cahill K, Stead LF, Lancaster T. Nicotine receptor partial agonists for smoking cessation. *Cochrane Database of Systematic Review* 2011;2:1–87.

Ebbert JO, Croghan IT, Sood A, Schroeder DR, Hays JT, Hurt RD. Varenicline and bupropion sustained release combination therapy for smoking cessation. *Nicotine Tob Res* 2009;11: 234–239.

Ebbert JO, Hays JT, Hurt RD. Combination pharmacotherapy for stopping smoking: what advantages does it offer? *Drugs* 2010;70:643–650.

Fiore MC, Jaen CR, Baker TB, et al. *Treating Tobacco Use and Dependence: 2008 Update. Clinical Practice Guideline.* Rockville, MD: US Department of Health and Human Services; 2008.

Gonzales D, Rennard SI, Nides M, et al. Varenicline, an alpha4beta2 nicotinic acetylcholine receptor partial agonist, vs sustained-release bupropion and placebo for smoking cessation: a randomized controlled trial. *JAMA* 2006;296:47–55.

Hertzberg MA, Moore SD, Feldman ME, Beckham JC. A preliminary study of bupropion sustained-release for smoking cessation in patients with chronic posttraumatic stress disorder. *J Clin Psychopharmacol* 2001;21:94–98.

Hughes JR, Stead LF, Hartman-Boyce J, Cahill K, Lancaster T. Antidepressants for smoking cessation. *Cochrane Database of Systematic Reviews* 2014;1:CD000031 pub4.

Hughes JR, Stead LF, Lancaster T. Antidepressants for smoking cessation. *Cochrane Database of Systematic Reviews* 2007;1:CD000031.

Jorenby DE, Hays JT, Rigotti NA, et al. Efficacy of varenicline, an alpha4beta2 nicotinic acetylcholine receptor partial agonist, vs placebo or sustained-release bupropion for smoking cessation: a randomized controlled trial. *JAMA* 2006;296:56–63.

Karam-Hage M, Cinciripini PM. Pharmacotherapy for tobacco cessation: nicotine agonists, antagonists, and partial agonists. *Curr Oncol Rep* 2007;9:509–516.

Karam-Hage M, Shah K, Cinciripini PM. Addition of bupropion-SR to varenicline alleviated depression and suicidal ideation: a case report. *Prim Care Companion J Clin Psychiatry* 2010;12:e1.

Lasser K, Boyd JW, Woolhandler S, Himmelstein DU, McCormick D, Bor DH. Smoking and mental illness: a population-based prevalence study. *JAMA* 2000;284:2606–2610.

Physicians' Desk Reference. 67th ed. Montvale, NJ: Thompson Publications; 2013.

Piper ME, Smith SS, Schlam TR, et al. A randomized placebo-controlled clinical trial of 5 smoking cessation pharmacotherapies. *Gen Psychiatry* 2009;66:1253–1262.

Silagy C, Lancaster T, Stead L, Mant D, Fowler G. Nicotine replacement therapy for smoking cessation. *Cochrane Database of Systematic Reviews* 2004;3:CD000146.

Smith SS, McCarthy DE, Janovitch S, et al. Comparative effectiveness of 5 smoking cessation pharmacotherapies in primary care clinics. *MD Arch Intern Med* 2009;169:2148–2155.

Tonstad S, Tonnesen P, Hajek P, et al. Effect of maintenance therapy with varenicline on smoking cessation: a randomized controlled trial. *JAMA* 2006;296:64–71.

US Centers for Disease Control and Prevention (CDC). Vital signs: current cigarette smoking among adults aged ≥18 years—United States, 2009. *MMWR Morb Mortal Wkly Rep* 2010;59:1135–1140.

US Centers for Disease Control and Prevention (CDC). State-specific trends in lung cancer incidence and smoking—United States, 1999–2008. *MMWR Morb Mortal Wkly Rep* 2011;60: 1243–1247.

US Centers for Disease Control and Prevention (CDC). Surveillance of demographic characteristics and health behaviors among adult cancer survivors—behavioral risk factor surveillance system, United States, 2009. *MMWR Morb Mortal Wkly Rep* 2012;61:1–23.

US Department of Health and Human Services. *Reducing Tobacco Use: A Report of the Surgeon General.* Atlanta, GA: US Department of Health and Human Services, Public Health Service, Centers for Disease Control, Centers for Chronic Disease Prevention and Health Promotion, Office on Smoking and Health; 2000.

US Food and Drug Administration (FDA). *Public Health Advisory: Important Information on Chantix (varenicline).* Rockville, MD: US Department of Health and Human Services; 2008.

Volkow ND, Fowler J, Wang G-J. Role of dopamine in drug reinforcement and addiction in humans: results from imaging studies. *Behav Pharmacol* 2002;13:355–366.

Chapter 16
Obesity and Exercise

Karen Basen-Engquist

Contents

Chapter Overview Physical inactivity and obesity are common problems among cancer survivors. Physical inactivity and obesity are risk factors for several forms of cancer, and weight gain and declines in physical activity often occur after a cancer diagnosis and during treatment. Low physical activity has been shown to lead to poor outcomes in breast and colon cancer survivors, and exercise interventions for survivors improve physical functioning and quality of life in several domains. Some evidence suggests that weight changes in breast cancer survivors may affect disease-free survival, but the evidence is conflicting on this point. Obesity can decrease cancer survivors' quality of life, as well as increase their risks for comorbid health problems. The American Cancer Society has recently published nutrition, physical activity, and weight management recommendations for cancer survivors. Survivorship care should include giving survivors access to this information.

L.E. Foxhall, M.A. Rodriguez (eds.), *Advances in Cancer Survivorship Management*,
MD Anderson Cancer Care Series, DOI 10.1007/978-1-4939-0986-5_16,
© The University of Texas M.D. Anderson Cancer Center 2015

In addition, encouraging survivors to adopt evidence-based behavioral strategies such as setting goals, monitoring themselves, changing their environment, and seeking social support can facilitate healthful behavior changes.

Introduction

Physical inactivity and obesity increase the risk of developing several cancers, including colon cancer, endometrial cancer, and postmenopausal breast cancer. Individuals often become less active as they go through treatment for cancer, even those who were previously active, because of symptoms and side effects of the treatment. Furthermore, weight gain is common in individuals who have been diagnosed with breast cancer, and evidence is emerging that weight gain is an issue for other cancer survivors as well, including survivors of testicular cancer (Sagstuen et al. 2005), prostate cancer treated with hormonal therapy (Kim et al. 2010), childhood brain tumors (Lustig et al. 2003), or childhood acute lymphoblastic leukemia treated with cranial radiation (Garmey et al. 2008). Thus, physical inactivity and obesity are prevalent in cancer survivor populations.

Physical inactivity and obesity are salient issues in survivorship care because they affect survivor quality of life and may put survivors at increased risk of developing recurrent disease (for breast and colon cancer) and certain second primary cancers. Providers should be aware of the implications of inactivity and obesity for cancer survivors and provide appropriate advice and counseling for behavioral change when warranted.

Exercise and Physical Activity in Cancer Survivors

Relationship to Disease Outcomes

Physical activity after diagnosis has been linked to decreased risk of recurrence and improved disease-specific and overall survival in breast and colorectal cancer survivors. These data are based on observational studies, including cohort studies of cancer survivors and clinical treatment trials in which participants' physical activity was measured and a secondary analysis was conducted to investigate the relationship between physical activity and outcomes. In all of these observational studies, physical activity was measured prior to assessment of the outcomes or endpoints.

A review of observational studies showed that breast cancer survivors who engaged in physical activity after diagnosis reduced their risk of breast cancer recurrence and breast cancer-related death compared with survivors who were inactive (Ballard-Barbash et al. 2012). Although one study showed no relationship between leisure time physical activity and breast cancer-related death, four studies have demonstrated a 35–51% reduction in breast cancer-related death among survivors who engaged in leisure time physical activity, and two have shown a trend in favor of reduced breast cancer-related death for those who engaged in leisure time physical activity.

For colorectal cancer, increased levels of physical activity are associated with reduced cancer-specific mortality and overall mortality. In one study of patients with stage III colorectal cancer, activity levels of 18 or more metabolic equivalent hours per week (equivalent to about 6 hours of moderate-intensity walking) were associated with a 47% improvement in disease-free survival rates (Meyerhardt et al. 2006). Observational studies have explored molecular modifiers of this effect, with results showing a relationship between postdiagnosis physical activity and disease-free survival only among colorectal cancer survivors who were positive for tumor alterations of cadherin-associated protein $\beta 1$ (Morikawa et al. 2011) or whose tumors showed loss of p27 (Meyerhardt et al. 2009).

Relationship to Quality of Life and Comorbidities

Exercise and physical activity have a range of other quality-of-life and health benefits for cancer survivors as well. Improvements in quality of life associated with exercise have been demonstrated in multiple randomized clinical trials, most of which compared outcomes in randomized groups of survivors participating in a supervised exercise intervention with outcomes in a control group of survivors who did not exercise or received the intervention after the final assessment.

Speck et al. (2010) published a systematic review of 82 randomized trials of exercise interventions published through November 2009, 66 of which were of sufficient quality to calculate effect sizes. Forty percent of the studies were conducted in patients during treatment and 60% were conducted after treatment. Eighty percent of the studies tested aerobic exercise interventions or aerobic exercise combined with other exercise modalities. Eighty-three percent of the studies involved breast cancer survivors. The exercise interventions, whether provided during or after treatment, were shown to increase physical activity levels, aerobic fitness, and upper and lower body strength, all very salient outcomes in cancer survivors, who are often in a deconditioned state after cancer treatment. Interventions conducted during treatment improved functional aspects of quality of life, anxiety, and self-esteem, and exercise interventions conducted after treatment positively influenced overall quality of life, breast cancer-specific aspects of quality of life, fatigue, self-reported mental confusion, and body image.

Exercise during and after treatment has also been shown to decrease body weight and body fat percentage. A recent Cochrane review of the quality-of-life benefits of exercise in cancer survivors showed that exercise programs improved quality of life in similar domains to those examined in the review by Speck et al. as well as sexuality, social functioning, and sleep disturbance (Mishra et al. 2012). Although the idea that exercise might improve cognitive functioning is intriguing, as has been observed in studies linking exercise in the elderly with improved cognitive functioning, the Cochrane review did not find sufficient evidence to determine whether exercise improved cognitive functioning in cancer survivors (Mishra et al. 2012).

Although only a few trials have examined resistance training interventions, this exercise modality has been shown to positively influence very salient quality-of-life issues in cancer survivors. Schmitz et al. (2009, 2010) conducted a randomized trial of a progressive weight training program for breast cancer survivors. The question of whether weight training is safe and beneficial for breast cancer survivors had been a controversial issue because of concerns that upper body exercise on the survivors' affected side could increase the risk of lymphedema. Participants in the progressive weight training program (154 of whom did not have lymphedema and 141 of whom had stable lymphedema) attended 90-minute small group sessions supervised by a fitness professional twice per week for 13 weeks. The first sessions started with 2 sets of 10 repetitions using low weight and gradually increased to 3 sets of 10 repetitions, and participants increased the weight if their symptoms did not increase. After the 13 weeks of supervised sessions, participants continued to do the exercises unsupervised twice per week. The intervention increased upper and lower body strength and was found to be safe for both participants with stable lymphedema at baseline and participants who did not have lymphedema. No significant difference was found between the weight training group and the control group in the proportion of patients who experienced a 5% or greater change in limb swelling. Among patients who had lymphedema, participants in the weight training group experienced fewer exacerbations of their lymphedema, and fewer and less severe symptoms, than did participants in the control group (Schmitz et al. 2009).

Exercise can also help improve health and quality of life in cancer survivors through its effects on comorbid health problems. This is important because, with advances in early detection and treatment, many survivors die of diseases other than cancer. In addition, some chronic diseases (e.g., arthritis) may not cause death but can decrease a survivor's health and physical functioning. Exercise has been shown to reduce the risk of cardiovascular disease and diabetes, as well as improve physical functioning among individuals with chronic conditions such as arthritis.

Obesity

Relationship to Disease Outcomes

Obesity may increase cancer survivors' risk of poor cancer outcomes, including recurrence and cancer-related death, especially among those with breast, prostate, and colon cancer (reviewed by Demark-Wahnefried et al. 2012). However, much of the negative effect of obesity appears to be related to body mass index at diagnosis, and it is unclear whether weight loss after diagnosis improves outcomes. Studies investigating whether weight loss improves outcomes are complicated by the fact that it is often unclear whether the weight loss was intentional or unintentional (e.g., weight loss caused by cachexia may indicate disease progression).

Weight gain is common among breast cancer survivors, and some studies have shown that this weight gain is linked to increased breast cancer-related death. Analyzing data from the Nurses' Health Study, Kroenke et al. (2005) found that among never-smokers, weight gain after a breast cancer diagnosis was associated with an increase in breast cancer-related death (65% increase among those who gained more than 2.0 kg/m^2). Nichols et al. (2009) analyzed a cohort of 3,993 breast cancer survivors and found that among women who gained more than 10 kg, all-cause mortality increased by 70% and breast cancer-related death increased by 78% compared with women whose weight was stable. Other observational studies have not shown a relationship between weight gain and risk of recurrence (Caan et al. 2008), although one study, which analyzed two cohorts of early-stage breast cancer survivors, showed a decreased risk of recurrence in women who lost a moderate amount of weight (5–10%) in one of the cohorts (Caan et al. 2006).

Additionally, findings from the Women's Intervention Nutrition Study indicated that among hormone receptor-negative breast cancer survivors who were randomized to receive a low-fat diet intervention, relapse-free survival improved by 24% compared with the control group (Chlebowski et al. 2006). The beneficial effect of the intervention may have been related to the weight loss that occurred in the low-fat diet group. In the Women's Healthy Eating and Living trial, in which breast cancer survivors were randomized to receive a high-fiber, low-fat diet high in vegetables and fruits or no intervention, no weight loss was observed in the intervention group and the intervention did not affect breast cancer event-free survival (Pierce et al. 2007a). However, secondary analyses to explore fruit and vegetable consumption in combination with exercise found that this combination led to a decreased risk of recurrence (Pierce et al. 2007b).

Relationship to Quality of Life

Obesity can also decrease cancer survivors' quality of life. Studies have shown that obesity in cancer survivors is related to increased fatigue and decreased physical functioning and quality of life (Basen-Engquist et al. 2009; Mosher et al. 2009). For example, in a survey of 753 survivors of breast, prostate, and colorectal cancer, Mosher et al. (2009) found that high body mass index was associated with poor physical aspects of quality of life, including increased pain, decreased physical functioning, increased fatigue, decreased self-perceived health, and increased limitations in fulfilling daily roles because of physical health problems. Studies have shown that weight loss interventions for cancer survivors involving exercise, dietary change, and behavioral techniques have also produced improvements in quality of life, particularly physical functioning (Morey et al. 2009; Basen-Engquist et al. 2010).

American Cancer Society Recommendations

The American Cancer Society has recently published guidelines on nutrition, exercise, and weight management for cancer survivors (Rock et al. 2012), which are summarized in Table 16.1. The recommendations emphasize eating a diet high in vegetables and fruits, eating whole grains instead of refined grains, and limiting intake of red meat and processed meats. Furthermore, to support achieving or maintaining a healthy weight, the American Cancer Society emphasizes limiting portion sizes of food and drinks and limiting the amount of high-calorie or energy-dense food consumed. At least 150 minutes of moderate- to vigorous-intensity physical activity per week is recommended, along with at least 2 days per week of strength training. Moderate-intensity exercise is equivalent to a brisk walk. Moderate-intensity activity should cause one to feel a bit out of breath but still able to talk. Strength training exercises should target all major muscle groups (i.e., upper body, lower body, and core).

Increasing Exercise Among Cancer Survivors

Opportunities have increased in the community for cancer survivors to find exercise programs specific to their needs. Through a partnership with the Livestrong Foundation, the YMCA offers Livestrong at the YMCA in many cities around the United States. This 12-week, supervised exercise program offered at the YMCA is provided to cancer survivors at no cost. The program varies somewhat from site to site, but all programs need to meet certain requirements, including extensive training of the staff in cancer-specific needs of survivors. A list of YMCA locations that

Table 16.1 American Cancer Society nutrition, physical activity, and weight management recommendations for cancer survivors

Domain	Recommendation
Nutrition	Choose whole grains instead of refined grain products.
	Eat at least 2.5 cups of vegetables and fruits per day.
	Choose foods and drinks in amounts that help you get to and maintain a healthy weight.
	Limit intake of processed meat and red meat.
Physical activity	Avoid inactivity; return to usual daily activities as soon as possible after diagnosis.
	Exercise at least 150 minutes per week.
	Do strength training exercises at least 2 days per week.
Weight management	Achieve and maintain a healthy weight.
	If overweight (body mass index ≥ 25 and <30) or obese (body mass index ≥ 30), increase physical activity and limit consumption of high-calorie, energy-dense foods.

offer the Livestrong program can be found at http://www.livestrong.org/What-We-Do/Our-Actions/Programs-Partnerships/LIVESTRONG-at-the-YMCA/LIVESTRONG-at-the-YMCA-Locations.

For survivors who do not live near a Livestrong at the YMCA program, but would like to start an exercise program with the assistance of a knowledgeable trainer, the American College of Sports Medicine now offers a certification for cancer exercise trainers. Individuals who are certified to be personal trainers in the general population can take an additional examination to test their expertise in issues facing cancer survivors specifically. A directory of certified cancer exercise trainers can be found at http://members.acsm.org/source/custom/Online_locator/onlineLocator.cfm.

Although specific programs for cancer survivors may be helpful to some survivors, especially those who want to start strength-training programs, emerging evidence shows that home-based exercise programs to increase moderate-intensity physical activity are safe and improve functioning and quality of life (Pinto et al. 2005; Basen-Engquist et al. 2006; Demark-Wahnefried et al. 2007; Morey et al. 2009). Walking at a moderate intensity is an excellent form of exercise, and one that most people can adopt without a great deal of cost or access to special facilities. Survivors starting a walking program need a comfortable pair of shoes that provide good support, as well as a place to walk. If walking in the neighborhood is not an option because of safety or weather concerns, many shopping malls open even before stores open, providing an excellent space for walking. Some malls even have organized walking groups. Schools and community centers also may have space that is available for walking at particular times. Survivors who have not been physically active should start with brief periods of walking (e.g., 10 minutes) and gradually increase the amount of time they spend walking. The 30 minutes per day does not have to be done all at once; walking three times per day for 10 minutes each time is also beneficial.

Weight Loss for Overweight and Obese Cancer Survivors

In general, survivors interested in weight loss should follow American Cancer Society diet and physical activity guidelines and manage portion sizes. Eating a diet that is high vegetables, fruits, and whole grains and low in energy-dense foods such as red meat, high-fat dairy products, and sugary beverages will help survivors consume a low-calorie diet and still feel satiated. In addition, survivors interested in weight management should take care to manage portion sizes. The "standard" portions to which many Americans have become accustomed are actually much larger than those on which recommendations are based. For example, a standard serving size for meat is 3–4 oz, which is approximately the size of a deck of cards, but many restaurants serve meat portions of 6–8 oz or larger. Many people are accustomed to pouring themselves a 2-cup serving of breakfast cereal. However, the appropriate portion size may be one-half to one cup, depending on the cereal. Guides to appropriate portion sizes, as well as other weight management information, can be found on the US Department of Agriculture Choose My Plate website (http://www.choosemyplate.gov/).

Behavioral Change Strategies

Evidence-based behavioral methods and strategies can help survivors make changes in their physical activity, eating behavior, and weight management. Consider encouraging survivors to use the following methods to support them in their behavioral change efforts.

Goal Setting

Behavioral change is facilitated by setting goals. A useful heuristic for developing goals is the acronym SMART: goals should be Specific, Measureable, Attainable, Relevant, and Time-specific. Specific goals (e.g., I will do three 10-minute walks on Monday, Tuesday, Thursday, Friday, and Saturday) are more effective than general goals (e.g., I will increase my walking next week). For cancer survivors, it is particularly important that goals be attainable and realistic. If a survivor is just starting an exercise program after finishing chemotherapy, she will likely not be able to do as much as she could before her diagnosis. Similarly, weight loss goals for overweight and obese survivors should target a modest loss of 1–2 pounds per week. Although achieving a normal body mass index would necessitate losing large amounts of weight for many survivors, which may be their initial goal, even losses of 5–10% of body weight are beneficial in terms of decreasing risk of or managing conditions such as hypertension and diabetes. In addition, some evidence suggests that focusing on behavioral change goals (eating behavior, physical activity) rather than weight goals may be beneficial to weight management because the behavior is more under a person's control than the person's actual weight (Bacon et al. 2005).

Self-Monitoring

Self-monitoring progress toward goals is one of the most effective strategies for behavioral change. Self-monitoring can be low-tech, such as noting exercise sessions on a calendar or keeping a food log, or it can involve the ever-expanding array of websites, smart phone apps, and devices that support self-monitoring. For example, the US Department of Agriculture Choose My Plate website has a tracker for monitoring physical activity and dietary intake (https://www.supertracker.usda.gov/default.aspx) that provides feedback on calories burned and consumed, as well as nutrient information. Survivors starting a walking program may benefit from using a pedometer to monitor their step counts (some pedometers also monitor minutes of activity by tracking the amount of time spent continuously moving for 10 minutes or more). Many pedometers are very affordable, and using a pedometer has been shown to effectively increase physical activity in randomized trials (Bravata et al. 2007).

Environmental Changes

Changing one's environment to facilitate positive behaviors (e.g., increasing physical activity and vegetable and fruit consumption) and discouraging behaviors that one aims to decrease (e.g., eating high-fat or high-sugar snacks and sitting for long periods of time) can promote desired behavioral changes. For example, setting out morning workout clothes the night before or bringing walking shoes to work can serve as a reminder to exercise as well as decrease the barriers to engaging in exercise. To encourage eating vegetables and fruits for snacks, one can make these items available at home and prepared ahead of time (e.g., washed and cut) so that they are easy choices when the urge to snack arises. When the aim is to cut back on high-calorie snacks, out of sight is out of mind: if such snacks are highly tempting, they should be put away in a cabinet or refrigerator where they are not easily seen, if they are purchased at all.

Social Support

Social support is critical for individuals making behavioral changes. Family support is especially critical, particularly for changes such as eating behavior that can affect the type of food served and available in the house. Health care provider support for behavioral changes is also important. Research shows that even a brief exercise recommendation from an oncologist can increase exercise behavior in survivors (Jones et al. 2004). In addition to seeking support from family and health care providers, survivors may find it useful to participate in group weight loss or exercise programs in the community to gain the support of others making similar changes.

Conclusion

Cancer survivorship can be seen as a teachable moment: a time when people are willing to re-examine their lifestyle and consider actions they can take to reduce their risk of disease and optimize their health and functioning. Exercise, nutrition, and weight management can influence quality of life and functioning, risk of other chronic diseases, and, for some types of cancer, recurrence and disease-specific survival. Cancer survivorship care should provide opportunities for survivors to obtain appropriate information about exercise, diet, and weight management, as well as ongoing support for making health-enhancing behavioral changes.

Key Practice Points

- Physical inactivity and obesity are prevalent in cancer survivors because these things are risk factors for certain cancers and because survivors of certain cancers are at risk for excess weight gain after diagnosis.
- Exercise and physical activity are associated with improved disease-free survival in breast and colon cancer survivors. Randomized studies have demonstrated that exercise interventions in cancer survivors improve overall quality of life, physical functioning, fatigue and other symptoms, psychological distress, body image, and other outcomes.
- Weight changes after a cancer diagnosis may be associated with an increased risk of breast cancer recurrence, but studies have shown mixed results. Obesity is associated with decreased quality of life in cancer survivors.
- Standard recommendations for nutrition, physical activity, and weight management for cancer survivors have been published by the American Cancer Society. Recommendations include maintaining a diet that emphasizes whole grains, fruits, and vegetables and limits red and processed meat; doing at least 150 minutes of moderate or intense physical activity and 2 days of strength training per week; and achieving and maintaining a healthy weight.
- Behavioral strategies such as setting goals, monitoring oneself, changing one's environment, and seeking social support are effective in helping cancer survivors increase their activity, improve their diet, and manage their weight.

Suggested Readings

Bacon L, Stern JS, Van Loan MD, Keim NL. Size acceptance and intuitive eating improve health for obese, female chronic dieters. *J Am Diet Assoc* 2005;105(6):929–936.

Ballard-Barbash R, Friedenreich CM, Courneya KS, Siddiqi SM, McTiernan A, Alfano CM. Physical activity, biomarkers, and disease outcomes in cancer survivors: a systematic review. *J Natl Cancer Inst* 2012;104(11):815–840.

Basen-Engquist K, Perkins H, Carmack C, et al. Test of weight gain prevention intervention in stage II and III breast cancer patients receiving neoadjuvant chemotherapy. *Cancer Epidemiol Biomarkers Prev* 2010;19(3):895–896.

Basen-Engquist K, Scruggs S, Jhingran A, et al. Physical activity and obesity in endometrial cancer survivors: associations with pain, fatigue, and physical functioning. *Am J Obstet Gynecol* 2009;200(3):288 e281–288.

Basen-Engquist K, Taylor CC, Rosenblum C, et al. Randomized pilot test of a lifestyle physical activity intervention for breast cancer survivors. *Patient Educ Couns* 2006;64(1–3):225–234.

Bravata DM, Smith-Spangler C, Sundaram V, et al. Using pedometers to increase physical activity and improve health: a systematic review. *JAMA* 2007;298(19):2296–2304.

Caan BJ, Emond JA, Natarajan L, et al. Post-diagnosis weight gain and breast cancer recurrence in women with early stage breast cancer. *Breast Cancer Res Treat* 2006;99(1):47–57.

Caan BJ, Kwan ML, Hartzell G, et al. Pre-diagnosis body mass index, post-diagnosis weight change, and prognosis among women with early stage breast cancer. *Cancer Causes Control* 2008;19(10):1319–1328.

Chlebowski RT, Blackburn GL, Thomson CA, et al. Dietary fat reduction and breast cancer outcome: interim efficacy results from the Women's Intervention Nutrition Study. *J Natl Cancer Inst* 2006;98(24):1767–1776.

Demark-Wahnefried W, Clipp EC, Lipkus IM, et al. Main outcomes of the FRESH START trial: a sequentially tailored, diet and exercise mailed print intervention among breast and prostate cancer survivors. *J Clin Oncol* 2007;25(19):2709–2718.

Demark-Wahnefried W, Platz EA, Ligibel JA, et al. The role of obesity in cancer survival and recurrence. *Cancer Epidemiol Biomarkers Prev* 2012;21(8):1244–1259.

Garmey EG, Liu Q, Sklar CA, et al. Longitudinal changes in obesity and body mass index among adult survivors of childhood acute lymphoblastic leukemia: a report from the Childhood Cancer Survivor Study. *J Clin Oncol* 2008;26(28):4639–4645.

Jones LW, Courneya KS, Fairey AS, Mackey JR. Effects of an oncologist's recommendation to exercise on self-reported exercise behavior in newly diagnosed breast cancer survivors: a single-blind, randomized controlled trial. *Ann Behav Med* 2004;28(2):105–113.

Kim HS, Moreira DM, Smith MR, et al. A natural history of weight change in men with prostate cancer on androgen-deprivation therapy (ADT): results from the Shared Equal Access Regional Cancer Hospital (SEARCH) database. *BJU Int* 2010;107(6):924–928.

Kroenke CH, Chen WY, Rosner B, Holmes MD. Weight, weight gain, and survival after breast cancer diagnosis. *J Clin Oncol* 2005;23(7):1370–1378.

Lustig RH, Post SR, Srivannaboon K, et al. Risk factors for the development of obesity in children surviving brain tumors. *J Clin Endocrinol Metab* 2003;88(2):611–616.

Meyerhardt JA, Heseltine D, Niedzwiecki D, et al. Impact of physical activity on cancer recurrence and survival in patients with stage III colon cancer: findings from CALGB 89803. *J Clin Oncol* 2006;24:3535–3541.

Meyerhardt JA, Ogino S, Kirkner GJ, et al. Interaction of molecular markers and physical activity on mortality in patients with colon cancer. *Clin Cancer Res* 2009;15(18):5931–5936.

Mishra SI, Scherer RW, Geigle PM, et al. Exercise interventions on health-related quality of life for cancer survivors. *Cochrane Database Syst Rev* 2012;8:CD007566.

Morey MC, Snyder DC, Sloane R, et al. Effects of home-based diet and exercise on functional outcomes among older, overweight long-term cancer survivors: RENEW: a randomized controlled trial. *JAMA* 2009;301(18):1883–1891.

Morikawa T, Kuchiba A, Yamauchi M, et al. Association of CTNNB1 (beta-catenin) alterations, body mass index, and physical activity with survival in patients with colorectal cancer. *JAMA* 2011;305(16):1685–1694.

Mosher CE, Sloane R, Morey MC, et al. Associations between lifestyle factors and quality of life among older long-term breast, prostate, and colorectal cancer survivors. *Cancer* 2009; 115(17):4001–4009.

Nichols HB, Trentham-Dietz A, Egan KM, et al. Body mass index before and after breast cancer diagnosis: associations with all-cause, breast cancer, and cardiovascular disease mortality. *Cancer Epidemiol Biomarkers Prev* 2009;18(5):1403–1409.

Pierce JP, Natarajan L, Caan BJ, et al. Influence of a diet very high in vegetables, fruit, and fiber and low in fat on prognosis following treatment for breast cancer: the Women's Healthy Eating and Living (WHEL) randomized trial. *JAMA* 2007a;298(3):289–298.

Pierce JP, Stefanick ML, Flatt SW, et al. Greater survival after breast cancer in physically active women with high vegetable-fruit intake regardless of obesity. *J Clin Oncol* 2007b;25(17):2345–2351.

Pinto BM, Frierson GM, Rabin C, Trunzo JJ, Marcus BH. Home-based physical activity intervention for breast cancer patients. *J Clin Oncol* 2005;23(15):3577–3587.

Rock CL, Doyle C, Demark-Wahnefried W, et al. Nutrition and physical activity guidelines for cancer survivors. *CA Cancer J Clin* 2012;62(4):243–274.

Sagstuen H, Aass N, Fossa SD, et al. Blood pressure and body mass index in long-term survivors of testicular cancer. *J Clin Oncol* 2005;23(22):4980–4990.

Schmitz KH, Ahmed RL, Troxel A, et al. Weight lifting in women with breast-cancer-related lymphedema. *N Engl J Med* 2009;361(7):664–673.

Schmitz KH, Ahmed RL, Troxel AB, et al. Weight lifting for women at risk for breast cancer-related lymphedema: a randomized trial. *JAMA* 2010;304(24):2699–2705.

Speck RM, Courneya KS, Masse LC, Duval S, Schmitz KH. An update of controlled physical activity trials in cancer survivors: a systematic review and meta-analysis. *J Cancer Surv* 2010;4(2):87–100.

Chapter 17
Nutrition

Sally Scroggs and Clare McKindley

Contents

Chapter Overview This chapter is designed to provide direction for health care providers looking for more education and training on the role nutrition plays in cancer risk reduction, specifically for cancer survivors. Nutrition guidelines from the most comprehensive research review are presented. Questions commonly asked by cancer survivors in a clinical setting are addressed. Because behavior change requires more than knowledge of guidelines, the chapter concludes with behavior change counseling tips and ideas on how to get survivors to apply the guidelines to their own plates. Finally, the chapter ends with a possible direction for nutrition guidelines in the future.

L.E. Foxhall, M.A. Rodriguez (eds.), *Advances in Cancer Survivorship Management*,
MD Anderson Cancer Care Series, DOI 10.1007/978-1-4939-0986-5_17,
© The University of Texas M.D. Anderson Cancer Center 2015

Introduction

Many cancer survivors proactively search for ways to reduce their risk of recurrence or metastasis. Lifestyle factors and behaviors, including nutrition, can play a role in reducing the risk of developing recurrent disease or a new primary cancer, as well as reducing comorbidities resulting from cancer treatment or preexisting health conditions. This chapter will focus on addressing the most common nutrition concerns expressed by survivors, from a clinical practice perspective.

Building the Recommendations

The most comprehensive research to date on the role of nutrition, food, and physical activity for cancer risk reduction is provided by the American Institute of Cancer Research/World Cancer Research Fund (AICR/WCRF 2006). AICR/WCRF provides a matrix that maps the associations between certain dietary and lifestyle components and the development of cancer at specific sites. AICR developed specific guidelines for cancer prevention and survivorship after analyzing more than 7,000 research articles. These guidelines use the terms *convincing increased/decreased risk*, *probable increased/decreased risk*, and *limited-suggestive increased/decreased risk* to define the strength of evidence that a dietary or lifestyle component is associated with cancer. The guidelines include eight quantifiable recommendations specific to cancer risk reduction and two special recommendations. One of these special recommendations specifically targets cancer survivors. Although limited research data are available from cancer survivor populations, AICR/WCRF recommends that survivors follow these guidelines to reduce the risk of developing recurrent disease or a new primary cancer.

The American Cancer Society (ACS) has published specific guidelines to help clarify the role of nutrition and physical activity after a cancer diagnosis. Revisions and updates to these guidelines occur approximately every 5 years, and the most recent update was published in 2012 (Rock et al. 2012). The guidelines contain four categories:

- Best practices from diagnosis to recovery and living with advanced cancer
- Guidelines for weight management, alcohol, and food safety
- Information on specific cancer sites
- Commonly asked questions and answers for cancer survivors

With these evidenced-based guidelines, health care providers can direct patients toward nutritional and lifestyle behaviors that can help reduce the risk of cancer.

Survivorship Challenges

According to the National Cancer Institute (2013), stress, depression, and anxiety are common during and after cancer therapy and can directly affect lifestyle behaviors, including nutritional intake. Directing survivors to support groups or physical activity groups, or using other appropriate methods, including encouraging survivors to work with mental health care professionals to aid in coping with symptoms and managing stress, may minimize negative behaviors or intake patterns that increase cancer risk.

According to the American Society of Clinical Oncology (2013), other latent side effects of cancer treatment may include the following:

- Lymphedema as a result of surgical excision of lymph nodes or radiation to the lymph nodes
- Heart disease or congestive heart failure as a result of the effects of radiation, the use of drugs such as doxorubicin (Adriamycin) or cyclophosphamide (Cytoxan, Clafen, or Neosar), or other cancer therapy
- Difficulty breathing or change in lung function after treatment with chemotherapy, radiation to the chest, or specific drugs such as bleomycin (Blenoxane), carmustine (BiCNU, Becenum, or Carmubris), prednisone, dexamethasone, or methotrexate
- Hormone alterations resulting from thyroidectomy, hysterectomy, steroid-induced hyperglycemia, or other changes to the endocrine or reproductive system
- Osteoporosis secondary to chemotherapy, steroid medications, hormone therapy, or a sedentary lifestyle (high-risk population: survivors of breast cancer, prostate cancer, or childhood leukemia)

Cancer survivors are not immune to comorbidities such as obesity, hypercholesterolemia, cardiovascular disease, diabetes, and other disease conditions. Clinicians working with recipients of stem cell transplantation have observed increasing rates of cardiovascular disease, dyslipidemia, steroid-induced hyperglycemia, and obesity. Gynecologic and breast cancer clinicians have observed similarly increasing trends.

Weight Management

AICR and ACS emphasize weight management as a priority because overweight and obesity increase the risk of cancer and overall mortality. Total body and abdominal fatness have been shown to increase the risk of developing cancer at a number of sites. According to ACS, a 5–10% weight reduction is likely to produce significant health benefits when achieved through physical activity and healthy eating behaviors. Additional research is needed among survivor populations to identify the ideal frequency, type, duration, and intensity of physical activity needed for the minimum and maximum possible reduction in cancer risk. Additionally, further evidenced-based research is needed to determine which dietary behaviors lead to the minimum and maximum health benefits in survivor populations.

For assessing cancer risk related to weight and fat distribution, the following cost-effective and noninvasive tools are available: body mass index (BMI) and waist circumference. BMI is a number determined by a person's weight and height that indicates total body fatness, calculated as weight (kg)/height $(m)^2$. Many online BMI calculators are available, including one from the US Centers for Disease Control and

Table 17.1 Body mass index (BMI) weight status categories for adults older than 20 years

BMI	Weight status
<18.5	Underweight
18.5–24.9	Normal
25–29.9	Overweight
≥30	Obese

Table 17.2 Health risk associated with waist circumference, for adults older than 20 years

	Waist circumference, inches	
Health risk	Men	Women
Low	≤40	≤35
High	>40	>35

Prevention (2011). An increased BMI (indicating overweight or obese; see Table 17.1) is associated with an increased risk for cancer at the following sites: colorectum, breast (in postmenopausal women), endometrium, esophagus, pancreas, gallbladder, kidney, and liver. However, BMI does have limitations. Overestimation of BMI is possible in highly muscular and lean individuals and underestimation of BMI is possible in elderly individuals or in those with muscular atrophy.

Waist circumference is used to estimate abdominal fat. People with either a high waist circumference (>40 inches in men or >35 inches in women; Table 17.2) or an increase in waist circumference over time are at increased risk for pancreatic, colorectal, breast (in postmenopausal women), and endometrial cancers. Waist circumference is measured by placing a tape measure around the waist, just above hip bone, without pressing the tape into the skin.

In the past, waist-to-hip ratio was used to estimate excess abdominal fat. However, recent research indicates that waist circumference is a more accurate tool (AICR/WCRF 2006; see chapter 6.1.1.2: http://www.dietandcancerreport.org/cancer_resource_center/downloads/chapters/chapter_06.pdf).

Guidelines for the Role of Nutrition and Food in Cancer Risk Reduction

Plant-Based Diet

A cancer-fighting diet consists of plant-based foods but does not exclude food from animal sources (meats, eggs, and dairy). Vegetables, fruits, whole grains, and legumes contain fiber, nutrients, and phytochemicals that may reduce the risk of cancer at a number of sites, including the mouth, pharynx, larynx, esophagus, stomach, lung, pancreas, and prostate. An easy visual measurement to design a meal is to fill two-thirds of a plate with these plant-based foods. The remaining third of the plate is for lean protein from animal sources, such as fish, poultry, and red meats.

Often, the recommended portion size for meats is equivalent to the size of a deck of cards. Non–animal-based protein sources include soy products, beans, peas, nuts, and seeds in combination with other plant foods such as whole grains.

Meats

Per AICR terms, evidence suggests a convincing increased risk for colorectal cancer associated with consumption of red meat, which includes beef, pork, lamb, and goat. There is a limited-suggestive increased risk for endometrial, esophageal, lung, and pancreatic cancer associated with consumption of red meat. The AICR/WCRF also notes a limited-suggestive increased risk for esophageal, lung, stomach, and prostate cancer associated with consumption of processed meat, and a convincing increased risk for colorectal cancer associated with consumption of processed meat (AICR/WCRF 2006; see http://www.aicr.org/reduce-your-cancer-risk/recommendations-for-cancer-prevention/recommendations_07_salt.html   and   the   AICR/WCRF Summary). Processed meat includes meat that is smoked, cured, or salted or has added chemical preservatives. AICR recommends a personal goal of consuming no more than 18 oz (500 g) of red meat per week. In 2011, the United States Department of Agriculture (USDA) reported that total per capita red meat consumption per week in the United States was 44 oz (USDA 2011). The current AICR/WCRF guidelines do not support a weight recommendation for processed meats; the guidelines recommend consuming "very little, if any" processed meat.

Red meat intake may increase exposure to carcinogenic material and promote increased production of n-nitroso compounds (NOCs) in the body. Carcinogenic chemicals of concern in red meats, in addition to NOCs, include heterocyclic amines (HCAs) and polycyclic aromatic hydrocarbons (PAHs). Heme iron in red meats, smoked meats, and cured meats and bacteria in the intestines and stomach are promoters of NOCs. Cooking meat at high temperatures, especially for lengthy time periods, and frying, grilling, and charbroiling meat (especially until it is well done) generate the highest levels of HCAs. PAHs are formed when juices from the meat drip onto the heat source, producing a smoke column. HCAs and PAHs are known carcinogens in animals and suspected carcinogens in humans.

Exposure to these carcinogens can be decreased by baking or marinating meats or using non-animal protein sources. Baking at temperatures of less than 400 °F and using foil reduce the formation of PAHs and HCAs by reducing the meat's exposure to smoke and high heat. Research has shown that marinating meat with herbs and spices containing polyphenolic antioxidants (such as carnosic acid, carnosol, and rosmarinic acid) can significantly reduce HCAs in grilled meats. Some of the spices that include these phytochemicals are rosemary, mint, oregano, and sage (Marcelous 2008; Smith et al. 2008).

Red meat intake can be reduced by limiting portions and frequency by choosing other animal protein sources such as fish, poultry, eggs, and dairy. Alternative non-animal protein sources include soy products, beans, peas, nuts, and seeds in combination with other plant foods or whole grains. Typically, protein needs can be met by consuming one to two servings of meat per day, with portions no larger than the size of a deck of cards.

Sodium

AICR recommends decreasing sodium intake to less than 2,400 mg daily. AICR/ WCRF cites probable increased risk of stomach cancer with the intake of salt and salted or salty foods, and limited-suggestive increased risk of nasopharyngeal cancer with the consumption of Cantonese-style salted fish. Salt is associated with an increased risk of stomach cancer because of direct damage to the stomach lining and because salt plays a role in the formation of endogenous NOCs, which enhance the action of carcinogens in the stomach and might facilitate *Helicobacter pylori* infections (AICR/WCRF 2006; see page 269).

Alcohol

Alcoholic beverages should be consumed in moderation, which means no more than two servings per day for men and one serving per day for women. A single serving is 12 oz of beer, 5 oz of wine, or 1.5 oz of 80-proof alcohol. Consuming alcohol has been linked to breast, colon, esophageal, head and neck, and liver cancer. When combined with smoking, alcohol consumption greatly increases the risk of head and neck cancer.

Frequently Asked Questions

Organic Foods

According to the USDA's National Organic Program (USDA Agricultural Marketing Service 2012), *organic* is a labeling term indicating that food was not grown or produced using chemical pesticides and herbicides, irradiation, hormones, antibiotics, genetic engineering, or other synthetic material. Other labels, such as *no added hormones*, *grass-fed*, and *cage-free*, often accompany an organic product. At this time, it is unknown whether organic foods are associated with a lower risk of cancer compared with conventional foods. Research is also inconclusive regarding the nutritional density of organically grown foods compared with conventionally grown foods. Regardless of the method of growth or production, following a diet rich in colorful vegetables, fruits, whole grains, and legumes is associated with convincing to suggestive decreased risk for cancer at several sites, as defined by the AICR/ WCRF (ACS 2012).

Vegetarian Diets

Vegetables and fruits have been shown to reduce the risk for cancers of the lung, pharynx, mouth, larynx, nasopharynx, esophagus, stomach, pancreas, colon, and rectum. As noted earlier, an easy visual measurement to design a meal is to fill two-thirds of the plate with these plant-based foods. However, some diet restrictions may increase risks for nutritional deficiencies or imbalance. Through the life cycle we all have different age- and sex-specific macronutrient and micronutrient demands to maintain general health. Micronutrients such as vitamin B12, zinc, iron, and calcium may not be present in doses to manage the body's individual requirements if products such as milk, eggs, and all animal products are not a part of the strict vegetarian diet pattern. However, it is still possible to achieve the recommended daily allowances for macronutrients and micronutrients with appropriate attention to the design of the diet. Supplementation may also be appropriate if whole food intake chronically produces insufficient levels of a micronutrient (ACS 2012).

Supplements

It is usually not necessary to consume additional vitamins, minerals, or antioxidants. However, supplementation may be indicated for certain cancer survivors; for example, calcium and vitamin D supplementation is used to maintain bone health in breast cancer survivors. In this population, osteopenia or osteoporosis often occurs as a side effect of chemoprevention when individuals are unable to consume adequate amounts of calcium or vitamin D in their diets. When possible, it is best to choose whole foods, with an emphasis on a colorful variety of plant-based menu selections, to obtain the recommended amount of nutrients. Some research has found that consuming single vitamins, minerals, or antioxidants in supplement form does not have the same health benefit as eating the whole food.

Vitamin D was recently evaluated by the Institute of Medicine's Food and Nutrition Board (Institute of Medicine 2010). The board proposed new reference ranges for vitamin D and detailed the health benefits of vitamin D and calcium in promoting bone matrix management. However, the research was inconclusive with regard to the role of vitamin D and calcium in cancer prevention. The new recommendations for vitamin D included a recommended dietary allowance of 600 International Units per day for most individuals and 800 International Units for those older than 70 years, and a new upper level of 4,000 International Units per day. The recommendations for calcium remained the same for those aged 19–50 years (recommended allowance of 1,000 mg/day; upper level 2,500 mg/day) and for men aged 51–70 years (1,000 mg/day; upper level 2,000 mg/day), but changed for women aged 51–70 years (1,200 mg/day; upper level 2,000 mg/day). For men and women older than 70 years, the recommendation remains at 1,200 mg/day (upper level 2,000 mg/day). The USDA's Food and Nutrition Information Center has an online tool for health care professionals to calculate daily dietary reference intakes (USDA, Interactive DRI 2013).

Soyfoods and Breast Cancer Survivors

Despite recent controversy regarding the protective or harmful properties of phy-toestrogens in soy, the 2012 ACS guidelines for breast cancer survivors state that "current evidence suggests no adverse effects on recurrence or survival from consuming soy and soy foods, and there is the potential for these foods to exert a positive synergistic effect with tamoxifen" (Rock et al. 2012). When choosing a soy product, aim to include the following: tofu, edamame, soy milk, miso, or tempeh. Soy is a complete protein and is an excellent option for a meatless meal. A serving of soy is as follows: one cup of soy milk, one-half cup of soy beans, one-third cup or 1 oz of soy nuts, one-half cup of edamame, or one-third cup (one-fourth of a block) of tofu (AICR 2012). Research remains inconclusive regarding appropriate intake levels of soy protein powders, textured vegetable proteins derived from soy, or supplemental soy protein in terms of cancer risk reduction (ACS 2012).

Eating a Rainbow

Adding an array of color to the diet provides a variety of phytochemicals and nutrients. Table 17.3 shows just a few examples of phytochemicals, organized by color.

Building two-thirds of the plate at a meal to contain plant-based foods is one method to support survivors in applying the cancer prevention recommendations relating to food intake. Another method is building off the ACS recommendation of consuming at least two and one-half cups of vegetables and fruits every day, with an emphasis on eating more vegetables than fruits. The USDA website (USDA, Choose my plate 2013) is a resource consumers may use for tracking cup-to-cup equivalents consumed.

Table 17.3 Phytochemicals found in foods of various colors

Color group	Foods	Phytochemical
Red	Tomatoes, watermelon, pink grapefruit	Lycopene
Red/purple	Grapes, eggplant, plums, blueberries	Anthocyanins
Orange	Sweet potatoes, carrots, apricots, mangos	Beta carotene
Orange/yellow	Nectarines, oranges, pineapples	Beta-cryptothanxin
Yellow/green	Spinach, avocados, corn	Lutein
Green	Broccoli, cauliflower, Brussels sprouts	Indole
White/green	Garlic, onions, celery, pears	Quercetin

Better Attitudes about Eating

Today's fast-paced culture often challenges mindful food attitudes and behaviors. Although we do gain energy and enjoyment from what we eat, we must remember that all foods influence the body. Encourage individuals to adopt the following food attitudes and behaviors:

- **Pay attention to physiologic signs of hunger and satiety**. Allow the body to guide decisions about when and how much to eat, rather than being swayed by advertisements, emotional hunger, or a busy schedule.
- **Choose a colorful variety of plant foods**. View meal times as opportunities to fill the body with disease-fighting and health-promoting foods. Aim for two-thirds of the meal or snack to come from a plant source, such as vegetables, fruits, beans, nuts, and whole grains.
- **Savor foods**. Eating slowly will increase the enjoyment of foods and help prevent overeating.
- **Focus on the meal**. Avoid eating while driving or performing other activities because this may increase intake of high-calorie, low-nutrient dense food choices and lead to overeating.

Future

In the future, new research in the area of nutrigenomics, the effect of nutrients on genes, and nutrigenetics, the effect of genes on nutrients, may help to explain varying results among individuals from the same nutrition research protocols. Dr. John Milner coined these terms when he was Chief of the Nutritional Science Research Group in the Division of Cancer Prevention of the National Cancer Institute. Learning about single-nucleotide polymorphisms in specific genotypes and how they affect metabolism and absorption will help health professionals gain insight into which individuals may need increased or decreased amounts of specific nutrients. Dr. Milner has mentioned the example of how polymorphisms in certain genotypes lead to different responses to calcium and vitamin D in terms of colon cancer risk reduction, which raises many questions:

- Will there always be a need for general nutrition guidelines or will we do away with them and have genotype-based intervention?
- Will this change behavior? Will providing an individual with specific genetic profile information enhance that individual's motivation to make changes in lifestyle and dietary patterns if there is a need for making the change, or will the individual view the information from a fatalist perspective, negating any attempt to change behavior?
- How will this research be used for health policies?

Take-Home Message

Regarding weight management, research states that overweight and obese individuals experience health benefits by reducing their body weight by 5–10%. Consequently, weight reduction should be the primary focus when treating patients at risk for overweight or obesity associated with increased fat weight. ACS guidelines state that "for survivors who are severely obese and have more pressing health issues, more structured weight loss programs or pharmacologic or surgical means may be indicated" (Rock et al. 2012). An interdisciplinary approach to weight management provides survivors with the opportunity to rethink health in terms of their diet and lifestyle patterns. By working with dietitians, exercise physiologists, counselors, and other ancillary health care providers, survivors can identify barriers for change and develop personal goals for disease prevention.

Key Practice Points

- With its work with the World Cancer Research Fund; more than 7,000 research articles relating to nutrition, food, and physical activity for cancer risk reduction; and the Continuous Update Project, the AICR serves as the most comprehensive review in the field of cancer and nutrition/physical activity. AICR's evidenced-based research helps practitioners provide the most up-to-date recommendations and guidelines in this field.
- Overweight and obesity may increase the risk of cancer and overall mortality; consequently, the ACS advocates for survivors, patients, and clients to achieve a healthy body weight, with an initial goal of 5–10% weight reduction from current overweight/obese status. BMI and waist circumference are two noninvasive assessment tools providers may use to set tangible benchmarks for clients to accomplish.
- A plant-based diet that includes at least 2.5 cups of vegetables and fruits in addition to fibrous whole grains and legumes will make nutrients and phytochemicals available to the body for disease prevention and may reduce the risk of cancer at numerous sites, including the mouth, pharynx, larynx, esophagus, stomach, lung, pancreas, and prostate.
- Red meat consumption is associated with a convincing increased risk for colon cancer; consequently, AICR advocates for consumers to limit intake to 18 oz or less weekly.
- Cancer organizations advise abstinence from alcohol; however, should one drink alcohol, one should do so in moderation (no more than two servings per day for men and one serving per day for women).
- Consuming dietary supplements is typically not necessary; however, side effects from cancer treatment and chemoprevention therapy may require

specific nutrient supplementation. Nutrition analysis and understanding of therapy provided to the survivor may determine the specific dietary supplement needs of the patient.

- Survivors' personalized health plans may be enhanced when they work with the physician as well as with other allied health professionals (e.g., counselors, dietitians, exercise physiologists, occupational therapists). The expertise of the allied health professionals will allow the survivor and the physician to focus on primary medical care.

Suggested Readings

American Cancer Society (ACS). ACS guidelines on nutrition and physical activity for cancer prevention. http://www.cancer.org/healthy/eathealthygetactive/acsguidelinesonnutritionphysical activityforcancerprevention/index. Published January 2012. Accessed April 12, 2013.

American Institute for Cancer Research (AICR). Soy. http://www.aicr.org/foods-that-fight-cancer/soy.html#intro. Updated December 4, 2012. Accessed April 12, 2013.

American Institute for Cancer Research/World Cancer Research Fund (AICR/WCRF). Food, nutrition, physical activity, and the prevention of cancer: a global perspective. Second expert report. http://www.dietandcancerreport.org/expert_report/report_contents/index.php. Updated June 2006. Accessed April 12, 2013.

American Society of Clinical Oncology. Late Effects. http://www.cancer.net/survivorship/late-effects. Accessed April 12, 2013.

Centers for Disease Control and Prevention. Body mass index. http://www.cdc.gov/healthyweight/assessing/bmi. Updated September 13, 2011. Accessed April 12, 2013.

Institute of Medicine. Dietary reference intakes for calcium and vitamin D. www.iom.edu/vitamind. Published November 30, 2010. Accessed April 12, 2013.

Kushner RF, Kushner N, Blatner DJ. Counseling overweight adults: the lifestyle patterns approach and toolkit. Chicago: American Diatetic Association; 2009.

Marcelous DG. Medical Toxicology of Natural Substances. New York: John Wiley & Sons; 2008.

National Cancer Institute. Follow-up care after cancer treatment. http://www.cancer.gov/cancertopics/factsheet/Therapy/followup. Accessed April 12, 2013.

Rock CL, Doyle C, Demark-Wahnefried W, et al. Nutrition and physical activity guidelines for cancer survivors. CA Cancer J Clin 2012;62(4):242–274.

Smith JS, Ameri F, Gadgil P. Effect of marinades on the formation of heterocyclic amines in grilled beef and steaks. J Food Sci 2008;73(6)T100–T105.

United States Department of Agriculture (USDA). Choose my plate. http://www.choosemyplate.gov/. Accessed April 12, 2013.

United States Department of Agriculture (USDA). Interactive DRI for healthcare professionals. http://fnic.nal.usda.gov/fnic/interactiveDRI/. Accessed April 12, 2013.

United States Department of Agriculture (USDA). Livestock and poultry: world markets and trade. http://www.fas.usda.gov/dlp/circular/2011/livestock_poultry.pdf. Published April 2011. Accessed April 12, 2013.

United States Department of Agriculture (USDA) Agricultural Marketing Service. National Organic Program. http://www.ams.usda.gov/AMSv1.0/ams.fetchTemplateData.do?template=TemplateC&navID=NationalOrganicProgram&leftNav=NationalOrganicProgram&page=NOPConsumers&description=Consumers&acct=nopgeninfo. Updated October 17, 2012. Accessed April 12, 2013.

Chapter 18
Screening for Second Primary Cancers

Therese B. Bevers

Contents

Chapter Overview Significant improvements in early detection and advances in cancer treatment in the past few decades have resulted in increasing numbers of cancer survivors. Given the major improvements in survival rates and durations, identification and characterization of the late sequelae of cancer and its treatment have become critical. It is well known that cancer survivors are at risk for recurrence of the primary cancer. The risk of developing a second primary cancer (SPC) is also increased. In view of the increasing number of cancer survivors, the development of SPCs has emerged as a significant problem that can affect quality of life and long-term survival. In addition to recurrence of the primary cancer, the diagnosis of a new cancer represents one of the most serious events experienced by cancer survivors. Interest in this area has increased owing to the potential for reducing the risk for SPCs through an understanding of genetic predispositions; lifestyle, behavioral, and environmental factors; and treatment-related effects that influence the development of SPCs. An understanding of the risks for SPCs can guide risk reduction strategies and cancer screening recommendations, with the goal of preventing SPCs or providing early detection and intervention.

L.E. Foxhall, M.A. Rodriguez (eds.), *Advances in Cancer Survivorship Management*, MD Anderson Cancer Care Series, DOI 10.1007/978-1-4939-0986-5_18, © The University of Texas M.D. Anderson Cancer Center 2015

Introduction

Survival from cancer has improved dramatically as a result of the early detection of cancer and advances in cancer treatment. As of 2007, about 12 million people in the United States were living with cancer. As the number of cancer survivors, as well as the duration of cancer survivorship, has increased, the incidence of second primary cancers (SPCs) has also increased. Accordingly, 1 in 6 cancer incidents (16%) reported to the National Cancer Institute's Surveillance, Epidemiology, and End Results (SEER) program is a SPC, making SPCs an important area of concern for patients and their physicians (Ries et al. 2006). Cancer survivors have approximately twice the probability of developing a new primary cancer compared with cancer-free individuals of the same age and risk (Krueger et al. 2008). In fact, excluding non-melanoma skin cancer, SPCs are now the fifth most common category of malignancy, behind lung, colorectal, breast, and prostate cancer (Rheingold et al. 2000).

It is important to recognize that SPCs are a by-product of medical success. If patients do not survive the primary cancer, they are not at risk for a SPC. In some patients, the prognosis is so poor with the primary cancer that there is little opportunity for the development of a SPC. As treatments improve, our understanding of the incidence of SPCs in patients with primary cancers that have a poor prognosis will naturally increase.

Definition of Second Primary Cancer

A seemingly straightforward definition of SPC is a new primary cancer in a person with a history of cancer. However, upon consideration, this definition is significantly more simplistic than originally realized, and it raises a number of questions. For example, are contralateral tumors in paired organs (e.g., breast, kidney) considered SPCs? What about second tumors within the same field (e.g., head and neck, colon)?

New malignancies that occur in the same site or organ as the primary cancer have been shown to account for 13.2% of the SPCs occurring among patients surviving 2 months or more; new tumors in the female breast (7.2%), colon (2%), and lung (1.8%) and melanoma of the skin (0.9%) made up most of these cases (Fraumeni et al. 2006). An additional 3.8% of SPCs originated in neighboring tissues or organs (e.g., within the head and neck, colorectum, or lower urinary tract), a result of a "field cancerization" process whereby carcinogenic exposures and susceptibility states contribute to multicentric tumors (Fraumeni et al. 2006). Molecular studies of some of these cancers indicated that multicentric involvement may actually result from the spread and implantation of a single clone of mutated cells and may involve effects of carcinogenic exposures or genetic factors over areas of tissue or organs.

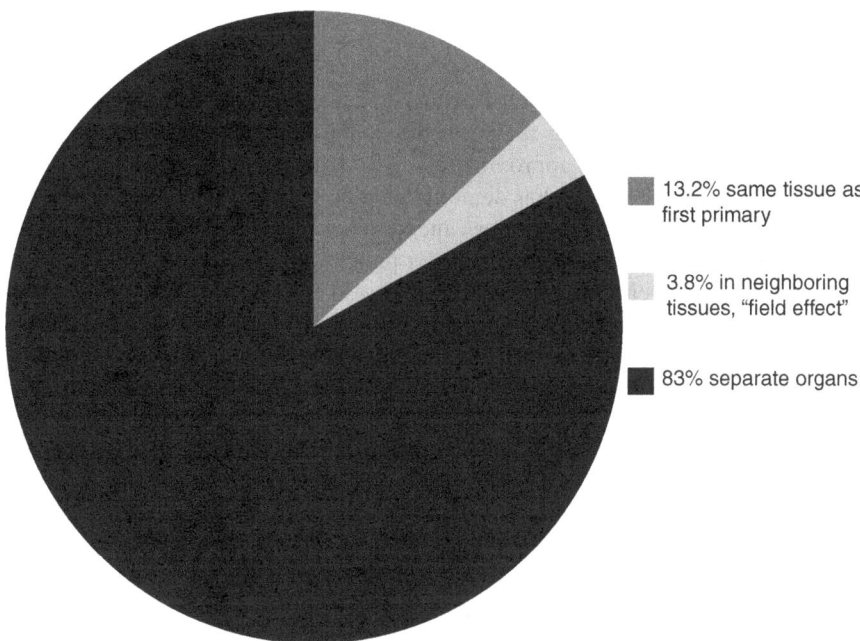

13.2% same tissue as first primary

3.8% in neighboring tissues, "field effect"

83% separate organs

Fig. 18.1 Location of second primary cancers (based on data from Fraumeni et al. 2006)

The oral cavity and pharynx site seems to be associated with the highest risk of multicentric tumors; ratios of observed SPCs in survivors to expected cancers in the general population (O/E ratios) at this site were 29.5 in women and 11.5 in men (Fraumeni et al. 2006).

However, 83% of SPCs reported in the SEER database arose in separate or independent organ systems (Fraumeni et al. 2006; Fig. 18.1). This constellation of cancers presents unique opportunities for primary prevention and may require the implementation of earlier or additional cancer screenings in cancer survivors to ensure early detection of disease outside of the primary cancer site. It is not uncommon for monitoring in cancer survivors to be focused on the site of the first primary cancer. The intent of this chapter is to identify cancer risks beyond the site of the first primary cancer. These risks may be related to the first primary cancer or independent of it, based solely on the aging of the survivor population. These risks present a unique opportunity to counsel survivors regarding risk reduction and screening strategies.

For the purposes of this chapter, the term SPCs refers to neoplasms that arise independently in a new site or tissue at least 2 months after the primary cancer is diagnosed (Krueger et al. 2008).

Incidence Patterns

The risks for SPCs vary by site of primary cancer, age at diagnosis, sex, and race. Analysis of large cancer registries has consistently revealed that the overall O/E ratio for SPCs is approximately 2.0 (Krueger et al. 2008). In some patient populations, research has demonstrated no increased risk for SPCs at all (e.g., among patients with prostate cancer). However, dramatically increased risks for SPCs have been reported in other patient populations (the O/E ratio is ~16 for tongue cancer after laryngeal cancer, ~34 for cancer of the small intestine after colorectal cancer, and ~14 for vaginal cancer after cervical cancer; Krueger et al. 2008). It is important to identify specific populations that are at increased risk for SPCs and require more intensive risk management and screening for SPCs.

Striking differences in the incidence of SPCs have been observed by age at diagnosis of the primary cancer; the risk for SPCs among survivors of childhood cancer (i.e., those diagnosed with a primary cancer between the ages of 0 and 17 years) is more than six times higher than in the general population (O/E = 6.13; Table 18.1). An age effect is further illustrated by the 2- to 3-fold increased risks for SPCs among patients diagnosed with the primary cancer as young adults (ages 18–39 years) compared with the 1.2- to 1.6-fold increased risks among those diagnosed at ages 40–59 years. In contrast, the observed number of SPCs is lower than expected among survivors whose primary cancer was diagnosed at age ≥80 years (O/E = 0.92). This is likely due to competing risks from comorbid conditions and shortened life expectancy in this population (Fraumeni et al. 2006).

Overall, women have a slightly higher risk of developing SPCs than men (O/E = 1.17 vs 1.11). This difference is likely due to the increased risk of developing a SPC in the breast and gynecologic organs among women, as well as the longer life expectancy of female cancer survivors (Krueger et al. 2008; Altekruse et al. 2010).

Table 18.1 Risk of developing a second primary cancer by age at diagnosis of primary cancer (n = 2,036,597)

Age at diagnosis of primary cancer	O/E ratio[a]
All ages	1.14
0–17 years	6.13
18–29 years	2.92
30–39 years	2.37
40–49 years	1.61
50–59 years	1.27
60–69 years	1.13
70–79 years	1.02
80–115 years	0.92

Adapted from Surveillance, Epidemiology, and End Results data, 1973–2000 (Curtis et al. 2006), for patients who survived at least 2 months after diagnosis of primary cancer between 1973 and 2000

[a]Ratio of observed subsequent primary cancers in survivors to expected primary cancers in the general population

However, the risk for SPCs in men consistently exceeded the risk for SPCs in women among patients whose primary cancer was diagnosed before the age of 60 years.

For all ages combined, black cancer survivors had a higher risk of developing a SPC than white cancer survivors (O/E = 1.13; Fraumeni et al. 2006).

Mechanisms

Although a certain fraction of SPCs in cancer survivors would be expected to develop at the same rate as primary cancers in the general population, the patterns of increased risk in cancer survivors are sufficiently distinctive to suggest that primary cancers and SPCs may share the same risk factors, or that cancer therapies may have potentially carcinogenic effects. Insights into carcinogenic pathways of SPCs can guide the approach to cancer screening and prevention among cancer survivors to reduce their risk for SPCs.

Three carcinogenic pathways have been outlined for SPCs (Krueger et al. 2008; Table 18.2):

1. Genetic factors involved in both the primary cancer and the SPC.
2. Lifestyle, behavioral, or environmental factors involved in both the primary cancer and the SPC.
3. Treatment-related (radiation therapy, chemotherapy, or hormonal therapy) effects from the primary cancer (essentially an iatrogenic effect).

Elevated risks for SPCs in cancer survivors may also be the result of closer follow-up by health care providers (i.e., overdiagnosis). In addition, cancer survivors are not immune to age-related cancer risks (e.g., for breast, prostate, or colorectal cancer). These cancer risks need to be considered along with the risks for SPCs identified above.

Genetic Predisposition

A number of well-described clinical genetic syndromes that are unique clinical entities predispose patients to SPCs. For example, the increased risk for cancers of the uterus, ovary, bile ducts, stomach, pancreas, and brain, as well as leukemia and

Table 18.2 Carcinogenic pathways of second primary cancers

Carcinogenic pathway	Examples
Genetic predisposition	Lynch syndrome, BRCA, Li Fraumeni syndrome, Cowden syndrome, and others
Lifestyle, behavioral, or environmental factors	Tobacco or alcohol consumption, obesity (poor diet and lack of exercise), sun exposure, infections (e.g., human papillomavirus, hepatitis B and C, human immunodeficiency virus, *Helicobactor pylori*)
Treatment-related effects	Radiation therapy, chemotherapy, hormonal therapy (e.g., tamoxifen)

lymphoma, following early-onset colon cancer suggests that the inherited mismatch repair genes causing the Lynch syndrome are also involved in the development of these SPCs (Lindor et al. 2008). Among young, premenopausal women with breast cancer, the remarkably high risks of contralateral breast and ovarian cancer are consistent with heritable syndromes associated with germline mutations of BRCA1/2, and the occurrence of breast cancer, sarcomas, and certain other cancers in children and young adults may reflect Li-Fraumeni syndrome, which is related mainly to germline mutations of p53 (Lindor et al. 2008).

Lifestyle, Behavioral, or Environmental Factors

Certain risk factors associated with the development of a primary cancer often play a role in the development of a SPC.

Tobacco and alcohol are major causes of cancer in the general population and also appear to account for a sizable proportion of the SPCs that occur in cancer survivors. Cancers associated with tobacco and alcohol use include cancers of the oropharynx, larynx, lung/bronchus, esophagus, bladder, renal ureter, pancreas, cervix, and stomach. Survivors with a history of one of these cancers and a history of tobacco or alcohol use are at increased risk of developing one of these cancers as a SPC.

Obesity has been linked to a number of cancers in the general population (endometrial, colon, esophageal, renal, pancreatic, and postmenopausal breast cancer) and is presumed to be a risk factor for SPCs as well. The relationship between SPCs and diet and physical inactivity is less clearly defined, but diet and physical inactivity clearly can be variables in obesity management. Reproductive factors may contribute to hormone-dependent cancers such as breast and uterine cancers.

There is a growing awareness that certain infectious agents (e.g., human papillomavirus [HPV], human immunodeficiency virus, human herpesvirus 8, Epstein-Barr virus, hepatitis B and C, *Helicobactor pylori*) may contribute to certain combinations of tumors. For example, individuals with one HPV-related cancer appear to be at risk for an HPV-related SPC (e.g., genital, anal, or oral cancers; Hisada and Rabkin 2005).

Treatment-Related Effects

SPCs can be attributable to the late effects of cancer therapy. One factor to be considered is the elapsed time between the completion of treatment for the primary cancer and the diagnosis of the SPC. Because carcinogenesis takes time, a SPC cannot be reasonably attributed to the treatment for the primary cancer if the interval was too short for the SPC to develop.

Treatment-related effects appear to be age-related. Cancer therapy has not been associated with a significant increase in risk for SPCs in adults. In contrast, children and young adults seem to be especially prone to the carcinogenic effects of intensive chemoradiation (Fraumeni et al. 2006).

Ionizing Radiation

Children and young adults are at increased risk for SPCs related to prior radiation therapy (Fraumeni et al. 2006). These risks begin to increase 10 years after radiation exposure, in keeping with the long latency typically observed with radiogenic solid tumors (Meadows et al. 1985). Elevated risks for breast, lung, and other cancers are especially pronounced among patients who underwent radiation therapy for Hodgkin lymphoma: the risk for breast cancer is approximately 3 times higher in young women who received radiation doses to the breast region, and the risk for lung cancer is approximately 6 times higher in both young men and young women, increasing with the dose of radiation received (Travis et al. 2002, 2003).

Although radiogenic cancers are uncommon following most adult-onset malignancies, increased risks for lung and esophageal cancer, as well as sarcomas, have been observed among adults who underwent radiation therapy for breast cancer (Curtis et al. 2006). Elevated risks have also been noted for acute leukemia and for solid tumors in heavily irradiated organs after pelvic radiation therapy for cervical or uterine cancer (Krueger et al. 2008).

Typically, SPCs occur within or at the margin of the irradiated field. Bone and soft tissue sarcomas are the most common SPCs following radiation therapy, but skin, brain, thyroid, and breast cancer can also occur. The risk is higher if the radiation exposure occurred during a period of rapid growth of the tissue, such as radiation therapy for a bone sarcoma during adolescence or for breast cancer during the second or third decade of life (Rheingold et al. 2009).

Certain factors may increase the carcinogenic effects of radiation. For example, smoking may act in a synergistic fashion with radiation, increasing the risk of lung cancer. This emphasizes the importance of primary prevention strategies such as smoking cessation (Rheingold et al. 2009).

Chemotherapy

Leukemia is the most common SPC following chemotherapy (Fraumeni et al. 2006). Although treatment-related acute myelogenous leukemia and myelodysplastic syndrome are the best-established types of chemotherapy-related SPCs, acute lymphoblastic leukemia and chronic myelogenous leukemia have also been reported. Chemotherapy-induced myeloid leukemias are relatively resistant to subsequent therapy (Neugut et al. 1990).

Treatment with alkylating agents (cyclophosphamide, ifosfamide, cisplatin, carboplatin, chlorambucil, busulfan, melphalan, nitrogen mustard, and procarbazine) increases the risk of developing leukemia almost 5-fold, and the risk increases almost 24-fold in patients receiving the highest doses (Tucker et al. 1987). Following treatment with alkylating agents, the risk for leukemia begins to increase at 1–2 years, peaks at 5–10 years, and then decreases (Travis 2006). Alkylating agents may potentiate the risk for secondary bone cancers when used with radiation therapy (Tucker et al. 1987).

Hormonal agents may also increase the risk of developing a secondary cancer. Among patients with breast cancer, treatment with tamoxifen has been associated with a 2-fold increase in the risk for uterine cancer, including rare tumors of the mixed Müllerian type (Fisher et al. 1994).

Management

As more cancer survivors have emerged, SPCs have been identified as a significant problem that can limit long-term survival and quality of life. However, it is not uncommon for oncologists and primary care physicians to become focused on surveillance for the primary cancer, neglecting risks for cancers at other sites (Earle and Neville 2004). Efforts to quantify and characterize the risks for SPCs related to the primary cancer have important implications for risk counseling, as well as risk reduction and screening recommendations. In addition, routine cancer screenings should be maintained because cancer survivors are not immune to the cancers commonly seen in the aging population.

A 3-point prevention strategy for cancer survivors at risk for SPCs has been outlined (Krueger et al. 2008):

1. Opt for the least carcinogenic therapeutic agents or regimens available.
2. Encourage patients to modify potential risk factors that have a behavioral component.
3. Maintain appropriate screening for SPCs to allow for early detection and treatment.

Minimizing Therapy-Related Risks

An improved understanding of therapy-related SPCs can inform modifications in regimens to minimize cytotoxic treatment exposure. When a SPC is an unfortunate by-product of the successful treatment of the primary cancer, it is important to look for safer cures in the future. Modification or reduction of existing regimens that have established efficacy, however, should not be conducted outside the setting of clinical trials. It may be difficult to moderate treatment for (and side effects related to) the primary cancer without decreasing the chance of cure. Moreover, it is important to keep in mind that treatment-related SPCs, although serious sequelae, do not occur unless patients survive the primary cancer. Thus, the survival benefits provided by many cancer treatments greatly outweigh the risks of developing SPCs.

Advances have been made in cancer treatments that minimize or eliminate the risk for SPCs. For example, lower radiation doses are administered to more targeted radiation fields, minimizing the exposure of regional organs to the radiation. Treatment with aromatase inhibitors, which do not increase the risk for uterine cancer as tamoxifen does, is now the standard hormonal therapy for postmenopausal women with invasive breast cancer.

Risk Reduction Through Lifestyle and Behavioral Changes

Preventive approaches that may decrease the risk for SPCs should be strongly advised. Survivors should be encouraged to implement practices consistent with a healthy lifestyle. More than 50% of deaths seen in a primary care practice can be prevented by tobacco avoidance or cessation, a healthy diet, limited alcohol intake, exercise, and avoidance of obesity. Presumably, the same factors apply to preventing some types of SPCs. A reduced risk for SPCs has been observed among survivors who changed their high-risk behaviors, most notably among those who ceased smoking and consuming alcohol.

Maintaining Appropriate Cancer Screening

The optimal screening strategies to reduce mortality from SPCs, including which screening modalities to use, age to initiate screening, and screening frequency, remain to be defined for most tumor sites. The goal is to detect any new cancer at an early stage when effective treatment is most possible. Sometimes, as in the case of pediatric cancer survivors, screening for SPCs needs to be maintained for decades. For example, young women exposed to thoracic radiation in their teens or 20s are recommended to begin breast cancer screening at age 25 years or 8–10 years after radiation exposure, whichever is later. This screening includes an annual breast MRI in additional to an annual mammogram, often done on a staggered schedule so that screening is performed every 6 months in this high-risk population (Bevers et al. 2009).

It is important to recognize that although cancer survivors have an increased risk for SPCs related to their primary cancer, they also have the same risks as the general population for other cancers. These risks are commonly related to aging and may be related to risks not associated with the primary cancer. For this reason, it is important to include routine cancer screening in the follow-up of cancer survivors. Women who have survived cancer should at least have routine breast, cervical, and colorectal cancer screening, using age- and risk-based guidelines. Men should undergo routine colorectal cancer screening and be counseled regarding the risks and benefits of prostate cancer screening.

Conclusion

Continued advances in early detection and cancer treatments have led to marked improvements in cure rates over the past 30 years. Although cancer survivors are at increased risk for recurrence of the primary cancer, they are also at increased risk for SPCs. SPCs have become an increasingly important concern in oncology over the past few decades.

Increased risks for SPCs related to the primary cancer can be a result of common risks, whether genetic or environmental, as well as treatment for the primary cancer. The evolving patterns of SPCs have important implications for patient counseling and recommendations for behavioral changes, prevention strategies, and cancer screening. Clearly, predictors of SPCs and more sensitive and specific screening strategies are needed.

Although cancer survivors may have an increased risk for SPCs related to their primary cancer, it is important to remember that they are also at risk for cancers seen in the general population, owing to age or risks unrelated to their primary cancer. Individuals should be educated about healthy lifestyle recommendations, and if efficacious screening methods (e.g., mammography, Pap smear and HPV testing, colonoscopy, and possibly prostate cancer screening) are available, this screening should be included in routine patient follow-up.

It is hard to quantify the psychological impact of developing a SPC after surviving the emotional experience of the primary cancer. Clearly, any effort that can minimize the development of a SPC is a worthwhile endeavor.

Key Practice Points

- SPCs are the fifth most commonly occurring cancers (excluding non-melanoma skin cancers).
- Risks for SPCs vary with the site of the primary cancer, age at diagnosis of the primary cancer (risks decrease with age), sex (women are at increased risk), and race (black patients are at increased risk).
- Three primary carcinogenic pathways have been identified: genetic predisposition; lifestyle, behavioral, or environmental factors; and treatment-related (radiation therapy, chemotherapy, or hormonal therapy) effects from the primary cancer (essentially an iatrogenic effect).
- Insights into carcinogenic pathways of SPCs can guide the approach to cancer surveillance and prevention among cancer survivors to reduce their risk of developing a SPC. Patients should be encouraged to modify potential risk factors that have a behavioral component. In addition, appropriate screening for SPCs should be maintained to allow for early detection and treatment, and the least carcinogenic therapeutic agents or regimens available should be used.

Suggested Readings

Altekruse SF, Kosary CL, Krapcho M, et al., eds. *SEER cancer statistics review, 1975–2007.* Bethesda, MD: National Cancer Institute; 2010. Based on November 2009 SEER data submission. Available at http://seer.cancer.gov/csr/1975_2007. Accessed November 19, 2012.

Bevers TB, Anderson BO, Bonaccio E, et al. NCCN clinical practice guidelines in oncology: breast cancer screening and diagnosis. *J Natl Compr Canc Netw* 2009;7(10):1060–1096.

Curtis RE, Ron E, Hankey BF, Hoover RN. New malignancies following breast cancer. In: Curtis RE, Freedman DM, Ron E, et al., eds. *New Malignancies among Cancer Survivors: SEER Cancer Registries, 1973–2000.* Bethesda, MD: National Cancer Institute; 2006.

Earle CC, Neville BA. Under use of necessary care among cancer survivors. *Cancer* 2004;101(8):1712–1719.

Fisher B, Costantino JP, Redmond CK, et al. Endometrial cancer in tamoxifen-treated breast cancer patients: findings from the National Surgical Breast and Bowel Project (NSABP) B-14. *J Natl Cancer Inst* 1994;86(7):527–537.

Fraumeni JF Jr, Curtis RE, Edwards BK, Tucker MA. Introduction. In: Curtis RE, Freedman DM, Ron E, et al., eds. *New Malignancies among Cancer Survivors: SEER Cancer Registries, 1973–2000.* Bethesda, MD: National Cancer Institute; 2006.

Hisada M, Rabkin CS. Viral causes of cancer. In: Shields PG, ed. *Cancer Risk Assessment.* Boca Raton, FL: Taylor & Francis; 2005.

Krueger H, McLean D, Williams D. *The Prevention of Second Primary Cancers. Progress in Experimental Tumor Research, vol. 40.* New York: Basel Karger; 2008.

Lindor NM, McMaster ML, Lindor CJ, et al. Concise handbook of familial cancer susceptibility syndromes. 2nd ed. *J Natl Cancer Inst Monogr* 2008;38:1–93.

Meadows AT, Baum E, Fossati-Bellani F, et al. Second malignant neoplasms in children: an update from the Late Effects Study Group. *J Clin Oncol* 1985;3(4):532–538.

Neugut AI, Robinson E, Nieves J, et al. Poor survival of treatment-related acute nonlymphocytic leukemia. *JAMA* 1990;264:1006–1008.

Rheingold SR, Neugut AL, Meadows AT. Secondary cancers: incidence, risk factors and management. In: Bast RC, Kufe DW, Pollock RE, et al., eds. *Cancer Medicine.* Hamilton, Ontario: BC Decker; 2000.

Rheingold SR, Neugut AI, Uldrick T, Meadows AT. Treatment-related secondary cancers. In: Hong WK, Bast RC, Hait WN, et al., eds. *Holland-Frei Cancer Medicine.* 8th ed. Shelton, CT: People's Medical Publishing House; 2009.

Ries LAG, Harkins D, Krapcho M, et al., eds. *SEER Cancer Statistics Review, 1975–2003.* Bethesda, MD: National Cancer Institute; 2006. Based on November 2005 SEER data submission. Available at http://seer.cancer.gov/csr/1975_2003/. Accessed August 22, 2013.

Travis LB. The epidemiology of second primary cancers. *Cancer Epidemiol Biomarkers Prev* 2006;15(11):2020–2025.

Travis LB, Gospodarowicz M, Curtis RE, et al. Lung cancer following chemotherapy and radiotherapy for Hodgkin's disease. *J Natl Inst* 2002;94:182–192.

Travis LB, Hill D, Dores GM, et al. Breast cancer following radiotherapy and chemotherapy among young women with Hodgkin's disease. *JAMA* 2003;290:465–475.

Tucker MA, D'Angio GJ, Boice JD Jr, et al. Bone sarcomas linked to radiotherapy and chemotherapy in children. *N Engl J Med* 1987;317(10):588–593.

Screening Algorithms

These cancer screening algorithms have been specifically developed for MD Anderson using a multidisciplinary approach and taking into consideration circumstances particular to MD Anderson, including the following: MD Anderson's specific patient population, MD Anderson's services and structure, and MD Anderson's clinical information. These algorithms are provided for informational purposes only and are not intended to replace the independent medical or professional judgment of physicians or other health care providers. Moreover, these algorithms should not be used to treat pregnant women.

Note: This algorithm is not intended for women with a personal history of breast cancer[1] Breast cancer screening may continue as long as a woman has a 10-year life expectancy and no co-morbidities that would limit the diagnostic evaluation or treatment of any identified problem. Women should be counseled about the benefits, risks and limitations of screening mammography.

RISK	AGE TO BEGIN SCREENING	SCREENING
Normal risk[2]	Age 20 - 39 years	• Consider clinical breast exam every 1-3 years[3] • Breast awareness[4]
	Age greater than or equal to 40 years	• Annual clinical breast exam • Annual screening mammogram[5] • Breast awareness[4]
Prior thoracic radiotherapy ages 10-30	Age less than or equal to 24 years	• Annual clinical breast exam • Breast awareness[4]
	Age greater than or equal to 25 years	• Annual screening mammogram[5] **plus** clinical breast exam every 6-12 months (Begin 8-10 years after radiotherapy or age 40, whichever first) • Consider MRI[6] as an adjunct to mammogram and clinical breast exam annually[7] • Breast awareness[4]
Increased risk 5-year risk of invasive breast cancer by Gail model calculation greater than or equal to 1.7% in women greater than 35 years[8]		• Annual screening mammogram[5] **plus** clinical breast exam every 6-12 months • Breast awareness[4]
Women who have a lifetime risk greater than or equal to 20 % as defined by models that are dependent on family history[8]	Age less than or equal to 24 years	• Annual clinical breast exam • Breast awareness[4]
	Age greater than or equal to 25 years	• Annual screening mammogram[5] **plus** clinical breast exam every 6-12 months (Begin 10 years prior to youngest case in the family but not younger than age 25) • Consider MRI[6] as an adjunct to mammogram and clinical breast exam annually[7] • Breast awareness[4]
Genetic predisposition[8]	Age less than or equal to 24 years	• Annual clinical breast exam • Breast awareness[4]
	Age greater than or equal to 25 years	• Annual screening mammogram[5] **plus** clinical breast exam every 6-12 months • MRI as an adjunct to mammogram and clinical breast exam annually[7] • Breast awareness[4]
Lobular Carcinoma In Situ[8]		• Annual screening mammogram[5] **plus** clinical breast exam every 6-12 months • Breast awareness[4]

1 Please see the Breast Cancer Treatment or Survivorship algorithms for the management of women with a personal history of breast cancer.
2 Women who do not meet one of the increased risk categories.
3 Effectiveness of clinical breast exams has not been assessed in women 20-39 years of age.
4 Women should be familiar with their breasts and promptly report changes to their healthcare provider.
5 Augmented breasts need additional views for complete assessment.
6 Risk of breast cancer begins to increase 8-10 years after thoracic exposure. The optimal age to begin MRI screening in this high risk population is not currently known.
7 Current practice at M. D. Anderson is to alternate the mammogram and breast MRI every 6 months. While there is no data to suggest that this is the optimal approach, it is done with the expectation that interval cancers may be identified earlier. Other screening regimens, such as breast MRI done at the time of the annual mammogram, are also acceptable.
8 For women at increased risk, see Risk Reduction Algorithm (currently in development).

Department of Clinical Effectiveness V4
Approved by The Executive Committee of Medical Staff 11/29/2011

Algorithm 18.1 Breast cancer screening

NOTE: It is critical that females who do not need annual cervical cancer screening, continue with annual appointments to obtain other appropriate preventive healthcare. Women with significant co-morbid or life-threatening illnesses may forego cervical cancer screening. This algorithm is not intended for women with a personal history of cervical cancer[1].

SCREENING

AGE TO BEGIN

Under 21 years of age → Screening not recommended

21 – 29 years of age → Liquid-based Pap Test (preferred) every 3 years[2]

30 - 65 years of age → Liquid-based Pap Test (preferred) and High Risk Human Papilloma Virus (HPV) testing (HPV testing is optional but preferred)[2,3]

- Pap Test normal and HPV testing negative → Repeat Liquid-based Pap Test (preferred) and HPV testing in 5 years
- Pap Test normal HPV testing not done → Repeat liquid-based Pap Test with or without HPV Testing in 3 years
- Abnormal Pap Test and/or HPV testing positive → See diagnostic guideline (currently in development)

Greater than 65 years of age → Screening not recommended[3,4,6]

Status post hysterectomy for benign disease → Screening not recommended[3,5,6]

[1] See the Cervical Cancer Treatment or Survivorship algorithms for the management of women with a personal history of cervical cancer.
[2] Women with certain risk factors (diethylstilbestrol exposure [DES] in utero, immunosuppression [e.g., Human Immunodeficiency Virus (HIV), organ transplant on immunosuppressive therapy]) should continue to be screened annually. Women with HIV should have cervical cytology screening twice in the first year after diagnosis and then annually.
[3] Women treated in the past for CIN2/3 or invasive cervical cancer require routine screening for at least 20 years.
[4] For women with no risk factors for cervical cancer (diethylstilbestrol exposure [DES] in utero, immunosuppression [e.g., Human Immunodeficiency Virus (HIV), organ transplant on immunosuppressive therapy]), if no abnormal Pap in the past 10 years and 3 consecutive negative Paps OR a negative Pap and negative HPV within the past 5 years, cervical cancer screening should be discontinued. Women with risk factors should continue to have screening as long as they are in good health. The screening should follow the 30-65 years age range.
[5] Women with supracervical hysterectomies should follow the guidelines as for women without a hysterectomy.
[6] If screening is stopped, it should not be restarted due to new sexual contact.
NOTE: Women who have received the Human Papilloma Virus Vaccine (HPV) should continue to be screened according to the above guideline.

Department of Clinical Effectiveness V4
Approved by the Executive Committee of the Medical Staff 03/26/2013

Copyright 2013 The University of Texas MD Anderson Cancer Center

Algorithm 18.2 Cervical cancer screening

Note: Screening for adults age 76 to 85 should be evaluated on an individual basis by their health care provider to assess the risks and benefits of screening. Colorectal cancer screening is not recommended over age 85.

PRESENTATION

RECOMMENDED SCREENING

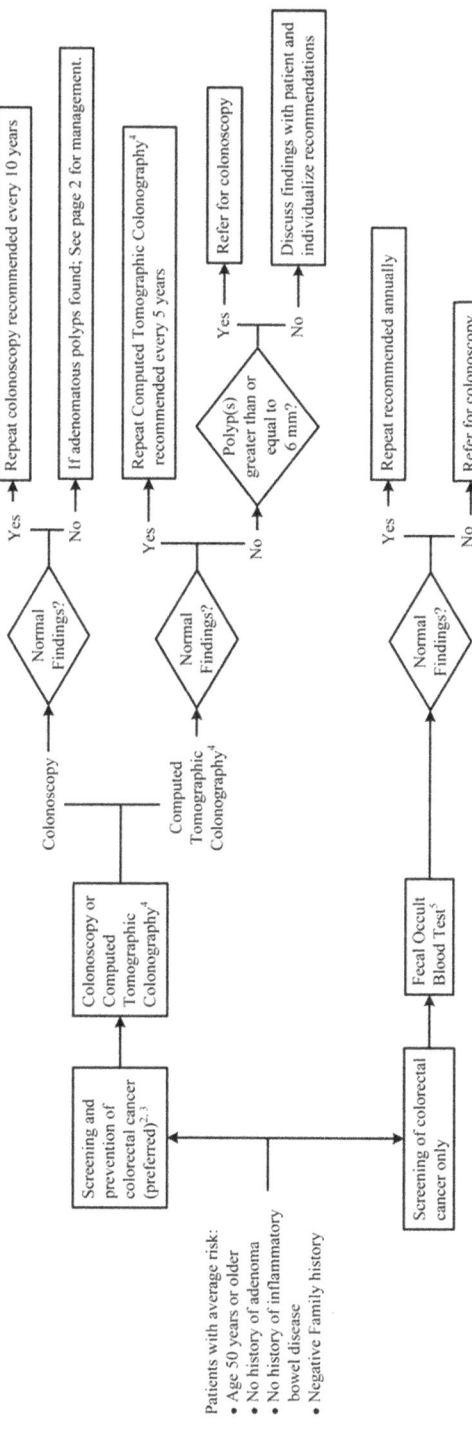

Patients with average risk:
• Age 50 years or older
• No history of adenoma
• No history of inflammatory bowel disease
• Negative Family history

[1] See the Colorectal Cancer Treatment or Survivorship algorithms for the management of individuals with a personal history of colorectal cancer.
[2] While there is good evidence to support Fecal Occult Blood Test, tests that both screen for and prevent colon cancer are the preferred screening modality. Annual Fecal Occult Blood Tests should not be performed if colonoscopy or CT colonography is used as the screening measure in an average-risk patient.
[3] Flexible sigmoidoscopy is an alternate option, but is not the preferred endoscopic modality as the entire colon is not visualized.
[4] Preauthorization with one's insurance carrier is always advised.
[5] High sensitivity Fecal Occult Blood Test (guaic-based or immunochemical).

Copyright 2011 The University of Texas MD Anderson Cancer Center

Department of Clinical Effectiveness V3
Approved by The Executive Committee of Medical Staff 11/29/2011

Algorithm 18.3 Colorectal cancer screening (average risk)

Note: Screening is only intended for asymptomatic individuals. Patient must be a candidate for and is willing to undergo curative treatment. Endometrial cancer screening may continue as long as a woman has a 10-year life expectancy and no co-morbidities that would limit the diagnostic evaluation or treatment of any identified problem.

PRESENTATION

RISK

SCREENING

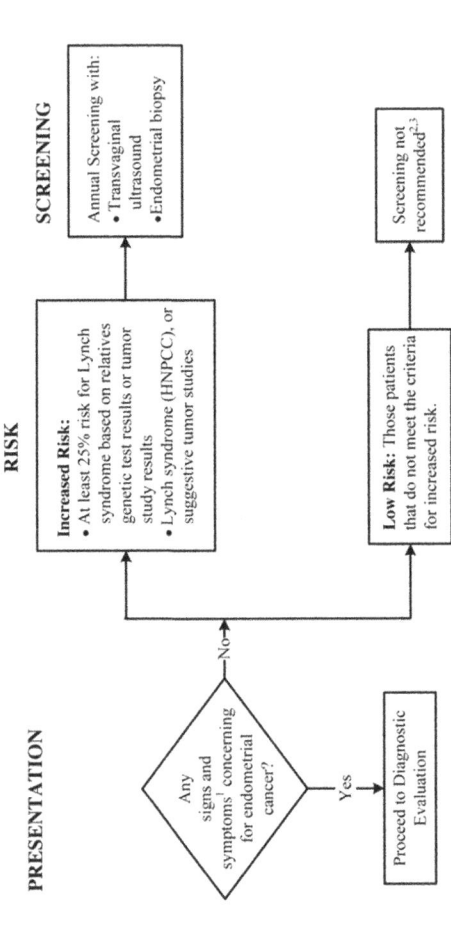

Increased Risk:
- At least 25% risk for Lynch syndrome based on relatives genetic test results or tumor study results
- Lynch syndrome (HNPCC), or suggestive tumor studies

Annual Screening with:
- Transvaginal ultrasound
- Endometrial biopsy

Low Risk: Those patients that do not meet the criteria for increased risk.

Screening not recommended[2,3]

Any signs and symptoms[1] concerning for endometrial cancer?

No

Yes

Proceed to Diagnostic Evaluation

[1] Signs and symptoms include:
   • abdominal vaginal bleeding • vaginal discharge • pelvic pressure
[2] While it is recognized that women who are overweight/obese, taking tamoxifen or with a prior history of pelvic radiation are at increased risk of endometrial cancer, screening is not recommended for these populations.
[3] Patients should have any gynecological symptoms promptly evaluated.

Copyright 2011 The University of Texas MD Anderson Cancer Center

Department of Clinical Effectiveness V1
Approved by the Executive Committee of the Medical Staff on 09/27/2011

Algorithm 18.4 Endometrial cancer screening

GENDER	AGE[5,6,7]	VACCINE[8,9,10,11]	VACCINE SCHEDULE[12,13,14]
Females	Target Age: 11-12 Years May start as early as 9 years of age Catch Up: 13-26 Years Optional: Greater than 26 years	HPV2[15] Or HPV4 (Preferred)[16]	Series of 3 vaccines[17] • Baseline • 1 to 2 months • 6 months
Males	Target Age: 11-12 Years May start as early as 9 years of age Catch Up: 13-26 Years Optional: Greater than 26 years	HPV4 (Preferred)[16]	Series of 3 vaccines • Baseline • 1 to 2 months • 6 months

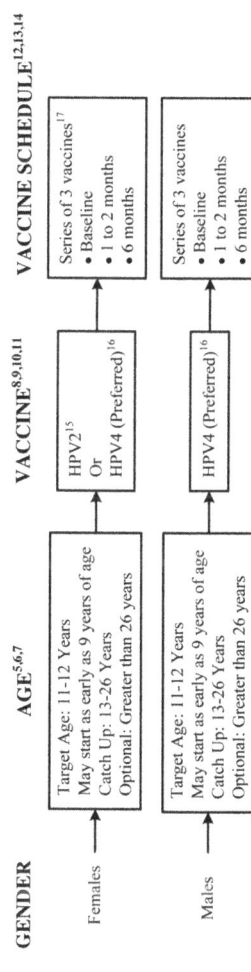

[1] MD Anderson strongly recommends that all females and males age 9-26 receive HPV vaccination.

[2] HPV2 and HPV4 are not live vaccines. HPV vaccination for immunocompromised patients should be delayed if possible until they are immunocompetent. If immunocompetency is unable to be achieved, proceed with administering HPV vaccination.

[3] Although primarily used to prevent cervical dysplasia, cervical cancer and genital warts, HPV vaccination may reduce the risk of other HPV-related premalignant and malignant lesions of the oropharynx, anus, penis, vagina and vulva.

[4] Vaccines for Children Program covers full HPV vaccination series for those that qualify.

[5] HPV2 and HPV4 are not FDA approved for use in males or females greater than 26 years of age; there is no information on the efficacy and prevention of outcomes for this population.

[6] Individuals over age 26 should be counseled regarding decreased effectiveness of the vaccine in individuals who are sexually active and already infected with one of the types of HPV in the vaccine.

[7] ACIP recommends a target age of 11-12 years.

[8] Efficacy of vaccine has been shown for ages 9-26 years.

[9] Absolute contraindications : anyone allergic to the vaccine or its delivery system.

[10] Relative contraindications: prior diagnosis of cervical cancer or dysplasia as the effectiveness of the vaccine is reduced.

Most common adverse events were mild or moderate and were most commonly injection site reactions. No deaths have been observed related to HPV vaccination.

[11] HPV vaccines are not recommended for use in pregnant women. If a woman is found to be pregnant after initiating the vaccination series, the remainder of the 3-dose series should be delayed until completion of pregnancy. Pregnancy testing is not needed before vaccination. If a vaccine has been administered during pregnancy, no intervention is needed.

[12] Those individuals who have not received the full series of 3 vaccinations should be counseled regarding possible decreased effectiveness of the vaccine.

[13] Minimum interval of 4 weeks between 1st and 2nd doses of vaccine. Minimum interval of 24 weeks between 1st and 3rd doses of vaccine. Doses received after a shorter-than-recommended dosing interval should be readministered.

[14] It is unknown if a booster vaccination is needed.

[15] Bivalent vaccine (Cervista®; GlaxoSmithKline) includes HPV 16 and 18.

[16] Quadrivalent vaccine (Gardasil®; Merck & Co) includes HPV 6,11, 16 and 18.

[17] Whenever feasible, the same HPV vaccine (HPV2 or HPV4) should be used for the entire vaccination series. However, if uncertain of type of prior HPV vaccine or it is unavailable, either HPV vaccine can be used to complete the series.

Department of Clinical Effectiveness V1
Approved by the Executive Committee of the Medical Staff on 04/30/2013

Algorithm 18.5 HPV vaccination for prevention of HPV-related cancers

Note: Patient must be a candidate for and is willing to undergo curative treatment.[1] The screening technique should be performed with a consistent technique and process.

RISK FACTORS   SCREENING

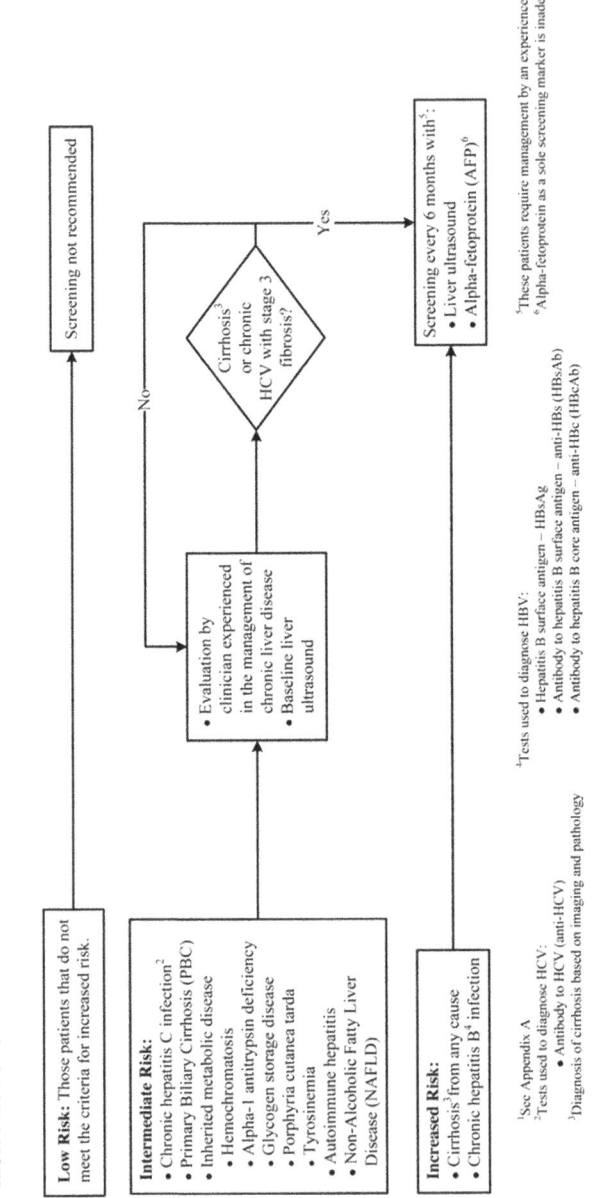

Low Risk: Those patients that do not meet the criteria for increased risk.

Intermediate Risk:
• Chronic hepatitis C infection[2]
• Primary Biliary Cirrhosis (PBC)
• Inherited metabolic disease
• Hemochromatosis
• Alpha-1 antitrypsin deficiency
• Glycogen storage disease
• Porphyria cutanea tarda
• Tyrosinemia
• Autoimmune hepatitis
• Non-Alcoholic Fatty Liver Disease (NAFLD)

Increased Risk:
• Cirrhosis[3] from any cause
• Chronic hepatitis B[4] infection

Screening not recommended

• Evaluation by clinician experienced in the management of chronic liver disease
• Baseline liver ultrasound

Cirrhosis[3] or chronic HCV with stage 3 fibrosis?

No

Yes

Screening every 6 months with[5]:
• Liver ultrasound
• Alpha-fetoprotein (AFP)[6]

[1]See Appendix A
[2]Tests used to diagnose HCV:
   • Antibody to HCV (anti-HCV)
[3]Diagnosis of cirrhosis based on imaging and pathology

[4]Tests used to diagnose HBV:
   • Hepatitis B surface antigen – HBsAg
   • Antibody to hepatitis B surface antigen – anti-HBs (HBsAb)
   • Antibody to hepatitis B core antigen – anti-HBc (HBcAb)

[5]These patients require management by an experienced clinician
[6]Alpha-fetoprotein as a sole screening marker is inadequate

Department of Clinical Effectiveness V1
Approved by the Executive Committee of the Medical Staff on 09/24/2013

Algorithm 18.6a Liver cancer screening (page 1)

APPENDIX A: CHILD-PUGH SCALE[1]

Chemical and Biochemical Parameters	Scores (Points) for Increasing Abnormality		
	1	2	3
Encephalopathy	None	1 - 2	3 - 4
Ascites	None	Slight	Moderate
Albumin	Greater than 3.5 g/dL	2.8 – 3.5 g/dL	Less than 2.8 g/dL
Prothrombin time prolonged	1 – 4 seconds	4 – 6 seconds	Greater than 6 seconds
Bilirubin	1 – 2 mg/dL	2 – 3 mg/dL	Greater than 3 md/dL
For primary biliary cirrhosis	1 – 4 mg/dL	4 – 10 mg/dL	Greater than 10 mg/dL

Class A = 5 to 6 points
Class B = 7 to 9 points
Class C = 10 to 15 points

[1]Class C are not candidates for screening for liver cancer given the high mortality associated with their cirrhosis.

Department of Clinical Effectiveness V1
Approved by the Executive Committee of the Medical Staff on 09/24/2013

Algorithm 18.6b Liver cancer screening (page 2)

APPENDIX B
Persons for Whom HBV Screening is Recommended

Individuals born in areas of high[1] and intermediate prevalence rates[2] for HBV including immigrants and adopted children[3,4]

- Asia: All countries
- Africa: All countries
- South Pacific Islands: All countries
- Middle East (except Cyprus and Israel)
- European Mediterranean: Malta and Spain
- The Arctic (indigenous populations of Alaska, Cabada, and Greenland)
- South America: Ecuador, Guyana, Suriname, Venezuela and Amazon regions of Bolivia, Brazil, Colombia and Peru
- Eastern Europe: All countries except Hungary
- Caribbean: Antigua and Barbuda, Dominica, Granada, Haiti, Jamaica, St. Kitts and Nevis, St. Lucia, and Turks and Calcos.
- Central America: Guatemala and Honduras

Other groups recommended for screening

- U.S. born persons not vaccinated as infants whose parents were born in regions with high HBV endemicity (greater than or equal to 8%)
- Household and sexual contacts of HBsAg-positive persons[4]
- Persons who have ever injected drugs[4]
- Persons with multiple sexual partners or history of sexually transmitted disease[4]
- Men who have sex with men[4]
- Inmates of correctional facilities[4]
- Individuals with chronically elevated ALT or AST[4]
- Individuals infected with HCV or HIV[4]
- Patients undergoing renal dialysis[4]
- All pregnant women
- Persons needing immunosuppressive therapy

[1]HBsAg prevalence 8%
[2]HBsAg prevalence 2%~7%
[3]If HBsAg-positive persons are found in the first generation, subsequent generations should be tested
[4]Those who are seronegative should receive hepatitis B vaccine

Copyright 2013 The University of Texas MD Anderson Cancer Center

APPENDIX C
Persons for Whom HCV Screening is Recommended

- Persons born during 1945-1965
- Persons who have injected illicit drugs in the recent and remote past, including those who injected only once and do not consider themselves to be drug users.
- Persons with conditions associated with a high prevalence of HCV infection including:
  - Persons with HIV infection
  - Persons with hemophilia who received clotting factor concentrates prior to 1987
  - Persons who have ever been on hemodialysis
  - Persons with unexplained abnormal aminotransferase levels
- Prior recipients of transfusions or organ transplants prior to July 1992 including:
  - Persons who were notified that they had received blood from a donor who later tested positive for HCV infection
  - Persons who received a transfusion of blood or blood products
  - Persons who received an organ transplant
- Children born to HCV-infected mothers
- Health care, emergency medical and public safety workers after a needle stick injury or mucosal exposure to HCV-positive blood
- Current sexual partners of HCV-infected persons[5]

[5]Although the prevalence of infection is low, a negative test in the partner provides reassurance, making testing of sexual partners of benefit in clinical practice.

Department of Clinical Effectiveness V1
Approved by the Executive Committee of the Medical Staff on 09/24/2013

Algorithm 18.6c Liver cancer screening (page 3)

Note: Screening is only intended for asymptomatic individuals. Individuals undergoing lung cancer screening should have a 10-year life expectancy and no co-morbidities that would limit the diagnostic evaluation or treatment of any identified problem. The screening technique should be performed with a consistent technique and process.

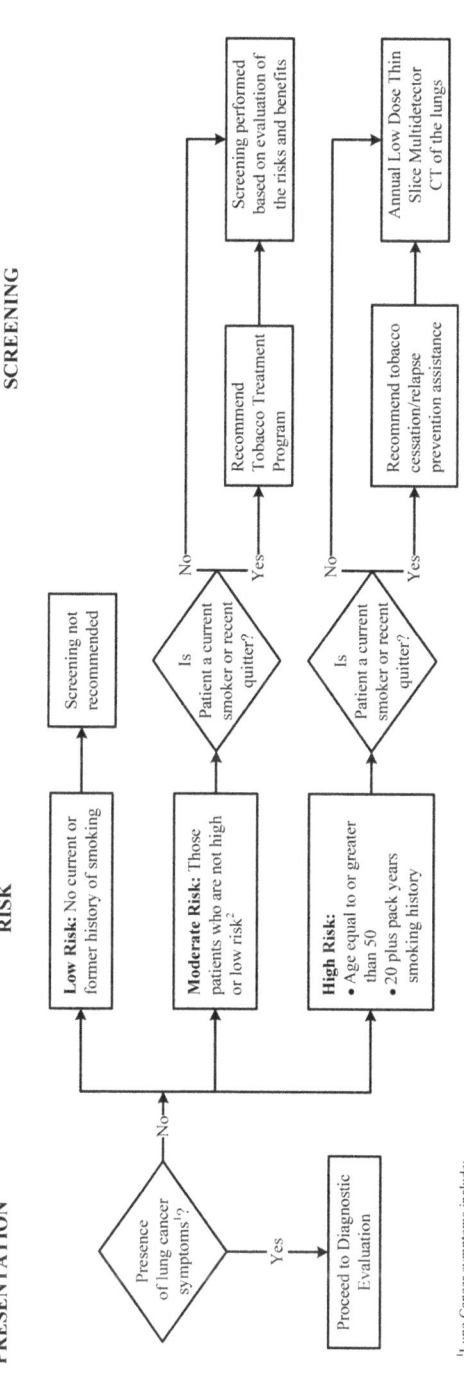

PRESENTATION   RISK   SCREENING

[1]Lung Cancer symptoms include:
• cough
• hoarseness
• unexplained weight loss
• Hemoptysis

[2]Examples of Moderate risk include but are not limited to:
• Significant second hand smoke exposure
• Previous history of other malignancies which would provide a higher risk for secondary lung cancer (e.g. patients with head and neck cancer related to smoking)
• Less than 20 pack years of smoking history

Department of Clinical Effectiveness V1
Approved by The Executive Committee of the Medical Staff on 08/30/2011

Algorithm 18.7 Lung cancer screening

Note: Screening is only intended for asymptomatic individuals. Patient must be a candidate for and is willing to undergo curative treatment. Ovarian cancer screening may continue as long as a woman has a 10-year life expectancy and no co-morbidities that would limit the diagnostic evaluation or treatment of any identified problem.

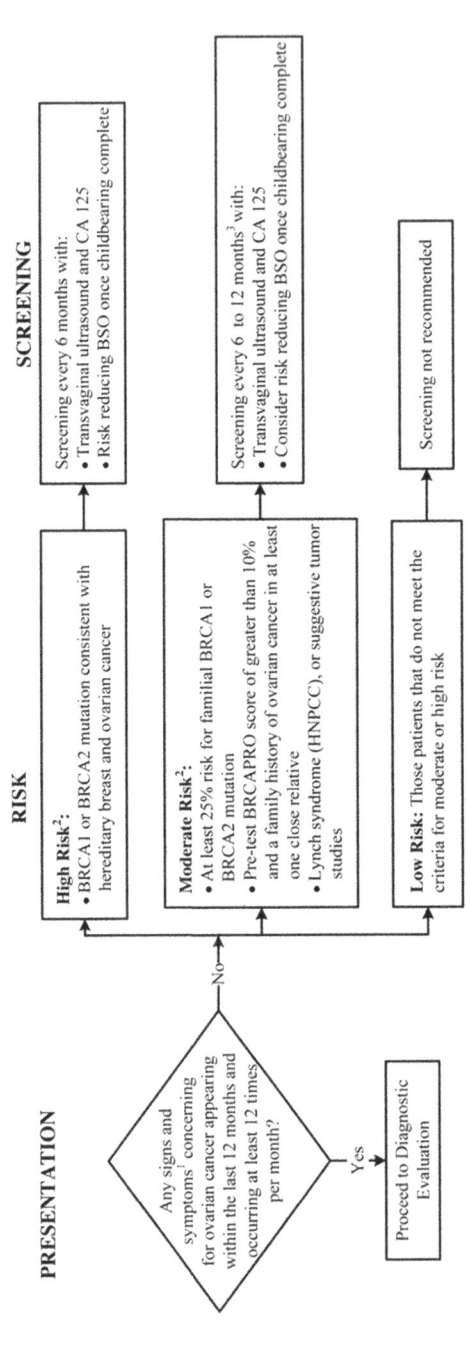

PRESENTATION

RISK

SCREENING

Any signs and symptoms[1] concerning for ovarian cancer appearing within the last 12 months and occurring at least 12 times per month?

Yes → Proceed to Diagnostic Evaluation

No →

High Risk[2]:
- BRCA1 or BRCA2 mutation consistent with hereditary breast and ovarian cancer

Moderate Risk[2]:
- At least 25% risk for familial BRCA1 or BRCA2 mutation
- Pre-test BRCAPRO score of greater than 10% and a family history of ovarian cancer in at least one close relative
- Lynch syndrome (HNPCC), or suggestive tumor studies

Low Risk: Those patients that do not meet the criteria for moderate or high risk

Screening every 6 months with:
- Transvaginal ultrasound and CA 125
- Risk reducing BSO once childbearing complete

Screening every 6 to 12 months[3] with:
- Transvaginal ultrasound and CA 125
- Consider risk reducing BSO once childbearing complete

Screening not recommended

[1] Signs and symptoms include:
- Pelvic or abdominal pain • Increased abdominal size/bloating • Difficulty eating/feeling full

[2] There is limited efficacy for ovarian cancer screening in moderate and high risk patients. Risk reducing surgery should be strongly considered once childbearing complete

[3] Beginning screening at age 35 or 5 to 10 years earlier than the earliest age of 1st diagnosis of ovarian cancer in the family

Department of Clinical Effectiveness V1
Approved by the Executive Committee of the Medical Staff on 09/27/2011

Algorithm 18.8 Ovarian cancer screening

Note: Screening is only intended for asymptomatic individuals. Patient must be a candidate for and is willing to undergo curative treatment.

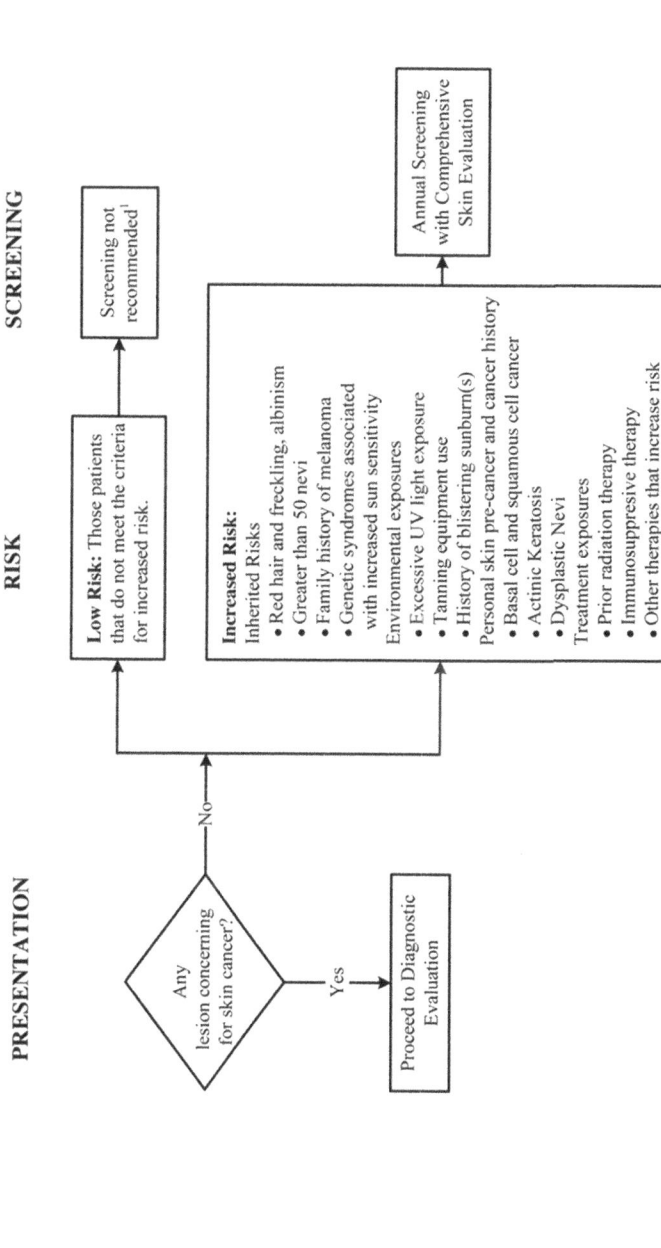

| PRESENTATION | RISK | SCREENING |

Any lesion concerning for skin cancer?

- **Yes** → Proceed to Diagnostic Evaluation
- **No** →

Low Risk: Those patients that do not meet the criteria for increased risk. → Screening not recommended[1]

Increased Risk:

Inherited Risks
- Red hair and freckling, albinism
- Greater than 50 nevi
- Family history of melanoma
- Genetic syndromes associated with increased sun sensitivity

Environmental exposures
- Excessive UV light exposure
- Tanning equipment use
- History of blistering sunburn(s)

Personal skin pre-cancer and cancer history
- Basal cell and squamous cell cancer
- Actinic Keratosis
- Dysplastic Nevi

Treatment exposures
- Prior radiation therapy
- Immunosuppresive therapy
- Other therapies that increase risk

→ Annual Screening with Comprehensive Skin Evaluation

[1]Patients should monitor their skin for any changes and seek prompt medical evaluation of any lesions concerning for Skin Cancer.

Department of Clinical Effectiveness V1
Approved by the Executive Committee of the Medical Staff on 09/27/2011

Algorithm 18.9 Skin cancer screening

.

Part IV
Long-Term and Late Effects

Chapter 19
Cardiovascular Issues

Michael S. Ewer

Contents

Chapter Overview Modern therapies for cancer are allowing increasing numbers of patients to enjoy long-term remission or cure of their disease. Unfortunately, the very modalities that help achieve these results cause injury to tissues or organs; these injuries may not be transient and may persist for the duration of survivorship. The heart, as a post-mitotic organ, does not regenerate after injury, and therefore is especially vulnerable to the long-term effects of a variety of treatment strategies for cancer. Although the future holds promise that new initiatives will allow organ or tissue regeneration, at present we must maximize protection of the heart at the time of exposure and minimize sequential stresses that might add to the cardiac burden during the period following the toxic injury. We now understand that cardiac injury may follow some forms of chemotherapy and biologic therapy as well as radiation therapy, and oncologists have learned to protect the heart to minimize the immediate damage. The burden of managing residual cardiac injury, however, migrates to the physician who provides care to cancer survivors, so that the late effects of treatment may be minimized. This chapter explores some of the strategies intended to improve quality of life for patients whose initial treatment for cancer resulted in cardiac injury.

L.E. Foxhall, M.A. Rodriguez (eds.), *Advances in Cancer Survivorship Management*,
MD Anderson Cancer Care Series, DOI 10.1007/978-1-4939-0986-5_19,
© The University of Texas M.D. Anderson Cancer Center 2015

Introduction

The heart is a focus of considerable concern for cancer survivors. Therapeutic interventions that have the potential to be curative can also result in cardiac injury that may be progressive, debilitating, and sometimes fatal. Although primary malignancies of the heart are unusual, and metastatic spread to cardiac tissue suggests advanced and often incurable disease, having a history of cardiac tumors is generally not of special concern during the period of survivorship. Cardiologists have learned to be proactive in minimizing the effects of cancer treatment. In addition, interventions most likely to result in cardiac injury have been identified, as have the patient populations in which the risk of cardiac complications is increased.

Nevertheless, cardiac effects remain a major concern for cancer survivors. Physicians caring for cancer survivors are aware that many of the late cardiac problems associated with cancer treatment become apparent only after years or even decades following the initial injury. The younger a patient is at the time of initial diagnosis or treatment, the more likely late manifestations are to appear during the years of survival. In one retrospective study examining the incidence of congestive heart failure, myocardial infarction, pericardial disease, and valvular disease among adult survivors of childhood cancers, significantly increased incidences of these complications (hazard ratios ranging from 4.8 to 6.3, and even higher hazard ratios when anthracyclines or radiation was used as part of the initial treatment) were found in cancer survivors compared with their siblings (Mulrooney et al. 2009). Additionally, another review focusing on adult survivors of childhood cancer who were treated with anthracyclines or radiation reported a significant dose-related increase in late cardiovascular effects (Tukenova et al. 2010).

Therefore, it is not surprising that the organ most commonly screened for adverse effects in patients prior to, during, and following treatment for cancer is the heart. The heart forms the basis of most preoperative evaluations or evaluations performed prior to starting chemotherapy; evaluation of possible cardiac involvement is sought during the course of many forms of chemotherapy or radiation therapy that encroaches on cardiac structures. Ongoing cardiac surveillance is part of the long-term care program for many cancer survivors, especially those who underwent treatment with anthracyclines, radiation, or a combination of both modalities.

At the present time, much of the effort devoted to cardiac screening or surveillance is intended to quantify, prevent, and recognize treatment-induced contractile dysfunction, often the result of either a loss of myocytes or impairment of their function. However, it should be noted that conditions beyond contractile dysfunction are often observed in this group of patients. In addition to the late effects mentioned above, cardiac dysrhythmia and conduction abnormalities can occur. Furthermore, a broader spectrum of ischemic responses, heart valve abnormalities, and various pericardial syndromes including constriction may be observed.

In addition, damage associated with treatment for cancer may be difficult to detect. The heart has substantial reserves and an astounding ability to compensate for injury, even in the face of substantial injury and loss of individual myocytes.

This compensation may make the initial presentation of the injury subtle enough that the injury is undetectable or underestimated. In some cases of cardiac injury, the full extent of the damage becomes evident only months or years after treatment is completed, when compensatory strategies have been exhausted. Even with the introduction of biomarkers and recently developed cardiac ultrasound techniques intended to detect cardiac damage early, currently available tools may be unable to detect or fully estimate cardiac damage at early stages.

This chapter will examine the ways in which the heart is affected by both cancer and its treatment and will provide some guidance in managing, following up, and treating cancer survivors who may have sustained cardiac stress or damage while they had cancer or were undergoing treatment for cancer.

Chemotherapy and Biological Agents

Contractile Dysfunction Following Treatment with Anthracyclines or Other Type I Agents

Concerns regarding contractile dysfunction following some forms of chemotherapy came to the attention of clinicians after the introduction of anthracyclines in the 1960s (Ritchie et al. 1970). Although the mechanisms of injury and the extent of the clinical spectrum of contractile dysfunction have, to a considerable degree, been elucidated, the problem of anthracycline-induced cardiotoxic effects remains one of considerable importance. Anthracyclines are now believed to damage the mitochondria and membrane integrity of myocytes at the time of administration. When the injury exceeds the threshold of reversibility, myocyte death ensues. Anthracyclines, as well as other agents that destroy myocytes, have now been classified as agents that cause *type I treatment-related cardiac dysfunction* (see Table 19.1). The cardiotoxicity of these agents is related to the cumulative dose; thus type I agents have a limited lifetime allowable cumulative dose. Type I agents are also associated with characteristic structural changes involving cellular organelles.

Loss of cardiac myocytes as a consequence of cardiotoxic chemotherapy with a type I agent affects all cancer survivors treated with such agents, regardless of the survivor's age at the time of treatment, preexisting cardiac status, or posttreatment cardiac burdens. However, preexisting cardiac stresses may lower the threshold of reversibility, and ongoing cardiac damage may exacerbate the effects of cell loss in patients who are cured of their malignancy. Survivors of cancer who have been treated with type I agents have decreased cardiac reserves, augmenting the effects of subsequent cardiac stress or injury.

However, huge differences exist among patients treated with type I agents, leading to considerable difficulty for clinicians in their attempts to estimate the degree of treatment-related injury. In addition, placing any given patient within a particular risk group may be problematic because preexisting cardiac status is not always

Table 19.1 Type I and type II treatment-related cardiac dysfunction

Characteristic	Type I treatment-related cardiac dysfunction (example: doxorubicin)	Type II treatment-related cardiac dysfunction (example: trastuzumab)
Primary functional mechanism	Cell death	Cell dysfunction
Reversibility	Symptoms may respond favorably to treatment, but the underlying cell damage is largely permanent and irreversible	Reversibility established for several agents, although controversy still exists
Cardiac biopsy results	Typical changes	No typical changes
Need for long-term treatment when associated with cardiac failure	Yes	Uncertain, especially in instances of full reversibility
Need for long-term follow-up	Probably prudent	Uncertain

Table 19.2 Stratification of risk for cardiac injury among patients who have received type I agents

Patient characteristics	Low risk	Intermediate risk	High risk
Cumulative dose of doxorubicin or equivalent	<300 mg/m^2	300–400 mg/m^2	>400 mg/m^2
Age at time of treatment	10–59 years	60–65 years	<10 or >65 years
Pretreatment cardiac ejection fraction	$>55\%$	50–55%	$<50\%$
Pretreatment conditions: hypertension not controlled or requiring more than 2 agents for control, hemodynamically significant valvular disorders, cardiac irradiation	None	1 or 2 conditions	More than 2 conditions
History of pretreatment cardiomyopathy of any cause	No	No	Yes
Obesity	No	Yes	Yes
Diabetes	No	Not insulin dependent	Insulin dependent

easily determined, the degree of damage caused in a particular patient by any identified cumulative dose varies, and the ability of a particular patient to compensate for cardiac damage depends on many factors that cannot always be integrated into the risk estimate. Nevertheless, some principles are well established and can influence decisions regarding surveillance of these patients in the years and decades following their type I agent exposure. Table 19.2 describes some characteristics of patients who have received type I agents and are considered to have a high, intermediate, or low risk of treatment-related cardiac injury. This stratification may help the physician caring for cancer survivors to estimate the need for surveillance, as well as avoid excessive cardiac follow-up that may have limited value.

The goal of cardiac surveillance following cure or control of malignancy is to maximize preservation of cardiac function in the face of decreased cardiac reserve and ongoing or sequential cardiac insults. To do this successfully, we must reduce cardiac stress to the maximal degree possible while preserving quality of life. The benefits of lifestyle modification may be under-recognized, but smoking cessation, achieving optimal body weight, and moderate exercise are general measures that, even in the absence of rigorous clinical studies to prove their specific benefit for patients who have received anthracyclines, remain a prudent strategy that is almost certainly effective. Optimal management of systemic or pulmonary hypertension and diabetes is also crucial in this setting.

Recognition that subclinical decreases in cardiac reserve are important, as well as awareness that cardiac ultrasound parameters are suboptimal, is crucial for effective cardiac surveillance. Ejection fraction (EF), which remains the mainstay of posttreatment cardiac surveillance, is geared toward early detection of subclinical cardiac abnormalities. As the heart loses its ability to compensate for injury, EF may decrease; such a decrease may predate the detection of any cardiac symptoms. EF, however, is not specific for posttreatment declines and may change as a result of any number of altered physiologic or metabolic states, including changes in the blood carrying capacity of oxygen or altered adrenergic states, or as a side effect of certain medications. Although a decline in EF should not be ignored, a clinician treating a patient who is a cancer survivor must recognize the frequency with which fluctuations in EF occur that are unrelated to prior cancer treatment and integrate the information from the functional test with other clinically available information. In some instances, confirmation of the drop in EF by a repeat study or a complementary study using a different modality may be prudent.

During the period of survivorship, 2 considerations regarding surveillance are relevant in patients who were previously treated with a type I agent: how often the patient should undergo cardiac evaluation, and at what threshold intervention should be considered. In the absence of strong clinical data, and on the basis of the risk stratification depicted in Table 19.2, reasonable cardiac surveillance might include documenting any cardiac problems occurring since completion of treatment, performing a physical examination, and estimating EF at 6 months after completion of treatment and yearly thereafter for those at high risk at the time of treatment, or 6 months after completion of treatment and every 2–3 years thereafter for those at intermediate or low risk. Intercurrent change in status should trigger additional evaluation. A confirmed drop in EF of more than 15 percentage points or more than 10 percentage points to a level below 50% should be deemed clinically relevant and should trigger the consideration of intervention. Long-term prospective studies demonstrating the utility of this strategy are not available, but in their absence, a general clinical consensus suggests that early diagnosis and intervention are prudent (Ewer and Ewer 2010).

In the setting of cardiac dysfunction related to prior treatment with a type I agent, we generally treat with a beta-adrenergic blocker, angiotensin-converting enzyme inhibitor, or angiotensin receptor blocker. One study strongly suggested that the progression of damage could be mitigated through early use of angiotensin-converting enzyme inhibitors and beta-adrenergic blockers (Cardinale et al. 2006). In refractory cases, spironolactone or judicious use of a loop diuretic may be considered. Standard dosing should be applied for all of these medications and long-term use is usually required.

Myocardial Dysfunction Following Treatment with Type II Cardiotoxic Agents

Type II agents, as noted in Table 19.1, cause decreased cardiac function through different mechanisms than those that cause cardiac dysfunction with type I agents; primary myocyte death is not characteristic of type II agent-related cardiac injury. Monoclonal antibodies and tyrosine kinase inhibitors fall within the category of type II agents. When myocyte death does occur, it may be related to previous use of a type I agent or to vulnerable cells experiencing oxidative stress. Interestingly, cardiac dysfunction following the use of several type II agents is largely reversible. Accumulating data suggest that long-term use of type II agents is safe, a fact that may alter the thresholds for routine surveillance in cancer survivors who were treated with these agents.

Cancer survivors who experience a mild transient decrease in EF after treatment with type II agents may not require specific cardiac treatment; however, those whose EF drops into the 40% range are usually treated, at least until the EF recovers to within the normal range. In contrast with patients who have experienced a cardiac event following treatment with a type I agent, who often require lifelong treatment for cardiac dysfunction, patients who experience transient decreases in EF following treatment with type II agents may not need lifelong treatment for cardiac dysfunction. The benefit of long-term treatment with agents to reduce cardiac workload in these patients is unknown. On the basis of the assumption that cell loss is not part of the primary injury, and considering recent findings from a clinical trial showing that patients treated with adjuvant trastuzumab survived up to 7 years without significant late events, a less aggressive treatment approach may be justified in cases in which the patient's EF has normalized following the use of a type II agent (Romond et al. 2012).

Cancer survivors who have received both type I and type II agents present a special dilemma; tests are currently not available to determine whether a subsequent event is the result of cell loss, which occurs with type I agents, or myocyte dysfunction, which occurs with type II agents. In such cases, thresholds for surveillance and treatment should follow those suggested for patients who have received type I agents.

Concerns Beyond Myocardial Dysfunction Related to Chemotherapy or Biological Agents

Most other cardiac adverse effects related to chemotherapy are temporally related to the administration of the treatment and are not concerns that extend into the period of survivorship. Spasm-induced ischemia can occur with 5-fluorouracil or capecitabine. Ischemia following the use of such agents is more common in patients with underlying coronary disease, and a history of such events may be a useful clue that surveillance for latent ischemia during survivorship is prudent. Similarly, dysrhythmia during administration of chemotherapy may alert the clinician to a reduced threshold for ectopy, suggesting the need for increased levels of scrutiny. Valvular sequelae in patients who have received chemotherapy or biologically active agents do not usually occur; however, underlying hemodynamically significant lesions should be followed during the period of survivorship because the timing of intervention may be more difficult to determine if the patient has reduced cardiac reserves. Although pericarditis may occur during the administration of some type I agents, chronic pericarditis does not occur as a late manifestation in these patients, and other etiologies should be sought in patients with ongoing pericardial problems.

Radiation Involving Cardiac Structures

Radiation remains an important therapeutic modality for many forms of cancer and is widely used in adjuvant treatment or as a potentially curative treatment for lung cancer, breast cancer, and lymphoma. In all of these instances, the heart may be exposed to levels of radiation that may cause significant late damage that could be of concern to cancer survivors; radiation at levels used for cancer treatment affects all cardiac structures. Although radiation-induced injury is dose-dependent, modern administration techniques now offer considerable protection of cardiac structures. Notwithstanding innovative strategies to spare the heart, many cancer survivors experience late radiation-induced injury, and radiation-induced injury is likely to occur among cancer survivors well into the future. Physicians caring for cancer survivors must also be aware that anthracycline-based chemotherapy and irradiation may cause "supra-additive cardiotoxicity" (Myrehaug et al. 2008).

The pericardium is the cardiac structure most commonly affected by radiation. Acute radiation-induced pericarditis is often self-limited and not associated with long-term sequelae; however, chronic pericarditis may extend into the period of survivorship and, rarely, may lead to constriction that may be severe or life-threatening. Patients who have experienced acute radiation-associated pericarditis are at increased risk for later pericardial problems, and recurrent episodes of pericarditis, often associated with minor infections, are common. Late pericardial pain during the survivorship period may mimic the pain associated with myocardial ischemia, but a history of pain exacerbated by the prone position rather than exertion, prompt response to a nonsteroidal anti-inflammatory agent, the presence of a pericardial friction rub, and typical electrocardiographic changes suggesting a pericardial origin may help to focus attention on the pericardium.

Although pericardial constriction may be disabling and life-threatening, the diagnostic criteria are sometimes confusing. Fluid retention, hepatomegaly, and low-output failure in a cancer survivor who has been treated with radiation to the chest should suggest the possibility of pericardial constriction. Cardiac ultrasound may show pericardial thickening, increased diastolic pressure, and reduced end-diastolic volume, but cardiac catheterization with analysis of pressure contours may be required for confirmation. Surgical intervention in the form of pericardial stripping is associated with considerable perioperative risk (Schwefer et al. 2009).

Radiation affects the cardiac vasculature; the coronary vessels may have a decreased luminal area and intimal thickening and ischemic cardiomyopathy may ensue (Wang et al. 2011). Microvascular involvement may lead to general fibrosis and cardiomyopathy. Involvement of larger vessels may cause a more characteristic pattern of ischemic heart disease that can be treated in the same manner as arteriosclerotic disease of the coronary vessels. The altered vasculature, however, presents special concerns with regard to surgical revascularization. Surgeons must be informed of the prior history of radiation that included a portion of the heart because surgery in the previously irradiated field may prove to be more difficult and the altered vasculature may impede optimal revascularization.

Clinically relevant radiation-related valvular disease is an infrequent finding, although altered valves are observed more frequently at autopsy in previously irradiated patients than in the general population. When observed in patients, valvular lesions are usually a late finding, and left-sided valves are more frequently involved than are right-sided valves. Thickened cusps or leaflets may be noted and, in more severe cases, calcification with a characteristic echocardiographic appearance may be observed. Treatment should follow the general guidelines for the management of valvular disease of other etiologies.

Radiation-associated disease of the conduction system is unusual. When it occurs, it may involve the bundle branches; right bundle branch blockage is more common than left bundle branch blockage. Varying degrees of atrioventricular nodal disease can also occur, and complete heart blockage, requiring pacing, has been reported in patients who were previously treated with radiation to the chest. Although some instances of conduction system involvement may be secondary to concomitant vascular injury, a direct effect of radiation on the conduction system itself is now considered likely. Physicians caring for cancer survivors must be aware of these entities; prompt intervention may prevent catastrophic or life-threatening events. Most radiation-induced cardiac damage presents highly rewarding opportunities for medical or surgical intervention.

Other Cardiac Considerations for Cancer Survivors

Although the heart responds to external toxic exposure over time in ways outlined above, it also experiences the burdens and stresses of everyday life that may include hypertension, infections, pregnancy, endocrine and metabolic disorders, other acute or chronic illnesses, and toxic or pharmacologic exposure. These stresses may diminish reserves further or temporarily stress the heart, causing an acute exacerbation that may result in frank decompensation. The heart of the cancer survivor, therefore, is not a static stable organ with diminished reserves, but an organ that responds, compensates, and adjusts to its environment to the extent that it can in the face of additive cardiac burdens. Added to this cardiac picture are the manifestations of treatment of the primary malignancy. In the case of a breast cancer survivor, these manifestations may be small, but in the case of a cancer survivor who has undergone a lung resection, they may be huge. Post-resection pulmonary hypertension, augmented by a history of tobacco use, may add additional cardiac stress in the form of cor pulmonale. Symptoms of fluid retention, shortness of breath, syncope, a prominent closure sound of the pulmonic valve (P2), and chest discomfort or chest pain should suggest cor pulmonale. Irradiation of the lungs may be an important contributing factor. Treatment may include calcium-channel blockers and sildenafil; diuretics may also be useful.

Endocrine disorders are common among cancer survivors and may be the underlying cause of a number of cardiac abnormalities, including dysrhythmia and high-output or other forms of cardiac failure. Although specific cardiac interventions may be useful during the acute phase of the illness, treating the underlying endocrine abnormality is essential for restoring homeostasis and improving quality of life.

Cardiac care in a cancer survivor who is pregnant presents special problems that may be best managed in conjunction with a physician who specializes in obstetric care of high-risk patients. Many cancer survivors undergo uncomplicated pregnancies following treatment of their malignancy, but careful monitoring may identify problems sufficiently early so that interventions can be instituted in a timely manner without compromising the well-being of either the mother or the child. Risks should be assessed on an individual basis and will be influenced by the degree of underlying cardiac damage.

Finally, cardiologists treating cancer survivors must be alert to the fact that these patients may have subtle or unusual presentations of various cardiac abnormalities. Cardiologists must also be aware that survivors require a broader view toward differential diagnosis. Early intervention makes an important difference for many survivors, and a focused approach to achieve early recognition of problems to minimize the extent of damage may be crucial. Controlling underlying risk factors through lifestyle modification and judicious use of medication can preserve cardiac function and may avoid or mitigate the long-term effects of curative therapeutic interventions. Notwithstanding the fact that some interventions may carry increased risks in cancer survivors, this expanding group of patients should not be denied consideration of any intervention that would be appropriate for the management of cardiac problems in the general population. Many cancer survivors have had meaningful improvement in their cardiac condition as well as their quality of life following revascularization, open-heart surgery, or implantation of simple or complex pacing and defibrillating devices; an increasing number of survivors have undergone successful cardiac transplantation.

Key Practice Points

- Anthracyclines are the class of anticancer agents with the greatest potential to cause cardiac damage, and that damage is related to the cumulative dose administered.

- Exposure to radiation in the heart affects all cardiac structures; the pericardium is especially vulnerable, but both small and large vessels are affected as well.
- The heart has extraordinary reserves to compensate for injury over long periods of time, and the injury may not come to the attention of either the patient or the physician until after compensatory mechanisms are exhausted.
- Protection of cardiac reserves after completion of treatment may delay or prevent clinically relevant cardiac sequelae from occurring.
- Reducing traditional risk factors for cardiac disease is especially important for patients who have been treated for cancer with cardiotoxic agents.
- The late effects of cancer treatment on the heart may be subtle, and surveillance during the posttreatment phase is important.
- When cancer patients at increased risk for cardiac disease are evaluated to determine the best course of treatment, communication between the oncologist and cardiologist may help minimize the extent of cardiac injury, thereby preserving cardiac function during the years of survivorship.

Suggested Readings

Cardinale D, Colombo A, Sandri M, et al. Prevention of high-dose chemotherapy-induced cardiotoxicity in high-risk patients by angiotensin-converting enzyme inhibition. *Circulation* 2006;114:2474–2481.

Ewer MS, Ewer SM. Cardiotoxicity of anticancer treatments: what the cardiologist needs to know. *Nat Rev Cardiol* 2010(10):564–575.

Mulrooney DA, Yeazel MW, Kawashima T, et al. Cardiac outcomes in a cohort of adult survivors of childhood and adolescent cancer: retrospective analysis of the Childhood Cancer Survivor Study cohort. *BMJ* 2009;339:b4606.

Myrehaug S, Pintilie M, Tsang R, et al. Cardiac morbidity following modern treatment for Hodgkin lymphoma: supra-additive cardiotoxicity of doxorubicin and radiation therapy. *Leuk Lymphoma* 2008;49:1486–1493.

Ritchie J, Singer J, Thorning D. Anthracycline cardiotoxicity: clinical and pathological outcome assessed by radionuclide ejection fraction. *Cancer* 1970;46:1109–1116.

Romond EH, Jeong H-H, Rastogi P, et al. Seven-year follow-up assessment of cardiac function in NSABP B-31, a randomized trial comparing doxorubicin and cyclophosphamide followed by paclitaxel (ACP) with ACP plus trastuzumab as adjuvant therapy for patients with node-positive, human epidermal growth factor receptor 2-positive breast cancer. *J Clin Oncol* 2012;30(31):3792–3799.

Schwefer M, Aschenbach R, Heidemann J, Mey C, Lapp H. Constrictive pericarditis, still a diagnostic challenge: comprehensive review of clinical management. *Eur J Cardiothorac Surg* 2009;36:502–510.

Tukenova M, Guibout C, Oberlin O, et al. Role of cancer treatment in long-term overall and cardiovascular mortality after childhood cancer. *J Clin Oncol* 2010;28:1308–1315.

Wang W, Wainstein R, Freixa X, Dzavik V, Fyles A. Quantitative coronary angiography findings of patients who received previous breast radiotherapy. *Radiother Oncol* 2011;100(2): 184–188.

Chapter 20
Cognitive Function

Christina A. Meyers

Contents

Chapter Overview Many cancer survivors suffer from neurocognitive, emotional, and behavioral symptoms that interfere with their academic, vocational, or social pursuits. These impairments commonly include problems with memory, attention, and speed of thinking. However, many cancer survivors can enjoy improved levels of functioning if properly diagnosed and provided with the right support. A number of interventions can lessen the adverse impact of neurocognitive impairments on cancer survivors' ability to function in daily life.

Introduction

Cancer patients experience a number of adverse symptoms, including cognitive impairment, fatigue, pain, sleep disturbance, and others, often in combination. Fortunately detailed symptom assessment is becoming increasingly recognized as a part of routine patient care by physicians, allied health care providers, and accrediting agencies. Cancer treatment may be considered successful only if these symptoms are managed, but successful management is hampered by insufficient knowledge of mechanisms. Interest in the mechanisms, patterns of symptoms, and interventions is growing as the survivorship

L.E. Foxhall, M.A. Rodriguez (eds.), *Advances in Cancer Survivorship Management*,
MD Anderson Cancer Care Series, DOI 10.1007/978-1-4939-0986-5_20,
© The University of Texas M.D. Anderson Cancer Center 2015

community grows and must deal with these adverse effects of cancer and cancer treatment.

Cognitive dysfunction occurs in most cancer patients who are receiving active therapy and is frequently a symptom that heralds the diagnosis. In addition, cognitive dysfunction persists in a substantial number of patients long after treatment is discontinued. This type of cognitive dysfunction is popularly termed "chemobrain" or "chemo fog." However, cognitive symptoms secondary to cancer and cancer treatment are part of a differential diagnosis of exclusion because a number of factors may be causal, and the specific intervention is based on the etiology of the cognitive dysfunction (Table 20.1).

In an effort to gather information directly from cancer survivors about their experience of "chemobrain" during and following treatment, an online survey conducted by the Hurricane Voices Breast Cancer Foundation specifically queried the impact of neurocognitive symptoms on a survivor's ability to work. Nearly two-thirds of the 471 survey respondents (most of whom were survivors of breast cancer) reported that cognitive changes had an adverse impact on their work functioning or relationships at work, and 10 respondents reported leaving jobs or being terminated. Nearly 300 of the 471 respondents felt that their cognitive symptoms warranted discussion with a medical professional; however, their concerns were met with mixed reactions. Fifty-five percent of respondents felt that their oncologist was understanding, but 42% felt that their oncologist's response was dismissive or indifferent. Only 10% were offered assistance; 6% of respondents had neuropsychological testing and less than 8% were referred for an intervention for their cognitive symptoms. The authors concluded that "Despite the pervasive impact on patients' lives, cognitive changes are not adequately acknowledged and addressed by healthcare providers" (Hurricane Voices Breast Cancer Foundation 2007). Oncologic professionals' lack of familiarity with research demonstrating that brain function is affected by treatment was cited as a potential factor responsible for the current state of affairs. However, assessment of cognitive function in cancer survivors is becoming more routine. For many patients, addressing cognitive problems that existed before the

Table 20.1 Potential causes of cognitive impairment in cancer survivors	
	Primary or metastatic cancer in the brain
	Indirect effects of non-brain cancer
	Neurotoxic effects of treatment
	Chemotherapy
	Radiation therapy
	Immunotherapy
	Hormonal therapy
	Surgery
	Effects of adjuvant medications
	Coexisting or preexisting neurologic and psychiatric illness
	Reactive mood and adjustment disorders
	Sensory impairment and general frailty
	Secondary gain

start of treatment is important, and the underlying cause can be proactively addressed. In addition, cognitive testing is increasingly becoming an endpoint in clinical trials. In this way, the effect of new agents or treatments on brain function can be evaluated.

Assessment of Cognitive Symptoms: The Role of the Neuropsychological Evaluation

For cancer survivors with treatment-related neurocognitive sequelae preventing or limiting successful return to work, neuropsychological assessment to examine strengths and weaknesses and to assist with intervention planning is indicated. Within the setting of oncology, neuropsychological evaluation provides a quantitative assessment of the cognitive and neurobehavioral symptoms that may arise as a consequence of cancer, treatment, or coexisting neurologic or psychiatric comorbidities. Brief screens of global neurocognitive dysfunction, such as those afforded by the Mini Mental Status Examination, are sensitive to profound cognitive impairment, which is rarely seen in cancer survivors. However, such screens are not sensitive to the types of neurocognitive disturbances most frequently seen in individuals with cancer, making them inappropriate when the purpose of the evaluation is to assist with decisions about returning to work and planning appropriate intervention strategies. Sole reliance on patient self-reporting is also problematic, because self-reported cognitive symptoms tend to correlate more significantly with indices of fatigue and mood than with objective evidence of cognitive impairment, as assessed by standardized neuropsychological testing.

Neuropsychological assessment in the setting of oncology is useful for (1) identifying any pretreatment neurocognitive deficits to allow more proactive intervention and to establish a baseline from which any neurotoxic effects of disease and treatment can be measured; (2) increasing understanding of the extent to which different treatment strategies improve neuropsychological functioning (secondary to improved tumor control) or have short-term or long-term neurotoxicities; (3) improving patient care and management by providing information to assist with treatment decisions, including differential diagnostic assessment; and (4) guiding interventions, such as pharmacologic and behavioral strategies aimed at reducing functional disabilities and improving quality of life.

Patterns of Cognitive Symptoms

The components of cognitive dysfunction vary as a result of the specific etiology, but several core cognitive domains appear to be differentially affected. Cancer patients with cognitive dysfunction often present with complaints of memory disturbance. They often describe everyday difficulties recalling something that they were told previously, forgetting or confusing details of recent events, forgetting to pass on a message, forgetting where they have placed things in their home or office, or forgetting dates and times of appointments. Other common patient complaints include "forgetting" words or the names of people or locations. In addition to these difficulties, patients may describe inefficiencies in attention, including trouble sustaining attention on a task for any length of time or a problem dividing attention between multiple tasks at the same time (i.e., "multitasking"). Thus, they may become overwhelmed when too much is happening at once. They are often easily distracted and find that they may go from project to project without getting any of them done. Cognitive processing speed is generally diminished, so that the patient is slower to perform their usual activities. Problems with organization or keeping up with conversations or occupational responsibilities owing to slowed mental processing speed are often described. Patients may describe their life in general as "no longer being on autopilot" and note that increased mental effort is required to perform even routine tasks. This contributes to the fatigue that is often a coexisting symptom.

Objective testing of memory generally demonstrates a restriction of working memory capacity (i.e., the patient is able to learn less information, and learning may be less efficient) and inefficient memory retrieval (i.e., spontaneous recall may be somewhat spotty). However, the ability to consolidate or store new information is generally intact, so that the memory disturbance observed in cancer patients is vastly different from that observed in those with neurodegenerative disorders such as Alzheimer disease, and the memory disturbance is often subtle and relative to the patient's pre-illness level of function. In general, reasoning and intellectual functions are not affected, but patients often have difficulty performing their normal work because of cognitive inefficiencies.

The impact of cognitive dysfunction on a cancer patient depends on the patient's developmental stage of life, line of work, and pre-illness lifestyle. For instance, the symptoms described above may not significantly affect the quality of life of an elderly retired person who can take things at his or her own pace. However, such symptoms may be disabling to an attorney in a courtroom setting and may necessitate changing jobs or claiming disability.

Etiology of Cognitive Symptoms

In adult patients with primary brain tumors or metastatic brain tumors from another cancer, the types of cognitive problems encountered are associated with the tumor location in the brain, tumor-related epilepsy, the speed of tumor growth, and the size of the tumor. In addition, most patients receive radiation treatment to the brain, which may also cause delayed cognitive symptoms.

In patients who have other types of cancer, studies have found that approximately one-third or more have cognitive symptoms before beginning treatment. However, most patients experience declines during or after treatment, and cognitive dysfunction may persist long after treatment is discontinued. The mechanisms by which chemotherapeutic agents affect brain function have only recently begun to be understood. A number of possible mechanisms are being studied, including the inflammatory response, autoimmune phenomena, hormonal influences, and direct neurotoxicity of specific agents. The development of animal models has increased understanding and will provide models to develop effective treatments. These findings are supported by imaging and electrophysiologic studies in cancer survivors that reveal alterations in metabolism, changes in brain anatomy, and alterations of brain electrical activity. In addition, cognitive dysfunction has been found to occur only in a subgroup of patients. Some survivors have no symptoms, most have mild to moderate symptoms, and very few have severe symptoms. This finding has provoked interest in identifying potential genetic risk factors that may underlie a given patient's vulnerability to develop cognitive side effects. Genes that alter the patient's ability to metabolize toxins, repair DNA, facilitate an inflammatory response, and other mechanisms are being studied.

Cognitive dysfunction in cancer patients can thus be conceptualized as a result of the interaction between the seed (cancer), the soil (the patient), and pesticides that are offered as treatment (Table 20.2). This is an exciting time for researchers who are interested in the effects of cancer and cancer treatment on brain function. Understanding the mechanisms of cognitive impairment and the development of efficacious interventions requires a multidisciplinary approach, including input from specialists in oncology, neuropsychology, cognitive neuroscience, genomics, proteomics, molecular epidemiology, functional neuroimaging, neuroimmunology, animal models, and drug discovery. Improved understanding of the pathophysiology of cognitive symptoms related to cancer treatment will guide the interventions to be offered to minimize the impact of cognitive dysfunction on patients' lives.

Table 20.2 Predictors of cognitive impairment

Host-related factors
   Genetic factors
   Immune reactivity
   Nutrition
   Cognitive reserve
Disease-related factors
   Tumor genetic mutations
   Paraneoplastic disorders
   Cytokines
Treatment-related factors
   Cytokines
   Poisons
   Specific mechanisms of action
Interactions between host, disease, and treatment-related factors

Interventions

There is a need to develop effective intervention techniques and programs for cancer patients and establish the efficacy of these interventions through clinical research. The loss of productivity, societal/economic demands, and psychological distress that are associated with cancer are highly significant. Advances in the treatment of cancer are being realized, and we must be ready to meet the needs of these survivors and their caregiving milieu. Effective and proactive assessment and treatment of cognitive dysfunction and other symptoms is a critical component throughout and following cancer treatment.

Fatigue, pain, sleep disturbance, and depression can make cognitive symptoms worse, and a multidisciplinary assessment, which includes treatment of all symptoms, a neuropsychological evaluation, and laboratory studies to rule out potentially reversible causes of cognitive problems, is optimal.

Stimulant therapies have proven effective in treating the cognitive dysfunction that commonly occurs in cancer patients, and other pharmacologic interventions commonly used to treat other diseases affecting cognitive function are currently being explored. Cognitive and behavioral intervention strategies that have been studied in the traditional rehabilitation literature concerning survivors of stroke and traumatic brain injury are becoming increasingly common. These interventions often focus on compensatory strategy training, stress management, energy conservation, and psychoeducation.

To provide a health care environment in which cancer survivors and their caregivers have access to best support practices requires a professional network that promotes evidence-based support practices throughout the continuum of care. Patient and family education is also extremely important. Potential neurobehavioral symptoms may not be explained to the patient, sometimes because the primary physician is not aware of the impact of even subtle symptoms on social and vocational functioning. Patients who experience these symptoms may wonder if they are mentally ill or may inaccurately attribute their symptoms to other causes. The more knowledgeable patients and their families are about the disease, treatment, and expected problems, the more effective the intervention process.

Conclusions

Cancer survivors who experience cognitive symptoms have the ability to improve their cognitive function at home and in vocational and leisure pursuits and enjoy an improved level of independence and quality of life, given the right support. We must be ready to meet the needs of these survivors and their caregiving milieu. Effective and proactive intervention strategies are a critical component throughout and following cancer treatment. As primary cancer therapies become more effective and more patients experience long-term remissions, assessing neurocognitive function and establishing effective treatment strategies will become even more important. Optimizing the quality of life of cancer patients is possible, essential, and should be on equal footing with antineoplastic therapy.

Key Practice Points

- Cognitive dysfunction is ubiquitous in cancer patients.
- The "seed" (cancer), the "soil" (patient), and the "pesticides" (treatments) all interact to cause symptom clusters that often include cognitive difficulties, fatigue, sleep disturbance, pain, affective distress, and other symptoms.
- Potential mechanisms by which persistent cognitive symptoms arise include inflammatory responses, hormonal influences, autoimmune phenomena, direct neurotoxicity of cancer drugs, and host genetic susceptibility.
- A number of intervention strategies, some borrowed from other neurological populations and some driven by our evolving understanding of the mechanisms of cancer-related cognitive dysfunction, can improve the function and quality of life of patients with cancer at all stages of their illness.

Suggested Readings

Hurricane Voices Breast Cancer Foundation. Cognitive Changes Related to Cancer Treatment. Published 2007. http://yourbrainafterchemo.com/PDFs/hv_cognitive_summary_final.pdf. Accessed October 8, 2013.

Meyers CA and Perry JR, eds. *Cognition and Cancer*. Cambridge: Cambridge University Press; 2008.

Rowland J, Hewitt M, Ganz P. Cancer survivorship: a new challenge in delivering quality cancer care. *J Clin Oncol* 2006;24:5101–5104.

Vargo MM, Smith RG, Stubblefield MD. Rehabilitation of the cancer patient. In: DeVita VT, Lawrence TS, Rosenberg SA, eds. *Cancer: Principles and Practice of Oncology*. Philadelphia, PA: Lippincott Williams & Wilkins; 2008:2857–2884.

Chapter 21
Endocrinologic Issues

Mimi I. Hu, Camilo Jimenez, Naifa L. Busaidy,
and Mouhammed Amir Habra

Contents

Introduction 344
Bone Metabolism Disorders 344
  Therapies Affecting Gonadal Function 344
    Selective Estrogen Receptor Modulators
    and Aromatase Inhibitors 345
    Gonadotropin-Releasing Hormone Agonists 346
    Bilateral Orchiectomy 346
    Chemotherapy-Induced Hypogonadism 346
  Other Factors Contributing to Bone Loss and Fractures 347
  Prevention and Management of Bone Loss in Cancer Patients 347
  Osteomalacia and Rickets 348
Metabolic Disorders 348
  Glucose Metabolism Disorders 348
  Lipid Disorders 349
    Hypertriglyceridemia 349
    Hypercholesterolemia 350
Thyroid Neoplasia and Dysfunction 350
  Thyroid Neoplasms 350
  Hyperthyroidism 351
  Hypothyroidism 351
Hypothalamic-Pituitary Dysfunction 352
  Hypopituitarism 352
  Central Diabetes Insipidus and Nephrogenic Diabetes Insipidus 354
  Syndrome of Inappropriate Antidiuretic Hormone Secretion 354
  Hyperprolactinemia 354
Adrenal Dysfunction 354
Gonadal System Disorders 355
Suggested Readings 357

Chapter Overview This chapter outlines the important and common late-onset, long-term endocrine disorders that occur as a consequence of cancer therapy in survivors: bone metabolism disorders, metabolic (i.e., glucose and lipid) disorders, thyroid neoplasia and dysfunction, hypothalamic-pituitary dysfunction, adrenal

L.E. Foxhall, M.A. Rodriguez (eds.), *Advances in Cancer Survivorship Management*,   343
MD Anderson Cancer Care Series, DOI 10.1007/978-1-4939-0986-5_21,
© The University of Texas M.D. Anderson Cancer Center 2015

dysfunction, and gonadal system disorders. Strategies for evaluating and managing these effects are included.

Introduction

Advances in targeted, antineoplastic therapies have positively influenced progression-free survival and cure rates in cancer survivors. However, long-term undesirable effects are recognized and often require a multidisciplinary approach for evaluation and management. Adverse effects of cancer therapy on the endocrine system can span from a subtle laboratory abnormality with limited clinical significance to an end-organ effect with significant morbidity.

Bone Metabolism Disorders

One of the most prevalent long-term health effects in cancer survivors is bone loss or osteoporosis. Osteoporosis is a systemic skeletal disorder defined by low bone mineral density (BMD) and deterioration of the bone tissue microarchitecture, which may result in an increased propensity to fracture.

Several groups of cancer survivors are recognized to be at particularly high risk of developing osteoporosis. Women with breast cancer and men with prostate cancer treated with modalities to decrease or suppress estrogen and testosterone levels are at high risk for excessive bone loss. A third group at risk for bone loss is patients with lymphoma, myeloma, or leukemia, because of their exposure to osteoclast-activating cytokines secreted by neoplastic cells and to high-dose glucocorticoids included in treatment regimens. In most cases, it is undetermined whether bone loss in cancer survivors arises directly from the therapy itself, from the underlying disease process (including the impact of cachexia, malnutrition, and poor calcium and vitamin D intake), or from a combination of the two. Declining BMD, with complications of fractures and pain, becomes more important with increased duration of survival. Developing strategies to monitor and prevent significant bone loss and to treat osteoporosis and insufficiency fractures in cancer survivors has become a prominent focus of clinical research.

Therapies Affecting Gonadal Function

Patients with breast and prostate cancer may develop osteoporosis as a consequence of therapeutic hypogonadism, an important strategy in controlling hormone-dependent growth in these cancers. Unfortunately, estrogen and testosterone deficiencies lead to increased bone resorption and diminished bone density owing to abnormally increased bone production of interleukin-1, interleukin-6, and tumor necrosis factor-alpha, as well as reduced bone synthesis of transforming growth factor-beta 1 (Janssens et al. 2005). Additionally, an abnormal increase in the ratio of RANKL (receptor activator of nuclear factor kappa-B ligand) to osteoprotegerin leads to increased osteoclastogenesis. Because estrogen- and androgen-deprivation therapies severely decrease hormone levels, similar or even worse microarchitectural abnormalities, manifesting clinically as osteoporosis or fractures, are expected in survivors of breast or prostate cancer compared with non–cancer survivors who have hormonal deficiencies.

Bone loss in the spine is more rapid and severe within the first year of various treatments for breast cancer (2.6–7.7%) than with natural menopause (averaging 2% per year for 5–10 years). More importantly, the annual incidence of vertebral insufficiency fractures is higher in patients with early-stage breast cancer than in the general population. Results from the Women's Health Initiative found that breast cancer survivors had a 15% higher rate of all fractures, regardless of the treatment they received, than women without any cancer history (Chen et al. 2005).

In patients with prostate cancer, androgen deprivation therapy (bilateral orchiectomy, leuprolide, or other gonadotropin-releasing hormone analogues), either alone or in combination with an antiandrogen therapy (e.g., flutamide, bicalutamide), causes profound hypogonadism characterized by loss of libido, muscle mass, and bone. Significant bone loss can occur in men within a year of castration or 6 months after initiating treatment with a gonadotropin-releasing hormone (GnRH) analogue. The annual incidence of osteoporotic fractures is higher in patients with prostate cancer treated with surgical or medical castration than in those who receive nonhormonal treatment or in healthy men (Melton et al. 2003). Fractures occur within 2 years of beginning androgen deprivation therapy and increase in frequency with the duration of the therapy. Importantly, skeletal fractures in patients with prostate cancer may be associated with decreased survival, independent of the pathologic stage of the cancer.

Selective Estrogen Receptor Modulators and Aromatase Inhibitors

In patients with breast cancer, selective estrogen receptor modulators (i.e., tamoxifen or raloxifene) have antagonistic effects in breast tissue, which supports the use of these agents as adjuvant therapy for patients at high risk for recurrence or as preventive therapy for healthy women at risk of developing breast cancer. However, both tamoxifen and raloxifene have antagonistic and agonistic effects on bone depending on the patient's menopausal status. Premenopausal women receiving tamoxifen or raloxifene can experience loss in bone mass attributable to antagonism of endogenous estrogen in bone. In contrast, postmenopausal women, who already have extremely low levels of bioavailable estrogen, typically exhibit increased bone density because the estrogen-like effect of a selective estrogen receptor modulator is sufficient to positively affect bone density (Vehmanen et al. 2006).

Aromatase inhibitors (AIs; e.g., anastrozole, letrozole, exemestane) have become preferred for postmenopausal women with hormone receptor–positive breast cancer.

By inhibiting the enzyme that mediates peripheral conversion of androgenic precursors (testosterone and androstenedione) of adrenal origin to estradiol and estrone, AIs can further suppress estrogen levels in postmenopausal women with breast cancer. Thus, AIs can lead to significant bone loss and increased fracture risk compared with placebo or tamoxifen (Baum et al. 2003; Howell 2006; Perez et al. 2006; Coleman et al. 2007). Interestingly, several studies revealed that patients with normal BMD at baseline did not become osteoporotic; in comparison, osteopenic patients experienced greater decreases in BMD after treatment with an AI (Perez et al. 2006; Coleman et al. 2007). Thus, surveillance and management of bone loss should be personalized to each patient on the basis of appropriate risk assessment.

Gonadotropin-Releasing Hormone Agonists

For premenopausal women, estrogen suppression is required for the treatment of hormone-sensitive breast cancer. This can be accomplished by bilateral oophorectomy, radiation-induced ovarian ablation, or administration of an agonist of GnRH or luteinizing hormone–releasing hormone (LHRH). Goserelin, an LHRH-agonist, in combination with tamoxifen is preferred over either treatment alone in premenopausal women with hormone-sensitive breast cancer. Consequently, BMD decreases substantially; however, BMD can recover partially within 1 year after cessation of treatment with goserelin.

In patients with prostate cancer, significant losses in BMD can occur in those treated with leuprolide or goserelin, in ranges higher than observed with normal male aging (Maillefert et al. 1999; Smith et al. 2001b). These losses in BMD are associated with abnormally increased bone turnover, in which bone destruction is predominant over bone formation.

Bilateral Orchiectomy

A significant reduction of BMD in both trabecular and cortical bone occurs in patients with prostate cancer 1–2 years after bilateral orchiectomy (Eriksson et al. 1995; Daniell 1997; Smith et al. 2001b). Fracture incidence is higher in patients treated with bilateral orchiectomy than in healthy, noncastrated cohorts (40% vs. 19%; Melton et al. 2003).

Chemotherapy-Induced Hypogonadism

Adjuvant systemic chemotherapy can induce ovarian failure in premenopausal women with early-stage breast cancer and can result in excessive bone loss in the first 12 months: 7% in the lumbar spine and 4.6% in the femoral neck. In addition, chemotherapy-induced menopause is a more important cause of osteoporosis than the direct effects of cytotoxic agents and glucocorticoids. Chemotherapy-induced amenorrhea is dependent on age (older than 40 years), dose, and medication type (e.g., cyclophosphamide, L-phenylalanine mustard, busulfan, chlorambucil, mitomycin-C). Patients with testicular cancer treated with cisplatin also develop hypogonadism.

Other Factors Contributing to Bone Loss and Fractures

Hematopoietic stem cell transplantation can lead to significant bone loss, most notably in the femoral neck, within the first 3–6 months after transplantation. In addition to increasing the risk of developing a hip fracture, reduced femoral neck BMD in patients undergoing transplantation is associated with avascular osteonecrosis.

Radiotherapy after surgical resection of breast, prostate, or gynecologic cancer can increase the risk of developing rib or pelvic insufficiency fractures. Exposure to high-dose corticosteroids used with systemic chemotherapy or to treat graft-versus-host disease exacerbates bone loss acutely. Other conditions, such as vitamin D deficiency or decreased physical activity during and after cancer therapy, may potentiate bone loss in this patient population.

Prevention and Management of Bone Loss in Cancer Patients

The National Comprehensive Cancer Center Network published guidelines on bone health surveillance in cancer patients. These guidelines incorporated fracture risk analysis by BMD, FRAX (an online calculation tool developed by the World Health Organization), and risk factors for bone loss, with guidance of pharmacologic therapy for low bone mass or osteoporosis (Gralow et al. 2009).

Prevention and treatment of bone loss in cancer patients has been best studied in breast cancer survivors receiving bisphosphonates for the prevention of bone loss related to chemotherapy, tamoxifen, and AIs (Gnant et al. 2008; Greenspan et al. 2008). Early initiation of bisphosphonate therapy may be beneficial in preventing or delaying bone loss. The clinical value of this practice will need to be validated, however, by demonstration of diminished fracture rates in longer follow-up studies of these patients. Very few trials have evaluated the effect of antiresorptive agents in patients with prostate cancer who undergo androgen deprivation therapy. For now, bisphosphonates remain the standard of care for men with osteoporosis.

Anabolic therapy with teriparatide, or parathyroid hormone 1-84, induces bone formation and prevents fractures in both men and women with severe osteoporosis. However, anabolic therapy induces production of growth factors that may theoretically induce tumor growth or tumor activation. Prior skeletal radiotherapy often precludes the use of teriparatide because of the perceived increased risk of developing osteosarcoma in these patients. These agents have not yet been investigated in patients with cancer; therefore, the risks and benefits of the use of anabolic agents should be considered carefully for cancer survivors (Hu et al. 2007).

Finally, denosumab, a fully human monoclonal antibody against RANKL to inhibit osteoclast activation, has been investigated in postmenopausal women with osteoporosis, cancer-related bone loss, and metastatic bone disease (Ellis et al.

2009; Smith et al. 2009; Stopeck et al. 2010; Boonen et al. 2011; Fizazi et al. 2011; Henry et al. 2011). Advantages of denosumab include the lack of nephrotoxicity and the reversibility of the suppressive effect on osteoclast activity.

Currently, no reports on the bone-protective effects of calcium and vitamin D in patients with cancer have been published. However, supplementation with vitamin D has been shown to reduce the risk for hip fractures in healthy ambulatory women. Evaluations of low bone mass are recommended to include an assessment of vitamin D status.

Osteomalacia and Rickets

Osteomalacia is a disorder of decreased bone mineralization of osteoid at sites of bone turnover, which can lead to bone pain, fracture, and difficulty walking or muscle weakness. In children, the abnormal mineralization and maturation of the growth plate at the epiphysis is called rickets. Vitamin D deficiency (related to poor nutritional intake, lack of sun exposure, or malabsorption) and renal wasting of phosphorus are common causes of osteomalacia, especially in cancer survivors. Other contributing factors include chronic kidney disease, exposure to aluminum in total parenteral nutrition, and systemic acidosis. Antineoplastic agents (e.g., ifosfamide, estramustine) can also cause or worsen osteomalacia. Treatment should include vitamin D replacement and correction of hypophosphatemia and hypocalcemia.

Metabolic Disorders

Glucose Metabolism Disorders

Glucocorticoids are used with many chemotherapy protocols and can have profound effects on glucose levels by increasing insulin resistance. Glucocorticoids can unmask preexisting prediabetic states by precipitating overt diabetes or make diabetes more difficult to control. The severity may range from asymptomatic hyperglycemia to nonketotic hyperosmolar coma. Most patients who are receiving glucocorticoids and have elevated glucose require insulin therapy to achieve blood glucose control, especially when given high-dose steroids.

Currently, there are no evidence-based, specific guidelines for the management of steroid-induced diabetes mellitus in patients with cancer. Long-acting and intermediate-acting insulin formulations are more effective at controlling glucose levels when they are combined with mealtime rapid-acting or short-acting insulin than with sliding-scale regimens that use short-acting insulin alone. Conflicting clinical study results concerning glargine and cancer have led to concerns that the mitogenic effect of insulin and insulin analogues, which cross-activate IGF-1 receptors, may promote malignancy. These concerns have drawn attention to the gap in knowledge about proper diabetic management strategies for cancer patients and survivors to maximize their survival (Eckardt et al. 2007; Hemkens et al. 2009; Home and Lagarenne 2009; Weinstein et al. 2009).

Temsirolimus, an inhibitor of mammalian target of rapamycin (mTOR), may cause secondary diabetes in 10–30% of patients with renal cell carcinoma. The mechanism by which temsirolimus leads to diabetes may be similar to that of tacrolimus, which decreases glucose-stimulated insulin release in the pancreatic islets.

L-asparaginase and pegylated asparaginase, used to treat hematologic malignancies, may cause hyperglycemia and occasionally diabetic ketoacidosis through unclear mechanisms (Gillette et al. 1972; Land et al. 1972). It has been postulated that inhibition of insulin, insulin receptor synthesis, or both may lead to a combined insulin deficiency and resistance syndrome. Pancreatitis, another known side effect, may contribute to hyperglycemia through islet cell destruction. Insulin therapy is frequently required to treat the hyperglycemia, which reverses upon discontinuation of treatment with L-asparaginase. Close monitoring for hypoglycemia is recommended after discontinuation of treatment with L-asparaginase. Long-term insulin therapy may not be needed in all cases of L-asparaginase-induced diabetes mellitus.

Streptozocin, used to treat malignant islet cell tumors and other neuroendocrine tumors, can lead to long-lasting impairment of pancreatic β-cells in the production and release of insulin; however, most of the effects of streptozocin are reversible upon discontinuation of treatment with the drug. Although the reported incidence of glucose intolerance varies from 6 to 60%, cases are often mild to moderate in severity.

Use of recombinant interferon-alpha (IFN-alpha-2a, -2b) to treat malignancies has been associated with the development of new-onset hyperglycemia, deterioration of glycemic control in diabetics, and diabetic ketoacidosis. Although the incidence of IFN-alpha–induced diabetes mellitus in patients with cancer is unclear, it arises in about 0.7% of patients treated for chronic active hepatitis C (Okanoue et al. 1996). The exact mechanism of IFN-alpha–induced diabetes is not well understood.

Lipid Disorders

Lipid disorders are seldom evaluated in the process of active anticancer therapy because patients are often encouraged to maintain a positive metabolic balance via liberal oral intake. Some lipid disorders may be short-lived without clear clinical consequences, but some may be of clinical importance and need to be detected and treated. In general, triglyceride levels higher than 1,000 mg/dL need to be treated urgently owing to serious potential complications, such as pancreatitis and visual impairment.

Hypertriglyceridemia

IFNs may induce hypertriglyceridemia (as high as 1,000 mg/dL) by increasing hepatic and peripheral fatty acid production and suppressing hepatic triglyceride lipase. In one case, a controlled diet and gemfibrozil had therapeutic effects despite continued treatment with IFN-alpha (Berruti et al. 1992).

All-trans retinoic acid (tretinoin) and other retinoic acid derivatives, which are used to treat several malignancies (e.g., head and neck cancer, acute promyelocytic leukemia), are well known to induce hypertriglyceridemia and hypercholesterol-emia (Marsden 1986; Castaigne et al. 1990; Vahlquist 1991; Fujiwara et al. 1995; Kanamaru et al. 1995). Hypertriglyceridemia is the most common drug-related adverse effect (79%) observed with bexarotene, a synthetic retinoid X receptor–selective retinoid used to treat cutaneous T-cell lymphoma (Duvic et al. 2001a, b). Cerebrovascular accidents and pancreatitis have been described in association with retinoid-induced hypertriglyceridemia. Retinoid-induced hyperlipidemia has been successfully treated with fibrates or fish oil.

mTOR inhibitors frequently cause hyperlipidemia owing to impaired clearance of lipids from the bloodstream, but often this issue disappears when treatment with the drug is discontinued.

Hypercholesterolemia

Dose-related hypercholesterolemia has been described in patients with adrenocorti-cal carcinoma treated with mitotane from inhibition of cholesterol oxidase (Vassilopoulou-Sellin and Samaan 1991). Patients with adrenocortical carcinoma usually have a poor prognosis, making mild to moderate elevation of cholesterol less clinically relevant. However, long-term survivors who continue to receive treat-ment with mitotane can experience early development of atherosclerotic disease. The benefits of treating mitotane-induced lipid abnormalities have not been estab-lished in long-term survivors.

Hypercholesterolemia is the second most common side effect of bexarotene (Duvic et al. 2001a, b). The long-term significance of this drug-induced hypercho-lesterolemia is unclear; however, atorvastatin has been successfully used to treat hypercholesterolemia in these patients at our institution.

Thyroid Neoplasia and Dysfunction

Thyroid Neoplasms

Ionizing radiation is the only well-established etiology of thyroid cancer, most com-monly the papillary subtype, through induction of DNA damage and formation of chromosomal rearrangements. A dose-response relationship between radiation exposure and relative risk of thyroid cancer occurs with radiation doses of ≤ 5 Gy (Ron et al. 1995). Female sex, age younger than 15 years when exposed to radiation, and a 20- to 30-year period since radiation exposure (even to areas outside of the head and neck) are associated with increased risk for thyroid cancer. Incidence of local invasion, multicentric disease, and distant metastasis at presentation is higher among patients with radiation-induced thyroid cancer than among patients with sporadic thyroid cancer. Thyroid carcinoma is most evident in long-term survivors of Hodgkin disease and non-Hodgkin lymphoma.

Chemotherapy is not a proven risk factor for thyroid carcinoma despite rare case reports to the contrary. The administration of radioactive iodine for diagnostic purposes does not seem to increase the risk of developing thyroid carcinoma.

Hyperthyroidism

Radiation-induced hyperthyroidism has been described but is far less common than radiation-induced hypothyroidism, which has long-term consequences. Thyroiditis-induced thyrotoxicosis occurs within 2 years of radiotherapy in most cases; several months later, hypothyroidism occurs. Risk of developing Graves disease also increases following radiotherapy. Patients with lymphoma treated with radiotherapy constitute the largest population to develop Graves disease after radiotherapy. Patients treated with radiation for nasopharyngeal, breast, or laryngeal carcinoma may also develop Graves disease.

Cytokine therapy (e.g., IFN-alpha, interleukin-2) has also been reported to lead to thyroid disease. IFN-alpha, via autoantibody production, can lead to autoimmune thyroid disease, specifically primary hypothyroidism, transient thyrotoxicosis, or, more rarely, Graves disease. Thyroid scans showing increased homogeneous uptake in the presence of hyperthyroidism are highly suggestive of Graves disease and warrant antithyroid medications. Treatment with interleukin-2 alone causes transient hyperthyroidism followed by hypothyroidism in about 50% of patients through an unclear mechanism (Vialettes et al. 1993).

Hypothyroidism

Head and neck radiotherapy, an important etiology of thyroid dysfunction, can induce primary hypothyroidism when administered in doses higher than 25 Gy to the region near the thyroid gland. Most cases of primary hypothyroidism occur about 5 years after radiotherapy. Subclinical hypothyroidism (elevated thyroid-stimulating hormone levels with normal thyroxine levels) without overt hypothyroidism occurs more often when doses of less than 40 Gy are administered. The probability of developing hypothyroidism increases with increasing radiation doses, increasing duration of follow-up after treatment, combined radiation and surgical treatments, and failure to shield midline structures. Other more immediate risk factors for hypothyroidism include thyroid resection during laryngectomy and disruption of the vascular supply of the thyroid gland during head and neck surgery.

Various agents used in cancer management have been associated with primary hypothyroidism: IFN-alpha, interleukin-2, cisplatin, bleomycin, dactinomycin, vinblastine, and etoposide. Newer antineoplastic agents such as targeted therapies or immunotherapies are associated with a variety of thyroid abnormalities. Autoimmune thyroid disease has been observed with the use of monoclonal antibodies against CD52 for chronic lymphocytic leukemia (alemtuzumab) and CTLA-4 for melanoma (ipilimumab; Hamnvik et al. 2011).

Tyrosine kinase inhibitors (imatinib, sorafenib, sunitinib, and pazopanib) can lead to increased levothyroxine requirements in patients who have undergone thyroidectomy, suggesting that tyrosine kinase inhibitors may accelerate the clearance of levothyroxine (Dora et al. 2008). Additionally, it has been hypothesized that the inhibition of vascular endothelial growth factor by tyrosine kinase inhibitors may decrease vascular supply to the thyroid gland. Prospective studies of sorafenib estimated that the risk of thyroid dysfunction with sorafenib reached 68%; however, only 6% had clinical symptoms requiring thyroid hormone replacement (Miyake et al. 2009). Similarly, 36% of patients treated with sunitinib had persistently elevated levels of thyroid-stimulating hormone, suggestive of primary hypothyroidism; this was especially evident in those who had received long-term treatment with sunitinib (Desai et al. 2006). Some patients were reported to present with thyrotoxicosis preceding hypothyroidism, which supports the theory that sunitinib leads to destructive thyroiditis (Faris et al. 2007; Grossmann et al. 2008). Impaired iodine uptake and inhibition of peroxidase activity were also suggested as potential mechanisms to explain hypothyroidism (Mannavola et al. 2007; Wong et al. 2007).

Hypothalamic-Pituitary Dysfunction

It is generally believed that chemotherapy alone does not induce hypothalamic-pituitary dysfunction, although Rose et al. (2004) showed that hypothalamic dysfunction could occur in survivors of non–central nervous system tumors who received chemotherapy instead of radiotherapy. Malignancies in the vicinity of the hypothalamic-pituitary axis are often treated with surgery or radiotherapy. The hypothalamus is more sensitive than the pituitary gland to the effects of radiation. Hypothalamic-pituitary dysfunction resulting from radiotherapy in the cranial region may be delayed and can linger for many years. Reports have suggested that the number of pituitary deficiencies increases with the length of time since the radiotherapy. Surgery to remove malignancies such as craniopharyngioma in the hypothalamic region may also result in hypothalamic dysfunction.

Hypopituitarism

Hypopituitarism is not as common for survivors of adult nonpituitary brain tumors as it is for survivors of childhood nonpituitary brain tumors (Agha et al. 2005). IFN has been associated with hypopituitarism (Concha et al. 2003; Chan and Cockram 2004). Besides surgery, radiotherapy is often used to treat malignancies in the craniospinal region. Hypopituitarism, one of the most common complications after radiotherapy to the hypothalamus-pituitary axis, has been reported to occur in 41% of survivors of nonpituitary brain tumors (Agha et al. 2005). After adjuvant radiotherapy for pituitary macroadenoma, 36% of patients developed partial pituitary hormone deficiency and 61% had panhypopituitarism; 87% needed hormone replacement therapy to alleviate symptoms (Langsenlehner et al. 2007). The prevalence of hypopituitarism increases with the duration of follow-up.

Hypophysitis is a rare immune-related side effect that has been reported in 1–6% of patients with melanoma treated with ipilimumab. Hypophysitis leads to headaches, visual disturbances, and panhypopituitarism, and it is usually visible on magnetic resonance imaging as a pituitary enlargement with thickening of the stalk. Patients should initially receive high doses of glucocorticoids along with thyroid hormone replacement therapy. The necessary duration of replacement therapy with physiologic doses of hydrocortisone and levothyroxine could be very long, and permanent substitution therapy may be required (Dillard et al. 2010).

Growth hormone (GH) deficiency, a commonly reported complication of childhood cancer and cancer treatment, is associated with increased adipose mass and decreased lean mass, as well as decreased strength, exercise tolerance, BMD, and quality of life. GH deficiency is the most frequently observed endocrine deficiency in long-term survivors of childhood cancer who received cranial radiotherapy, and the effects are related to the dose of radiation received (Gleeson and Shalet 2004). After receiving radiotherapy to the brain, 90% of patients can become GH deficient within 10 years after treatment (Borson-Chazot and Brue 2006). Chemotherapy has also been implicated in GH deficiency. Findings from a study of children treated with or without adjuvant chemotherapy after radiotherapy for medulloblastoma revealed that the addition of chemotherapy may intensify the adverse effects of radiotherapy on GH secretion (Olshan et al. 1992). In addition, glucocorticoids can completely suppress the secretion of GH.

Gonadotropin deficiency refers to either the absence or loss of luteinizing hormone and follicle-stimulating hormone. This deficiency has been recognized as an effect of surgery in the hypothalamic region, chemotherapy, and radiotherapy. In adults, gonadotropin deficiency may cause sex steroid hormone deficiency, amenorrhea, loss of libido, erectile dysfunction, and infertility. Radiation doses greater than 35 Gy to the hypothalamus-pituitary axis may result in gonadotropin deficiency in 27–61% of patients (Constine et al. 1993; Agha et al. 2005; Cohen 2005). The incidence of gonadotropin deficiency increases with time since radiotherapy, with a cumulative incidence of 20–50% reported in patients at long-term follow-up, making it the second most common anterior pituitary hormone deficiency (Rappaport et al. 1982).

The frequency of pituitary or hypothalamic hypothyroidism and hypoadrenalism in patients who undergo radiotherapy for brain tumors not involving the pituitary gland is generally less than 5% (Constine et al. 1987).

Central Diabetes Insipidus and Nephrogenic Diabetes Insipidus

Nephrogenic diabetes insipidus (DI) may result from the effects of ifosfamide or streptozocin on tubular reabsorption of water (Murray-Lyon et al. 1971; Delaney et al. 1987; Rossi et al. 1995; Negro et al. 1998). Although both ifosfamide and streptozocin produce cytotoxic effects on renal tubular cells, the cellular mechanism of nephrogenic DI is not clearly outlined. To the best of our knowledge, no new reports on nephrogenic DI from antineoplastic drugs have been published in the past decade.

Unlike anterior pituitary dysfunction, central DI has not been diagnosed in survivors of childhood tumors who underwent radiotherapy to the hypothalamic-pituitary axis (Gleeson and Shalet 2004). Central DI frequently occurs as a result of pituitary or hypothalamic malignancies and from surgery or cranial radiotherapy to these regions.

Syndrome of Inappropriate Antidiuretic Hormone Secretion

Toxicity or nerve impairment to the posterior pituitary gland may result in the inappropriate production and secretion of antidiuretic hormone (ADH). Syndrome of inappropriate ADH secretion (SIADH) has long been associated with cancer therapy. Cytotoxic treatments that may cause SIADH include vinca alkaloids, cisplatin, cyclophosphamide, and melphalan (Sorensen et al. 1995; Otsuka et al. 1996; Brougham et al. 2002; Ishii et al. 2002; Kusuki et al. 2004). SIADH may also present as an endocrine paraneoplastic syndrome in which excessive ADH is secreted by tumors, usually of neuroendocrine origin (Robinson et al. 1980).

Hyperprolactinemia

Hyperprolactinemia is also a common disorder of the hypothalamic-pituitary axis (Karasek et al. 2006). Dopamine from the hypothalamus normally inhibits prolactin secretion from the pituitary gland. Cranial radiotherapy may interfere with this inhibition, especially with high doses of radiation (>50 Gy), resulting in hyperprolactinemia (Constine et al. 1987). Hyperprolactinemia has been described in both sexes and at all ages, but it occurs most frequently in young women after intensive radiotherapy and is usually subclinical.

Adrenal Dysfunction

The adrenal gland is often overlooked in terms of screening and testing for endocrine disruption. Symptoms of adrenal insufficiency may include malaise, fatigue, weakness, anorexia, nausea, vomiting, weight loss, abdominal pain, diarrhea, hypothermia or hyperthermia, hypotension, altered mental status, and coma. Such symptoms often overlap with symptoms of cancer or cancer therapy and adrenal deficiency may be overlooked. Numerous medications prescribed to patients with cancer may lead to adrenal dysfunction.

Mitotane can induce primary adrenal insufficiency through its adrenolytic activity, thus supporting its role in the treatment of adrenocortical carcinoma. Because mitotane must be administered in large doses to be therapeutic, it may destroy both normal and malignant adrenocortical cells. Suppressed glucocorticoid secretion and increased glucocorticoid and mineralocorticoid liver metabolism may also occur (Allolio and Fassnacht 2006; van Ditzhuijsen et al. 2007).

Various other antineoplastic agents have been associated with adrenal insufficiency, including busulfan (Ward et al. 1965; Smalley and Wall 1966) and suramin (Dorfinger et al. 1991). Although adrenal toxicity has been observed in animals treated with sunitinib, no overt, clinically significant adrenal suppression has been reported in humans receiving the drug. However, physicians are encouraged to monitor their patients for potential subclinical adrenal toxic effects.

Prolonged glucocorticoid exposure in the context of primary cancer treatment or supportive care (such as in graft-versus-host disease) is the most common cause of secondary adrenal insufficiency in cancer survivors. Long-term suppression of the hypothalamic-pituitary axis by exogenous glucocorticoids may render the adrenals atrophic (Howard and Pui 2002; Allolio and Fassnacht 2006). Slow tapering of high-dose steroids is required to allow resumption of normal adrenal function. Megestrol acetate is a progestational agent used to treat patients with endometrial and breast cancer and to improve appetite in patients with wasting syndromes. This agent has steroid activity that may suppress pituitary ACTH production, and abrupt withdrawal may cause central adrenal insufficiency.

Gonadal System Disorders

With advances in cancer treatment leading to prolonged survival, female and male survivors may be at risk for the development of reproductive disorders as a consequence of radiotherapy to the gonadal or hypothalamic regions, cytotoxic chemotherapy, or surgical resection of gonadal organs. It is important to discuss fertility issues before initiating treatments that carry significant risks for ovarian and testicular dysfunction or central hypogonadism (as described in a previous section).

In women, the effects of pelvic radiotherapy on the ovaries differ depending on the patient's age, the radiation dose, and the field of treatment. Radiation doses as low as 6 Gy can lead to ovarian failure and infertility in prepubertal girls and women older than 40 years (Lushbaugh and Casarett 1976; Howard 1991). Permanent infertility in women younger than 40 years usually occurs after radiation doses of greater than 20 Gy (Lushbaugh and Casarett 1976). Primary gonadal dysfunction in men after radiation exposure is also dose-dependent. Low-dose testicular radiotherapy leads to a transient suppression of sperm counts with a recovery time proportional to the radiation dose. Permanent infertility occurs with fractionated radiation doses of more than 2 Gy (Howell and Shalet 2002).

As discussed above, cytotoxic chemotherapy can lead to either primary or secondary hypogonadism. Alkylating agents (e.g., chlorambucil, melphalan, busulfan, cyclophosphamide, procarbazine) are not cell cycle–specific drugs, thereby making them generally highly gonadotoxic (Freckman et al. 1964; Ezdinli and Stutzman 1965; Bokemeyer et al. 1996; Meirow and Nugent 2001). Etoposide has been associated with transient and permanent ovarian failure (Choo et al. 1985; Wong et al. 1986). In men, alkylating agents, such as cyclophosphamide and chlorambucil, are associated with reversible but prolonged azoospermia. A high rate of permanent testicular dysfunction has been reported with procarbazine use (Charak et al. 1990). Dose-related impairment of spermatogenesis has been reported during treatment for testicular carcinoma with cisplatin, etoposide, and bleomycin (Petersen et al. 1994).

Consultation with a fertility preservation specialist is recommended after determining that a patient is at risk for treatment-induced infertility and is interested in fertility preservation options. Options include ovarian suppression, donor eggs or sperm, or ovarian or testicular tissue cryopreservation prior to initiating gonadotoxic therapy (Jeruss and Woodruff 2009).

Key Practice Points

- Because bone loss is one of the most prevalent endocrine adverse effects in cancer survivors, appropriate assessment (bone densitometry, vitamin D measurement, and FRAX assessment) should be performed for patients at risk.
- Hyperglycemia and dyslipidemia related to cancer treatments may be mild to severe, warranting medical treatment; however, long-lasting morbidity is not well established.
- A primary thyroid malignancy can develop in long-term cancer survivors who received radiotherapy to the neck during childhood.
- Thyroid dysfunction (hyperthyroidism, hypothyroidism) can occur after exposure to many different cancer treatments; symptoms suggestive of thyroid dysfunction warrant a good physical examination and laboratory testing.
- Hypopituitarism is most common in survivors of childhood nonpituitary brain tumors who received radiotherapy to the craniospinal region.
- Central hypogonadism from cancer treatments (e.g., craniospinal radiotherapy or surgical resection) and primary hypogonadism can lead to very uncomfortable symptoms and temporary or permanent infertility.
- Education regarding potential endocrine complications related to cancer treatments must be provided to patients, oncologists, and primary caregivers so that timely and appropriate evaluation, referrals to specialists, and management can be initiated.

Suggested Readings

Agha A, Sherlock M, Brennan S, et al. Hypothalamic-pituitary dysfunction after irradiation of nonpituitary brain tumors in adults. *J Clin Endocrinol Metab* 2005;90:6355–6360.

Allolio B, Fassnacht M. Clinical review: adrenocortical carcinoma: clinical update. *J Clin Endocrinol Metab* 2006;91:2027–2037.

Baum M, Buzdar A, Cuzick J, et al. Anastrozole alone or in combination with tamoxifen versus tamoxifen alone for adjuvant treatment of postmenopausal women with early-stage breast cancer: results of the ATAC (Arimidex, Tamoxifen Alone or in Combination) trial efficacy and safety update analyses. *Cancer* 2003;98:1802–1810.

Berruti A, Gorzegno G, Vitetta G, et al. Hypertriglyceridemia during long-term interferon-alpha therapy: efficacy of diet and gemfibrosil treatment. A case report. *Tumori* 1992;78: 353–355.

Bokemeyer C, Berger CC, Kuczyk MA, et al. Evaluation of long-term toxicity after chemotherapy for testicular cancer. *J Clin Oncol* 1996;14:2923–2932.

Boonen S, Adachi JD, Man Z, et al. Treatment with denosumab reduces the incidence of new vertebral and hip fractures in postmenopausal women at high risk. *J Clin Endocrinol Metab* 2011;96:1727–1736.

Borson-Chazot F, Brue T. Pituitary deficiency after brain radiation therapy. *Ann Endocrin (Paris)* 2006;67:303–309.

Brougham MF, Kelnar CJ, Wallace WH. The late endocrine effects of childhood cancer treatment. *Pediatr Rehabil* 2002;5:191–201.

Castaigne S, Chomienne C, Daniel MT, et al. All-trans retinoic acid as a differentiation therapy for acute promyelocytic leukemia. I. Clinical results. *Blood* 1990;76:1704–1709.

Chan WB, Cockram CS. Panhypopituitarism in association with interferon-alpha treatment. *Singapore Med J* 2004;45:93–94.

Charak BS, Gupta R, Mandrekar P, et al. Testicular dysfunction after cyclophosphamide-vincristine-procarbazine-prednisolone chemotherapy for advanced Hodgkin's disease. A long-term follow-up study. *Cancer* 1990;65:1903–1906.

Chen Z, Maricic M, Bassford TL, et al. Fracture risk among breast cancer survivors: results from the Women's Health Initiative Observational Study. *Arch Intern Med* 2005;165:552–558.

Choo YC, Chan SY, Wong LC, et al. Ovarian dysfunction in patients with gestational trophoblastic neoplasia treated with short intensive courses of etoposide (VP-16-213). *Cancer* 1985;55: 2348–2352.

Cohen LE. Endocrine late effects of cancer treatment. *Endocrinol Metab Clin North Am* 2005;34: 769–789.

Coleman RE, Banks LM, Girgis SI, et al. Skeletal effects of exemestane on bone-mineral density, bone biomarkers, and fracture incidence in postmenopausal women with early breast cancer participating in the Intergroup Exemestane Study (IES): a randomised controlled study. *Lancet Oncol* 2007;8:119–127.

Concha LB, Carlson HE, Heimann A, et al. Interferon-induced hypopituitarism. *Am J Med* 2003;114:161–163.

Constine LS, Rubin P, Woolf PD, et al. Hyperprolactinemia and hypothyroidism following cytotoxic therapy for central nervous system malignancies. *J Clin Oncol* 1987;5:1841–1851.

Constine LS, Woolf PD, Cann D, et al. Hypothalamic-pituitary dysfunction after radiation for brain tumors. *N Engl J Med* 1993;328:87–94.

Daniell HW. Osteoporosis after orchiectomy for prostate cancer. *J Urol* 1997;157:439–444.

Delaney V, de Pertuz Y, Nixon D, et al. Indomethacin in streptozocin-induced nephrogenic diabetes insipidus. *Am J Kidney Dis* 1987;9:79–83.

Desai J, Yassa L, Marqusee E, et al. Hypothyroidism after sunitinib treatment for patients with gastrointestinal stromal tumors. *Ann Intern Med* 2006;145:660–664.

Dillard T, Yedinak CG, Alumkal J, et al. Anti-CTLA-4 antibody therapy associated autoimmune hypophysitis: serious immune related adverse events across a spectrum of cancer subtypes. *Pituitary* 2010;13:29–38.

Dora JM, Leie MA, Netto B, et al. Lack of imatinib-induced thyroid dysfunction in a cohort of non-thyroidectomized patients. *Eur J Endocrinol* 2008;158:771–772.

Dorfinger K, Niederle B, Vierhapper H, et al. Suramin and the human adrenocortex: results of experimental and clinical studies. *Surgery* 1991;110:1100–1105.

Duvic M, Hymes K, Heald P, et al. Bexarotene is effective and safe for treatment of refractory advanced-stage cutaneous T-cell lymphoma: multinational phase II-III trial results. *J Clin Oncol* 2001a;19:2456–2471.

Duvic M, Martin AG, Kim Y, et al. Phase 2 and 3 clinical trial of oral bexarotene (Targretin capsules) for the treatment of refractory or persistent early-stage cutaneous T-cell lymphoma. *Arch Dermatol* 2001b;137:581–593.

Eckardt K, May C, Koenen M, et al. IGF-1 receptor signalling determines the mitogenic potency of insulin analogues in human smooth muscle cells and fibroblasts. *Diabetologia* 2007;50: 2534–2543.

Ellis GK, Bone HG, Chlebowski R, et al. Effect of denosumab on bone mineral density in women receiving adjuvant aromatase inhibitors for non-metastatic breast cancer: subgroup analyses of a phase 3 study. *Breast Cancer Res Treat* 2009;118:81–87.

Eriksson S, Eriksson A, Stege R, et al. Bone mineral density in patients with prostatic cancer treated with orchidectomy and with estrogens. *Calcif Tissue Int* 1995;57:97–99.

Ezdinli EZ, Stutzman L. Chlorambucil therapy for lymphomas and chronic lymphocytic leukemia. *JAMA* 1965;191:444–450.

Faris JE, Moore AF, Daniels GH. Sunitinib (sutent)-induced thyrotoxicosis due to destructive thyroiditis: a case report. *Thyroid* 2007;17:1147–1149.

Fizazi K, Carducci M, Smith M, et al. Denosumab versus zoledronic acid for treatment of bone metastases in men with castration-resistant prostate cancer: a randomised, double-blind study. *Lancet* 2011;377:813–822.

Freckman HA, Fry HL, Mendez FL, et al. Chlorambucil-prednisolone therapy for disseminated breast carcinoma. *JAMA* 1964;189:23–26.

Fujiwara H, Umeda Y, Yonekura S. Cerebellar infarction with hypertriglyceridemia during all-trans retinoic acid therapy for acute promyelocytic leukemia. *Leukemia* 1995;9:1602–1603.

Gillette PC, Hill LL, Starling KA, et al. Transient diabetes mellitus secondary to L-asparaginase therapy in acute leukemia. *J Pediatr* 1972;81:109–111.

Gleeson HK, Shalet SM. The impact of cancer therapy on the endocrine system in survivors of childhood brain tumours. *Endocr Relat Cancer* 2004;11:589–602.

Gnant M, Mlineritsch B, Luschin-Ebengreuth G, et al. Adjuvant endocrine therapy plus zoledronic acid in premenopausal women with early-stage breast cancer: 5-year follow-up of the ABCSG-12 bone-mineral density substudy. *Lancet Oncol* 2008;9:840–849.

Gralow JR, Biermann JS, Farooki A, et al. NCCN task force report: bone health in cancer care. *J Natl Compr Canc Netw* 2009;7:S1–S35.

Greenspan SL, Brufsky A, Lembersky BC, et al. Risedronate prevents bone loss in breast cancer survivors: a 2-year, randomized, double-blind, placebo-controlled clinical trial. *J Clin Oncol* 2008;26:2644–2652.

Grossmann M, Premaratne E, Desai J, et al. Thyrotoxicosis during sunitinib treatment for renal cell carcinoma. *Clin Endocrinol (Oxf)* 2008;69:669–672.

Hamnvik OP, Larsen PR, Marqusee E. Thyroid dysfunction from antineoplastic agents. *J Natl Cancer Inst* 2011;103:1572–1587.

Hemkens LG, Grouven U, Bender R, et al. Risk of malignancies in patients with diabetes treated with human insulin or insulin analogues: a cohort study. *Diabetologia* 2009;52:1732–1744.

Henry DH, Costa L, Goldwasser F, et al. Randomized, double-blind study of denosumab versus zoledronic acid in the treatment of bone metastases in patients with advanced cancer (excluding breast and prostate cancer) or multiple myeloma. *J Clin Oncol* 2011;29:1125–1132.

Home PD, Lagarenne P. Combined randomised controlled trial experience of malignancies in studies using insulin glargine. *Diabetologia* 2009;12:2499–2506.

Howard GC. Fertility following cancer therapy. *Clin Oncol (R Coll Radiol)* 1991;3:283–287.

Howard SC, Pui CH. Endocrine complications in pediatric patients with acute lymphoblastic leukemia. *Blood Rev* 2002;16:225–243.

Howell A. The 'Arimidex', Tamoxifen, Alone or in Combination (ATAC) trial: a step forward in the treatment of early breast cancer. *Rev Recent Clin Trials* 2006;1:207–215.

Howell SJ, Shalet SM. Effect of cancer therapy on pituitary-testicular axis. *Int J Androl* 2002;25: 269–276.

Hu MI, Gagel RF, Jimenez C. Bone loss in patients with breast or prostate cancer. *Curr Osteoporosis Rep* 2007;5:170–178.

Ishii K, Aoki Y, Sasaki M, et al. Syndrome of inappropriate secretion of antidiuretic hormone induced by intraarterial cisplatin chemotherapy. *Gynecol Oncol* 2002;87:150–151.

Janssens K, ten Dijke P, Janssens S, et al. Transforming growth factor-beta1 to the bone. *Endocr Rev* 2005;26:743–774.

Jeruss JS, Woodruff TK. Preservation of fertility in patients with cancer. *N Engl J Med* 2009;360: 902–911.

Kanamaru A, Takemoto Y, Tanimoto M, et al. All-trans retinoic acid for the treatment of newly diagnosed acute promyelocytic leukemia. Japan Adult Leukemia Study Group. *Blood* 1995;85: 1202–1206.

Karasek M, Pawlikowski M, Lewinski A. [Hyperprolactinemia: causes, diagnosis, and treatment]. *Endokrynol Pol* 2006;57:656–662.

Kusuki M, Iguchi H, Nakamura A, et al. The syndrome of inappropriate antidiuretic hormone secretion associated with chemotherapy for hypopharyngeal cancer. *Acta Otolaryngol Suppl* 2004:74–77.

Land VJ, Sutow WW, Fernbach DJ, et al. Toxicity of L-asparginase in children with advanced leukemia. *Cancer* 1972;30:339–347.

Langsenlehner T, Stiegler C, Quehenberger F, et al. Long-term follow-up of patients with pituitary macroadenomas after postoperative radiation therapy: analysis of tumor control and functional outcome. *Strahlenther Onkol* 2007;183:241–247.

Lushbaugh CC, Casarett GW. The effects of gonadal irradiation in clinical radiation therapy: a review. *Cancer* 1976;37:1111–1125.

Maillefert JF, Sibilia J, Michel F, et al. Bone mineral density in men treated with synthetic gonadotropin-releasing hormone agonists for prostatic carcinoma. *J Urol* 1999;161: 1219–1222.

Mannavola D, Coco P, Vannucchi G, et al. A novel tyrosine-kinase selective inhibitor, sunitinib, induces transient hypothyroidism by blocking iodine uptake. *J Clin Endocrinol Metab* 2007;92:3531–3534.

Marsden J. Hyperlipidaemia due to isotretinoin and etretinate: possible mechanisms and consequences. *Br J Dermatol* 1986;114:401–407.

Meirow D, Nugent D. The effects of radiotherapy and chemotherapy on female reproduction. *Hum Reprod Update* 2001;7:535–543.

Melton LJ 3rd, Alothman KI, Khosla S, et al. Fracture risk following bilateral orchiectomy. *J Urol* 2003;169:1747–1750.

Miyake H, Kurahashi T, Yamanaka K, et al. Abnormalities of thyroid function in Japanese patients with metastatic renal cell carcinoma treated with sorafenib: a prospective evaluation. *Urol Oncol* 2009;5:515–519.

Murray-Lyon IM, Cassar J, Coulson R, et al. Further studies on streptozotocin therapy for a multiple-hormone-producing islet cell carcinoma. *Gut* 1971;12:717–720.

Negro A, Regolisti G, Perazzoli F, et al. Ifosfamide-induced renal Fanconi syndrome with associated nephrogenic diabetes insipidus in an adult patient. *Nephrol Dial Transplant* 1998;13:1547–1549.

Okanoue T, Sakamoto S, Itoh Y, et al. Side effects of high-dose interferon therapy for chronic hepatitis C. *J Hepatol* 1996;25:283–291.

Olshan JS, Gubernick J, Packer RJ, et al. The effects of adjuvant chemotherapy on growth in children with medulloblastoma. *Cancer* 1992;70:2013–2017.

Otsuka F, Hayashi Y, Ogura T, et al. Syndrome of inappropriate secretion of antidiuretic hormone following intra-thoracic cisplatin. *Intern Med* 1996;35:290–294.

Perez EA, Josse RG, Pritchard KI, et al. Effect of letrozole versus placebo on bone mineral density in women with primary breast cancer completing 5 or more years of adjuvant tamoxifen: a companion study to NCIC CTG MA.17. *J Clin Oncol* 2006;24:3629–3635.

Petersen PM, Hansen SW, Giwercman A, et al. Dose-dependent impairment of testicular function in patients treated with cisplatin-based chemotherapy for germ cell cancer. *Ann Oncol* 1994;5:355–358.

Rappaport R, Brauner R, Czernichow P, et al. Effect of hypothalamic and pituitary irradiation on pubertal development in children with cranial tumors. *J Clin Endocrinol Metab* 1982;54: 1164–1168.

Robinson C, Jeffries RC, Walsh GC. Inappropriate ADH secretion caused by oat cell carcinoma and relieved by lung resection. *Thorax* 1980;35:635–637.

Ron E, Lubin JH, Shore RE, et al. Thyroid cancer after exposure to external radiation: a pooled analysis of seven studies. *Radiat Res* 1995;141:259–277.

Rose SR, Schreiber RE, Kearney NS, et al. Hypothalamic dysfunction after chemotherapy. *J Pediatr Endocrinol Metab* 2004;17:55–66.

Rossi R, Godde A, Kleinebrand A, et al. Concentrating capacity in ifosfamide-induced severe renal dysfunction. *Ren Fail* 1995;17:551–557.

Smalley RV, Wall RL. Two cases of busulfan toxicity. *Ann Intern Med* 1966;64:154–164.

Smith MR, Egerdie B, Hernandez Toriz N, et al. Denosumab in men receiving androgen-deprivation therapy for prostate cancer. *N Engl J Med* 2009;361:745–755.

Smith MR, McGovern FJ, Fallon MA, et al. Low bone mineral density in hormone-naive men with prostate carcinoma. *Cancer* 2001a;91:2238–2245.

Smith MR, McGovern FJ, Zietman AL, et al. Pamidronate to prevent bone loss during androgen-deprivation therapy for prostate cancer. *N Engl J Med* 2001b;345:948–955.

Sorensen JB, Andersen MK, Hansen HH. Syndrome of inappropriate secretion of antidiuretic hormone (SIADH) in malignant disease. *J Intern Med* 1995;238:97–110.

Stopeck AT, Lipton A, Body JJ, et al. Denosumab compared with zoledronic acid for the treatment of bone metastases in patients with advanced breast cancer: a randomized, double-blind study. *J Clin Oncol* 2010;28:5132–5129.

Vahlquist C. Effects of retinoids on lipoprotein metabolism. *Curr Probl Dermatol* 1991;20: 73–78.

van Ditzhuijsen CI, van de Weijer R, Haak HR. Adrenocortical carcinoma. *Neth J Med* 2007;65: 55–60.

Vassilopoulou-Sellin R, Samaan NA. Mitotane administration: an unusual cause of hypercholesterolemia. *Horm Metab Res* 1991;23:619–620.

Vehmanen L, Elomaa I, Blomqvist C, et al. Tamoxifen treatment after adjuvant chemotherapy has opposite effects on bone mineral density in premenopausal patients depending on menstrual status. *J Clin Oncol* 2006;24:675–680.

Vialettes B, Guillerand MA, Viens P, et al. Incidence rate and risk factors for thyroid dysfunction during recombinant interleukin-2 therapy in advanced malignancies. *Acta Endocrinol (Copenh)* 1993;129:31–38.

Ward HN, Konikov N, Reinhard EH. Cytologic dysplasia occurring after busulfan (myleran) therapy. A syndrome resembling adrenocortical insufficiency and atrophic bronchitis. *Ann Intern Med* 1965;63:654–660.

Weinstein D, Simon M, Yehezkel E, et al. Insulin analogues display IGF-I-like mitogenic and anti-apoptotic activities in cultured cancer cells. *Diabetes Metab Res Rev* 2009;25:41–49.

Wong E, Rosen LS, Mulay M, et al. Sunitinib induces hypothyroidism in advanced cancer patients and may inhibit thyroid peroxidase activity. *Thyroid* 2007;17:351–355.

Wong LC, Choo YC, Ma HK. Primary oral etoposide therapy in gestational trophoblastic disease. An update. *Cancer* 1986;58:14–17.

Chapter 22
Fatigue

Carmen P. Escalante and Ellen F. Manzullo

Contents

Chapter Overview Fatigue is a common symptom experienced by cancer survivors. It is important for the clinician to question the patient about the presence of this symptom because patients are often hesitant to mention it. In addition, cancer-related fatigue (CRF) commonly clusters with other symptoms, such as sleep disturbance, pain, depression, and anxiety. Patients with moderate to severe CRF should undergo a comprehensive evaluation that includes a history, physical examination, laboratory evaluation, and an assessment of their fatigue and possible associated symptoms. Nonpharmacologic interventions for the treatment of CRF include psychosocial interventions, activity enhancement, dietary management, and sleep management; pharmacologic interventions include agents such as stimulants. Further research is needed to elucidate the actual pathophysiology of CRF and better tailor treatment strategies.

L.E. Foxhall, M.A. Rodriguez (eds.), *Advances in Cancer Survivorship Management*,
MD Anderson Cancer Care Series, DOI 10.1007/978-1-4939-0986-5_22,
© The University of Texas M.D. Anderson Cancer Center 2015

Introduction

As strides have been made with earlier diagnosis of and more effective treatments for cancer, the number of cancer survivors has increased. Clinicians in both academic and community settings are more frequently seeing patients who have been treated for cancer with a variety of modalities, including surgery, chemotherapy, and radiotherapy. Although these patients are considered free of cancer, they often present with sequelae resulting from their treatment. One of the most common and distressing symptoms these patients experience is fatigue. Cancer-related fatigue (CRF) is defined as a distressing, persistent, and subjective sense of physical, emotional, or cognitive tiredness or exhaustion related to cancer or cancer treatment that is not proportional to recent activity and interferes with usual functioning (Mock et al. 2000). Cancer patients as well as survivors can experience CRF to such an extent that it interferes with their everyday life. The prevalence of CRF among cancer survivors is 17–21%, using the ICD-10 criteria for diagnosis. However, if other criteria are used, such as fatigue scale scores, the prevalence may be as high as 33–53%.

CRF is an important symptom that has often been overlooked for several reasons. First, clinicians working in an outpatient setting are usually very busy and experience time constraints related to assessing CRF. In addition, clinicians often lack knowledge related to the evaluation and formulation of a treatment plan for this common symptom. Moreover, cancer survivors may be hesitant to mention CRF for fear that it could indicate disease recurrence or that it is simply an expected treatment effect. As a result, the clinician must make a definite effort to inquire about CRF with cancer survivors. Health care providers should also be familiar with methods of assessing and treating CRF. Cancer survivors and their families should be advised that if this symptom is present, they should alert their physician so that an evaluation can be done and a treatment plan can be formulated. CRF may decrease the cancer survivor's overall quality of life and ability to maintain a career or fulfill other responsibilities.

CRF rarely occurs alone. In fact, CRF commonly occurs with other symptoms. It is important to assess the patient for the presence of other symptoms, as well as the severity of the symptoms. In the CRF Clinic at MD Anderson, patients with severe CRF have also been found to have increased levels of sleep disturbance, pain, depression, and anxiety (Escalante et al. 2010).

Etiology and Proposed Mechanisms of Cancer-Related Fatigue

Because of the high prevalence of fatigue among cancer patients and survivors, better understanding of the causal mechanism of CRF is needed. Unfortunately, the etiology of CRF is poorly understood. Several possible mechanisms have been proposed:

1. Serotonin dysregulation: cancer or cancer treatment leads to an increase in brain serotonin levels or upregulation of 5-HT receptors, resulting in reduced somatomotor drive, modified hypothalamic-pituitary-adrenal axis function, and a feeling of reduced capacity due to physical work.

2. Disturbance of the hypothalamic-pituitary-adrenal axis: cancer or cancer treatment alters the hypothalamic-pituitary-adrenal axis, resulting in endocrine changes, such as low cortisol levels, that result in fatigue.
3. Circadian rhythm disruption: changes in circadian function result in alteration of endocrine function and metabolic processes, as well as sleep disorders.
4. ATP dysfunction: cancer or cancer treatment leads to a defect in the regeneration of ATP in skeletal muscle, thereby resulting in decreased ability to perform mechanical tasks.
5. Peripheral release of neuroactive agents: release of these agents leads to activation of vagal afferent nerves, resulting in suppression of somatic muscle activity and "sickness behavior."
6. Dysregulation of cytokines: dysregulated levels of cytokines such as tumor necrosis factor-alpha or interleukin-beta can lead to increased fatigue.

A patient's CRF could be caused by any or all of these potential mechanisms. Further research on the causes of CRF is needed so that better prevention and treatment modalities may be established.

Fatigue Measurement

It is important to screen cancer survivors for CRF so that if it is present, an appropriate evaluation may be performed and an individualized treatment program may be created. The National Comprehensive Cancer Network recommends the following screening question: How would you rate your fatigue on a scale of 0–10 over the past 7 days? Mild fatigue is scored as 1–3; moderate fatigue, 4–6; and severe fatigue, 7–10. The National Comprehensive Cancer Network recommends using the words none, mild, moderate, and severe to describe fatigue for patients who are unable to assign a number to it. In the CRF Clinic at MD Anderson, we use the Brief Fatigue Inventory (Mendoza et al. 1999), which consists of nine questions. This inventory evaluates the patient's present, usual, and worst levels of fatigue and its impact on the patient's daily life. Answers to the questions are scored as described above and individual question scores are summed and averaged to produce a final score. The scoring system for the final scores is as follows: mild fatigue, <4; moderate fatigue, 4–6; severe fatigue, ≥7.

Evaluation

When a clinician evaluates a cancer survivor with CRF, the clinician must obtain a complete history and perform a physical examination. It is vital to note the patient's cancer diagnosis and the treatment received, such as surgery, chemotherapy, radiotherapy, bone marrow transplantation, or hormonal treatment, in the patient's history. Cancer survivors should also be assessed during the clinic visit for the presence of comorbid conditions and other factors contributing to CRF. It is important

Table 22.1 Factors contributing to cancer-related fatigue

Medical issues
Anemia
Endocrine dysfunction
Hypothyroidism
Hypogonadism
Diabetes mellitus
Adrenal insufficiency
Neurologic dysfunction
Cardiac dysfunction
Pulmonary dysfunction
Hepatic dysfunction
Renal dysfunction
Rheumatologic disorders
Physical function changes
Physical inactivity
Physical deconditioning
Nutritional imbalances
Medications
Sedating agents (e.g., hypnotics, narcotics, neuropathic agents)
Beta-blockers
Other (drug interactions and other medication side effects)
Cancer treatment effects
Chemotherapy
Radiotherapy
Surgery
Bone marrow transplantation
Biologic response modifiers
Hormonal treatment
Sleep dysfunction
Obstructive sleep apnea
Restless leg syndrome
Narcolepsy
Insomnia
Symptom burden
Pain
Anxiety and depression
Stress

to keep in mind that a multitude of comorbid conditions may result in fatigue. For example, cardiac disease, pulmonary dysfunction, hepatic disease, renal insufficiency, hypothyroidism, and anemia are just a few of the medical issues that may contribute to the patient's fatigue (Table 22.1).

Another important component of the patient's history is a thorough evaluation of medications the patient is taking. Certain medications such as sedating agents and beta blockers may add to increased fatigue. Another key aspect of medication review is an assessment of any over-the-counter medications the patient may be taking, including vitamins, supplements, and herbal therapy. Polypharmacy and drug interactions may also be a factor in the CRF. Additionally, inquiry into alcohol and illicit drug usage is necessary. These behaviors may impact the patient's overall medical condition.

A complete review of systems is also necessary because this can provide valuable clues to the presence of comorbid conditions that have not been diagnosed or are being inadequately treated. For instance, questions regarding sleep quality may aid in the assessment of sleep disturbances such as insomnia, narcolepsy, restless leg syndrome, and obstructive sleep apnea.

A detailed history regarding the patient's CRF should also be attained. It may be very helpful to establish when the patient began to experience fatigue, its pattern over time, factors that have alleviated the fatigue or made it worse, and its overall impact on the patient's daily life. By asking a patient to describe a typical day, the clinician may begin to assess the patient's overall activity level. It is important to inquire whether employed patients are having difficulty fulfilling their job duties and whether the patient is or has recently been on short-term or long-term disability.

Inquiries should be made regarding whether the patient exercises; regular daily exercise can be beneficial to many patients with CRF. Finally, a complete physical examination is required for those with moderate to severe fatigue. The National Comprehensive Cancer Network has developed a practice guideline for CRF that may be helpful to practitioners (Mock et al. 2007).

At MD Anderson, a clinic is dedicated to the evaluation, treatment, and long-term follow-up of cancer patients and survivors with CRF. During the initial clinic visit, patients undergo a complete history and physical examination as detailed above. In addition, patients are required to complete a packet of survey tools in an effort to assess not only the severity of the fatigue, but also the presence and degree of other symptoms that normally cluster with fatigue, such as pain, anxiety, depression, stress, and poor sleep quality. Each patient undergoes an initial workup that includes a complete blood count, chemistry panel, and tests to measure electrolyte levels and thyroid-stimulating hormone levels. The thyroid-stimulating hormone test should be performed within 6 months of the initial clinic visit and the additional tests within 2 months of the visit, especially in patients who have not recently undergone diagnostic testing. Further studies may need to be requested to determine whether comorbid conditions may be a factor in the patient's CRF. Then, an initial treatment plan is formulated and a subsequent visit is arranged.

Treatment Interventions

All cancer patients should be educated on general strategies for the management of CRF, regardless of the patient's level of fatigue. These approaches are often helpful to patients and families. General strategies for managing CRF include energy conservation and distraction. Examples of energy conservation include setting priorities, delegating activities, and scheduling activities at times of peak energy. Distraction may include playing games, working on puzzles and listening to music, or visiting family or friends.

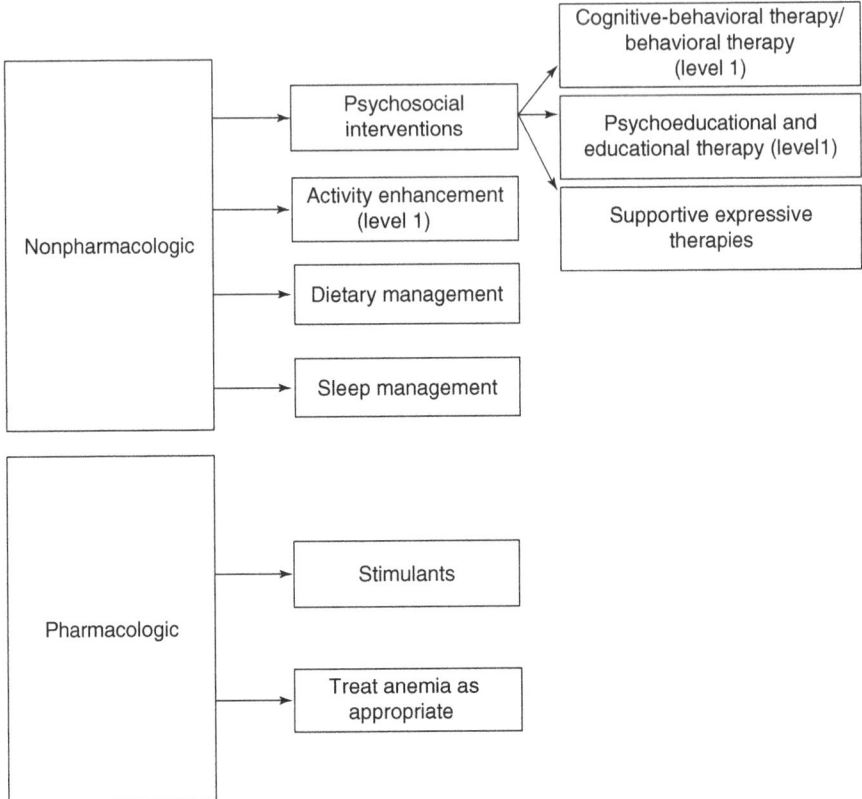

Fig. 22.1 Cancer-related fatigue treatment interventions (level 1 indicates National Comprehensive Cancer Network Category 1: the recommendation is based on high-level evidence [e.g., randomized, controlled trials] and there is uniform consensus in the National Comprehensive Cancer Network)

In addition, it is often helpful for the patient to self-monitor fatigue levels, noting activities that both improve and worsen levels of fatigue. For instance, writing in a daily diary may be helpful for identifying fatigue patterns.

CRF treatment interventions are organized into two major categories: nonpharmacologic and pharmacologic (Fig. 22.1).

Nonpharmacologic Treatment Interventions

Nonpharmacologic treatment interventions are divided into four categories: psychosocial interventions, activity enhancement, dietary management, and sleep management. Psychosocial interventions and activity enhancement have the most supportive evidence that they benefit cancer patients with CRF.

Psychosocial Interventions

Cancer survivors commonly experience stress, anxiety, and depression following completion of their active treatment. Often, these symptoms are associated with fatigue and should be surveyed during the initial medical evaluation. Evidence from clinical trials and meta-analyses demonstrates the effectiveness of a diverse group of nonpharmacologic psychoeducational interventions. Improvements in CRF following these types of interventions have been noted to persist for as long as 2 years.

Types of psychosocial interventions include educational activities, support groups and individual counseling, comprehensive coping methods, stress management training, and personal behavioral intervention. Cognitive-behavioral therapy has benefited some patients with fatigue. Cognitive-behavioral therapy includes aspects of self-care management; aid with information, decision-making, and problem-solving; communication with health care providers; and counseling and support. Self-care management includes behaviors such as taking brief naps early in the day or listening to guided imagery tapes daily. Psychosocial interventions may not be effective in all patients with CRF, especially if we assume that CRF has a biologic mechanism.

Activity Enhancement

Strong data support the efficacy of activity enhancement (exercise) in managing CRF. Although the exact mechanism of exercise that improves CRF is not clearly elucidated, one hypothesis relates to improvement in functional capacity, thus leading to a decreased effort in performing daily activities and, therefore, less fatigue.

A variety of studies, involving various types of patients and cancer diagnoses, have shown that exercise decreases levels of CRF. Many of these studies are limited by small size, variable methodologies, diverse exercise interventions, and differences in study follow-up time. Despite these limitations, all studies have consistently shown that exercise decreases levels of CRF. Exercise interventions assessed have included use of bed-cycle ergometers, walking programs, stationary biking, strength and resistance training, flexibility training, routine stretching, yoga, and seated exercise, as well as choice of an aerobic-type exercise.

Each patient should be carefully evaluated prior to instituting an exercise program, with consideration of age and functional status, condition of any underlying comorbidities, prior cancer treatment received, and any residual treatment side effects that may interfere with an exercise program. An individualized approach should be taken. Some patients with poor physical conditioning may need a physical therapy or rehabilitation program initially. Others with significant comorbidities may need a more in-depth medical evaluation prior to recommendation of any specific exercise intervention.

Dietary Management

Nutritional issues are very common in cancer survivors. The most common problems include malabsorptive syndromes, especially in patients who have undergone surgical interventions for gastrointestinal malignancies, and electrolyte disorders resulting from renal tubular dysfunction. Some patients have more poorly controlled diabetes, or develop diabetes, with weight gain after treatment. This may be particularly prominent in breast cancer survivors who are receiving hormonal therapy. In addition, discussion of weight management measures in overweight or obese cancer survivors should be a priority. Other patients with poor oral intake may require nutritional support with feeding tube placement or total parenteral nutrition. Dietary assessment in patients complaining of CRF should be performed, and patients with significant nutritional issues should undergo a more in-depth review.

Sleep Management

Various sleep dysfunctions, from the extremes of insomnia to hypersomnia, are often present in patients with CRF, and these dysfunctions are frequently challenging to remedy. A number of factors may cause or contribute to the sleep dysfunction, including anxiety and depression, the amount of sleep the patient gets, day napping, medication side effects, nutritional characteristics, and night awakenings. Patients with symptoms of obstructive sleep apnea may benefit from further workup, including a sleep study. Cognitive-behavioral therapy has also been used to treat sleep dysfunctions, with an emphasis on stimulus control, sleep restriction, and sleep hygiene.

Complementary Therapies

Complementary therapies that have been studied for the treatment of CRF include acupuncture, aromatherapy, adenosine triphosphate infusions, healing touch, hypnosis, lectin-standardized mistletoe extract, levocarnitine, massage, mindfulness-based stress reduction, polarity therapy, relaxation, and Tibetan yoga. Presently, insufficient data support the routine use of these interventions for the treatment of CRF. Larger, randomized trials are necessary to establish evidence of the efficacy of complementary therapies for CRF (Molassiotis et al. 2007; Sood et al. 2007; Vickers et al. 2004). Results of these preliminary trials suggest a potential benefit of these therapies for the treatment of CRF, but further study is needed.

Pharmacologic Treatment Interventions

The most commonly used pharmacologic agents for the treatment of CRF include stimulants and antidepressants. Although these two groups of agents have been most studied, data are still scant. The studies are often poorly designed, include a

Table 22.2 Commonly used stimulants for the treatment of cancer-related fatigue

Name (trade name)	Preparation type	FDA approval	Starting dose	Maximum dose	Common side effects
Methylphenidate (Ritalin)	Short-acting	ADHD, narcolepsy	5 mg orally, morning and noon	1 mg/kg per day	Jitteriness, headache
Methylphenidate (Concerta)	Long-acting	ADHD, narcolepsy	18 mg orally, morning only	54 mg per day	Jitteriness, headache
Modafinil (Provigil)	Short-acting	Narcolepsy, OSAHS, SWSD	100 mg orally, morning and noon	200 mg orally, morning and noon (400 mg per day)	Headache, nausea, nervousness
Armodafinil (Nuvigil)	Long-acting	Narcolepsy, OSAHS, SWSD	150 mg orally, morning only	250 mg per day	Headache, nausea, dizziness

FDA indicates US Food and Drug Administration, *ADHD* attention deficit hyperactivity disorder, *OSAHS* obstructive sleep apnea/hypopnea syndrome, *SWSD* shift work sleep disorder

relatively small number of patients, and are difficult to compare and interpret. Larger, better-designed clinical trials are needed to provide stronger evidence.

Stimulants

The most frequently used stimulants to treat CRF include methylphenidate, modafinil, and armodafinil, none of which are approved by the US Food and Drug Administration for the treatment of CRF (Table 22.2).

Methylphenidate has both short-acting and long-acting preparations. This drug has been available for many years and is commonly used in children for the treatment of attention deficit hyperactivity disorder. It is a controlled substance in the United States and requires triplicate prescription. Usually, the starting dose for the treatment of CRF for the short-acting preparation is 5 mg in the morning and 5 mg at noon. Short-acting methylphenidate may require dose titration, with a usual maximum dose of 1 mg/kg per day. For most patients with CRF, minimal improvement is observed with doses of more than 20 mg per day. Doses of the long-acting preparation start at 18 mg daily in the morning. The dose titration can begin within 2–3 days following use of the stimulant because the effect is usually observed fairly quickly. Side effects frequently become more prevalent with higher doses. These may include jitteriness or nervousness, tachycardia, insomnia, headache, and anorexia.

The short-acting preparation of methylphenidate has a short plasma half-life (2 hours), with a rapid onset of action and duration of action lasting 3–6 hours. The long-acting preparation has a 12-hour duration of action. Whether a short-acting or long-acting stimulant is prescribed depends on the patient's preference. The long-acting preparation is taken only once daily and may improve compliance in patients who have difficulty adhering to a twice-daily medication schedule. However, the twice-daily medication plan may lend itself to more specific titration at particular times of the day. For example, a patient with more fatigue in the afternoon may take a larger dose of the short-acting preparation at noon compared with the morning dose. This feature may be attractive to some patients.

One study of methylphenidate for the treatment of CRF used a dosing schedule that allowed patients to repeat doses of 5 mg every 2 hours as needed, up to 20 mg daily. Results of this study showed significant improvements in fatigue at the end of the first week compared with baseline in patients in both the placebo group and the methylphenidate group. The benefits may be attributable to contact with the study personnel on a daily basis or the placebo effect (Bruera et al. 2006). No trials have been conducted comparing stimulants for the treatment of CRF. Often a patient not benefiting from one stimulant changes to another and reports improvement.

Modafinil is a nonamphetamine central nervous system stimulant that has received US Food and Drug Administration approval for the treatment of narcolepsy, obstructive sleep apnea/hypopnea syndrome, and shift work sleep disorder. Modafinil has been used to treat fatigue related to multiple sclerosis. Studies of modafinil for the treatment of CRF have shown conflicting results. A large study showed reductions in CRF only in a subgroup of patients with high baseline levels of CRF (Jean-Pierre et al. 2010). Two smaller pilot studies composed of 27 patients and 20 patients demonstrated statistically significant reductions in CRF for most patients treated with modafinil. These pilot studies also demonstrated that modafinil led to reduced sleepiness during the day, reduced depression and anxiety, and improved performance status (Blackhall et al. 2009; Spathis et al. 2009).

Modafinil has a peak plasma concentration after 2–4 hours, with a half-life of 15 hours. The initial dose is 100–200 mg in the morning. Modafinil is short-acting and requires a second dose around noon, depending on the time of the first dose. The maximum dose is 400 mg per day.

Dextroamphetamine is approved by the US Food and Drug Administration for the treatment of narcolepsy and attention deficit hyperactivity disorder. Fifty patients with advanced cancer and fatigue were studied in a placebo-controlled trial of dextroamphetamine, with a dose of 10 mg twice daily (Auret et al. 2009). Patients were treated for 8 days and showed no benefit. This outcome may be attributable to the population studied (poor performance status), the short treatment time, or interactions with the various other medications that patients in this group were taking during the study period. More study is needed to determine whether this agent may be beneficial for patients with CRF.

Armodafinil is a long-acting stimulant currently approved for the treatment of narcolepsy and shift work sleep disorder. It is also approved for the treatment of obstructive sleep apnea/hypopnea syndrome. The exact mechanism of action of armodafinil is unknown. Armodafinil is the R-enantiomer of modafinil, and it has a half-life elimination of 15 hours, a time to peak plasma of 2 hours, and a steady state of approximately 7 days. Armodafinil is taken once daily in the morning, at a dose of either 150 mg or 250 mg. The maximum daily dose is 250 mg. Armodafinil has been studied in human immunodeficiency virus (HIV)-related fatigue in a placebo-controlled randomized trial and was effective and well-tolerated in HIV-positive patients (Rabkin et al. 2011). The response rate to armodafinil was 75%, compared with 25% in the placebo group. Patients reported substantially improved energy. Although there is interest in using this agent to treat CRF, data are not currently available to endorse its routine use.

Antidepressants

Fatigue and depression are highly correlated and may be viewed as overlapping in some cases. However, 3 placebo-controlled randomized trials of selective serotonin reuptake inhibitors (paroxetine, sertraline) in cancer patients have demonstrated that fatigue and depression differ and are each a distinct entity. These trials did not demonstrate improvement in fatigue with treatment, although improvement in depressive symptoms was observed (Auret et al. 2009; Morrow et al. 2008).

Bupropion has been studied in cancer patients with CRF with or without moderate to severe levels of depression (Moss et al. 2006). Both groups of patients showed improvements in fatigue and depression, suggesting that bupropion could be a potential treatment for CRF. However, the study was limited by a small number of patients and open-label methodology. Larger, randomized trials are needed to validate preliminary findings.

The varied findings thus far in the study of antidepressants as a treatment for CRF may be related to the assorted classes of antidepressants and their related mechanisms of action.

Other Agents

Other agents studied for the treatment of CRF have been wide-ranging. Steroids have been studied primarily in patients with CRF at the end of life and not in cancer survivors (Bruera et al. 1985). Other outcome measures (strength, weakness, activity level) were substituted for CRF in these trials. No agreement has been established that these metrics are correct substitutes for fatigue. In addition, side effects limit the routine use of steroids in other cancer populations.

Donepezil is a selective acetyl cholinesterase inhibitor approved for the treatment of Alzheimer disease. It was evaluated for the treatment of CRF in a randomized, placebo-controlled trial of 142 cancer patients (Bruera et al. 2007). Patients received 5 mg of donepezil or a placebo daily for 7 days. During week 2, all patients were offered open-label donepezil. No benefit was found for donepezil over placebo in the management of CRF.

In another double-blind randomized crossover trial, multivitamins were studied against placebo in 40 breast cancer patients undergoing radiotherapy (de Souza et al. 2007). Lower levels of fatigue were noted in the placebo arm.

Twenty-nine cancer patients with carnitine deficiency participated in a double-blind phase followed by an open-label phase trial of L-carnitine lasting 2 weeks (Cruciani et al. 2009). No improvement in CRF was noted with L-carnitine.

Hematopoietic growth factors, erythropoietin, and darbopoietin have been used to treat chemotherapy-induced anemia in cancer patients, and some studies have shown improvements in fatigue when anemia is corrected (Lyman and Glaspy 2006; Gabrilove et al. 2007). Because of thromboembolic events, increased mortality rates, and other adverse cancer outcomes related to these agents, guidelines regarding appropriate use, including specific recommendations based on tumor diagnosis and hemoglobin levels, have resulted in less use of these agents.

In summary, few well-designed, large clinical trials of pharmacologic agents to treat CRF have been done, and no trial thus far has focused on cancer survivors with CRF.

Key Practice Points

- CRF is different from the fatigue commonly experienced by healthy adults.
- CRF can be physical, mental, and emotional.
- Not only patients, but also their caregivers and health care professionals should be educated about CRF.
- Research focusing on the pathophysiology of CRF is in its infancy. Further studies are needed so that more effective interventions can be developed.
- Tools such as questionnaires that quantify the severity of a patient's CRF are valuable for a patient's initial evaluation and long-term follow-up.
- Patients with moderate to severe CRF require a detailed evaluation so that an individualized treatment plan can be formulated.
- Treatment interventions can be nonpharmacologic or pharmacologic. Activity enhancement (exercise) and psychosocial interventions are supported by the most evidence and are category 1 recommendations (National Comprehensive Cancer Network Clinical Practice Guidelines in Oncology: CRF).
- Stimulants may be used to treat CRF, although they lack data to support a category 1 recommendation.
- Antidepressants should be considered only if depression is present with CRF. Data are lacking to support antidepressants for primary treatment of CRF.

Suggested Readings

Auret KA, Schug SA, Bremner AP, Bulsara M. A randomized, double-blind, placebo-controlled trial assessing the impact of dexamphetamine on fatigue in patients with advanced cancer. *J Pain Symptom Manage* 2009;37(4):613–621.

Blackhall L, Petroni G, Shu J, Baum L, Farace E. A pilot study evaluating the safety and efficacy of modafinal for cancer-related fatigue. *J Palliat Med* 2009;12(5):433–439.

Bruera E, El Osta B, Valero V, et al. Donepezil for cancer fatigue: a double-blind, randomized, placebo-controlled trial. *J Clin Oncol* 2007;25:3475–3481.

Bruera E, Roca E, Cedaro L, Carraro S, Chacon R. Action of oral methylprednisolone in terminal cancer patients: a prospective randomized double-blind study. *Cancer Treat Rep* 1985; 69(7–8):751–754.

Bruera E, Valero V, Driver L, et al. Patient-controlled methylphenidate for cancer fatigue: a double-blind, randomized, placebo-controlled trial. *J Clin Oncol* 2006;24(13):2073–2078.

Cruciani RA, Dvorkin E, Homel P, et al. L-carnitine supplementation in patients with advanced cancer and carnitine deficiency: a double-blind, placebo-controlled study. *J Pain Symptom Manage* 2009;37(4):622–631.

Escalante CP, Kallen MA, Valdres RU, et al. Outcomes of a cancer-related fatigue clinic in a comprehensive cancer center. *J Pain Symptom Manage* 2010;39(4):691–701.

Gabrilove JL, Perez E, Tomita DK, Rossi G, Cleeland CS. Assessing symptom burden using the MD Anderson symptom inventory in patients with chemotherapy-induced anemia: results of a multicenter, open-label (SURPASS) of patients treated with darbepoetin-alpha at a dose of 200 micrograms every 2 weeks. *Cancer* 2007;110(7):1629–1640.

Jean-Pierre P, Morrow GR, Roscoe JA, et al. A phase 3 randomized, placebo-controlled, double-blind, clinical trial of the effect of modafinil on cancer-related fatigue among 631 patients receiving chemotherapy: a University of Rochester Cancer Center Community Clinical Oncology Program Research base study. *Cancer* 2010;116(14):3513–3520.

Lyman GH, Glaspy J. Are there clinical benefits with early erythropoietic intervention for chemotherapy-induced anemia? A systematic review. *Cancer* 2006;106(1):223–233.

Mendoza TR, Wang XS, Cleeland CS, et al. The rapid assessment of fatigue severity in cancer patients: use of the Brief Fatigue Inventory. *Cancer* 1999;85(5):1186–1196.

Mock V, Atkinson A, Barsevick A, et al. NCCN practice guidelines for cancer-related fatigue. *Oncology (Williston Park)* 2000;14(11A):151–161.

Mock V, Atkinson A, Barsevick A, et al. Cancer-related fatigue. Clinical practice guidelines in oncology. *J Natl Compr Canc Netw* 2007;5(10):1054–1078.

Molassiotis A, Sylt P, Diggins H. The management of cancer-related fatigue after chemotherapy with acupuncture and acupressure: a randomised controlled trial. *Complement Ther Med* 2007;15(4):228–237.

Morrow GR, Jean-Pierre P, Roscoe JA, et al. A phase III randomized, placebo-controlled, double-blind trial of a eugeroic agent in 642 cancer patients reporting fatigue during chemotherapy: a URCC CCOP study (abstract). *J Clin Oncol* 2008;504s.

Moss E, Simpson JS, Pelletier G, et al. An open-label study of the effects of bupropion SR on fatigue, depression and quality of life of mixed-site cancer patients and their partners. *Psychooncology* 2006;15:259–267.

Rabkin J, McElhiney MC, Rabkin R. Treatment of HIV-related fatigue with armodafinil: a placebo-controlled randomized trial. *Psychosomatics* 2011;52(4):328–336.

Sood A, Barton DL, Bauer BA, Loprinzi CL. A critical review of complementary therapies for cancer-related fatigue. *Integr Cancer Ther* 2007;6(1):8–13.

de Souza F, Bensi C, Trufelli DC, et al. Multivitamins do not improve radiation therapy-related fatigue: results of a double-blind randomized crossover trial. *Am J Clin Oncol* 2007;30: 432–436.

Spathis A, Dhillan R., Booden D, Forbes K, Vrotsou K, Fife K. Modafinil for the treatment of fatigue in lung cancer: a pilot study. *Palliat Med* 2009;23(4):325–331.

Vickers AJ, Straus DJ, Fearon B, Cassileth BR. Acupuncture for postchemotherapy fatigue: a phase II study. *J Clin Oncol* 2004;22(9):1731–1735.

Chapter 23
Immunologic Issues

Kenneth V.I. Rolston

Contents

Chapter Overview Patients with cancer frequently develop immunologic impairment as a result of the underlying malignancy and its treatment. Each immunologic deficit is associated with a specific spectrum of infection, although there is some overlap. Multiple risk factors may be present in the same patient, increasing the risk of and widening the spectrum of infection. Some nonimmunologic factors also play a role in the predisposition to infection. Increased survival durations among patients with solid tumors and hematologic malignancies and those who have undergone hematopoietic stem cell transplantation have resulted in a growing population of patients who remain at risk for the development of serious infections for sustained periods of time. This chapter discusses the immunologic defects commonly encountered in subgroups of cancer patients, focusing on the risk factors, infectious complications, and other features unique to each subgroup. A brief discussion of immune reconstitution in hematopoietic stem cell transplantation recipients is included. The stem cell transplantation specialists at MD Anderson perform more hematopoietic stem cell transplantations than at any other institution in the United States. Finally, the chapter concludes with a brief discussion of

L.E. Foxhall, M.A. Rodriguez (eds.), *Advances in Cancer Survivorship Management*,
MD Anderson Cancer Care Series, DOI 10.1007/978-1-4939-0986-5_23,
© The University of Texas M.D. Anderson Cancer Center 2015

antimicrobial stewardship, which has become an important and (in the opinion of the author) mandatory strategy in the overall management of infection in cancer patients, particularly long-term survivors.

Introduction

Infection is a common problem in patients with cancer, both during active treatment and in the survivorship phase. Patients develop significant impairment of host defenses as a result of either the underlying disease or its treatment. Host defense mechanisms can be immunologic or nonimmunologic. Immunologic host defenses, which respond to specific microbial antigens, include phagocytosis (carried out primarily by polymorphonuclear leukocytes and cells of the monocyte-macrophage lineage), cell-mediated immunity (primarily a function of T-cells), humoral immunity and antibody production (primarily a function of B-cells), and the complement system. Nonimmunologic host defenses include anatomic barriers such as the skin and mucous membranes, gastric acid, epithelial ciliary function, tears, and even intestinal peristalsis. This chapter will focus primarily on immunologic host defenses and the infectious complications associated with them.

Neutropenia

Neutropenia, defined as an absolute neutrophil count of $\leq 500/mm^2$, is the most common predisposing factor for infections (Rolston and Bodey 2010). Both the degree and the duration of neutropenia influence the development of infection. Bacterial infections are common during the initial phase of neutropenia, and fungal infections are encountered more frequently as neutropenia persists. Fever is the most common, and sometimes the only, manifestation of infection in neutropenic patients. Some patients with adequate numbers of neutrophils may still be susceptible to infection owing to impaired neutrophil function (e.g., neutrophil migration, phagocytosis).

Impaired Cellular Immunity

Defects in the T lymphocyte or mononuclear phagocytic system also result in an increased susceptibility to infection. Cell-mediated immunity plays a primary role in protecting against intracellular pathogens. T-4 lymphocytes, however, can influence all aspects of immunity as a consequence of their ability to induce specific immune responses in other cells. T lymphocyte function is impaired in a variety of disorders, such as Hodgkin disease and chronic or acute lymphocytic leukemia.

Immunosuppressive therapy with agents such as corticosteroids and tacrolimus and treatment with purine analogs such as fludarabine and clofarabine, monoclonal antibodies such as alemtuzumab or rituximab, and alkylating agents such as temozolomide also produce lymphocytopenia and prolonged suppression of lymphocyte function (Samonis and Kontoyiannis 2001; Su et al. 2004; Martin et al. 2006).

Impaired Humoral Immunity

The immune response mediated by antibodies is referred to as humoral immunity. B lymphocytes are responsible for antibody production. In disorders such as multiple myeloma, Waldenström macroglobulinemia, and the various "heavy chain diseases," malignant proliferation of plasma cells or their precursors occurs at the expense of normal plasma cells, resulting in low levels of normal immunoglobulins (Karlsson et al. 2011). Hypogammaglobulinemia is also present in 30–40% of patients with chronic lymphocytic leukemia. Patients with impaired humoral immunity are particularly susceptible to infections caused by encapsulated organisms such as *Streptococcus pneumoniae*. Common infection-causing organisms associated with the various immunologic deficits are listed in Table 23.1.

Patients with Hematologic Malignancies

The predominant risk factor for infection in patients with hematologic malignancies is neutropenia (Crawford et al. 2004). Severe and prolonged neutropenia (absolute neutrophil count $\leq 500/mm^3$ for >10 days) occurs when normal bone marrow is replaced by malignant cells and as a result of cytotoxic chemotherapy. Bacterial, fungal, and some viral infections are common in neutropenic patients (Table 23.1). Neutropenia, however, is not the only risk factor for infection in patients with hematologic malignancies. Impaired cell-mediated immunity occurs in patients with Hodgkin disease and those treated with corticosteroids. Immunosuppressive drugs such as purine analogs and monoclonal antibodies produce defects in cell-mediated immunity and humoral immunity, and the risk and spectrum of infection may resemble that observed in recipients of allogeneic stem cell transplantation. Additionally, patients with a hematologic malignancy requiring splenectomy develop prolonged impairment of antibody production.

Hematopoietic Stem Cell Transplantation Recipients

Recipients of myeloablative hematopoietic stem cell transplantation experience profound and prolonged periods of pancytopenia and immunosuppression. Although the degree of myelosuppression is milder following nonmyeloablative regimens, the

Table 23.1 Common
pathogens in patients
with cancer

Neutropenia
Gram-positive bacteria
Coagulase-negative staphylococci
Staphylococcus aureus (including MRSA)
Viridans group streptococci
Enterococcus species (including VRE)
Beta-hemolytic streptococci
Gram-negative bacteria
Escherichia coli
Klebsiella species
Pseudomonas aeruginosa
Stenotrophomonas maltophilia
Fungi
Candida species
Aspergillus species
Zygomycetes
Fusarium species
Cellular Immune Dysfunction
Bacteria
Listeria monocytogenes
Rhodococcus species
Salmonella species
Mycobacteria
Nocardia species
Legionella species
Fungi
Aspergillus species
Cryptococcus neoformans
Histoplasma capsulatum
Coccidioides immitis
Pneumocystis jiroveci
Helminths
Strongyloides stercoralis
Humoral Immune Dysfunction
Streptococcus pneumoniae
Haemophilus influenzae

MRSA indicates methicillin-resistant *Staphylococcus aureus*, *VRE* vancomycin-resistant *Enterococcus*

degree and duration of lymphodepletion and resultant immunosuppression tends to be similar. Following transplantation, neutrophil recovery occurs first, followed by monocyte, natural killer cell, platelet, and red cell recovery. B-cell recovery generally takes 6–12 months to occur, and patients remain at risk for infections caused by encapsulated bacteria during this time. Humoral immune competence following transplantation can be reliably assessed only by documenting adequate increases in specific antigens following vaccination or infection. T-cells are the last to recover, and their recovery is greatly affected by several factors, including graft-versus-host disease (GVHD), age, other comorbidities, and infectious exposure prior to transplantation. Full immune competence is defined as the ability to safely receive live vaccines. This occurs at approximately 24 months after transplantation in patients who do not have active GVHD and who are not receiving immunosuppressive therapy.

Patients receiving myeloablative preparatory regimens develop infections in three distinct phases (Mir and Battiwalla 2009). Phase I is the pre-engraftment phase, which generally lasts for 15–45 days after the transplantation. During this phase, severe neutropenia and breaches in the mucocutaneous barriers increase the risk for bacterial infections and infections caused by *Candida* species. As neutropenia persists, infections with *Aspergillus* species and other molds begin to emerge. Herpes simplex virus reactivation also occurs during this phase. Phase II is the postengraftment phase (30–100 days after the transplantation). During this phase, infections related to impaired cell-mediated immunity predominate. GVHD and immunosuppressive therapy can greatly increase the occurrence of infections during this phase. Infections with herpes viruses (especially cytomegalovirus), *Pneumocystis jiroveci*, and *Aspergillus* species are common during this phase. Phase III is the late phase (>100 after the transplantation). Patients with chronic GVHD and alternative donor transplantation recipients remain at risk for infection during this phase. Infections with cytomegalovirus, varicella zoster virus, and encapsulated bacteria, such as *Streptococcus pneumoniae*, are most common. A detailed description of the clinical features, diagnosis, treatment, and prevention of these various infections is beyond the scope of this chapter (Tomblyn et al. 2009; Freifeld et al. 2011).

Patients with Solid Tumors

Infections in patients with hematologic malignancies and hematopoietic stem cell transplantation recipients have been studied extensively, and many of the principles for the management of infections in patients with cancer have been developed in this group of patients. Solid tumors, however, account for most cancers in adults, and most cancer survivors have or had solid tumors. The American Cancer Society estimates that approximately 1.4 million new solid tumors are diagnosed each year in the United States.

Risk Factors for Infection

Several factors contribute to the risk of infection in patients with solid tumors (Table 23.2). Unlike patients with hematologic malignancies, patients with solid tumors usually have normally functioning neutrophils, and conventional

Table 23.2 Risk factors for infection in patients with solid tumors

Risk factor	Contributing factors
Neutropenia	Chemotherapy; other agents (e.g., ganciclovir); radiation; tumor infiltration of bone marrow
Disrupted anatomic barriers	Chemotherapy; radiation; surgical procedures; catheters and other medical devices
Tumor obstruction	Primary or metastatic tumor in the airways, biliary tract, urinary tract, or bowel
Certain procedures and devices	Vascular access catheters; shunts; prosthetic devices; percutaneous endoscopic gastrostomy tubes; diagnostic and therapeutic surgical procedures
Miscellaneous	Loss of gag reflex/cord compression; impaired micturation; age; malnutrition; antibiotics

chemotherapy rarely produces severe neutropenia that lasts for more than 7–10 days. Thus, the "at risk" period is short, and many neutropenic patients with solid tumors are considered to have a low risk of developing an infection (Klastersky et al. 2000).

Anatomic barriers (intact skin and oropharyngeal, respiratory, gastrointestinal, and genitourinary mucosal surfaces) provide an important defense mechanism against invasion by microorganisms. Chemotherapy often damages mucosal surfaces, increasing the risk of infection. Mucosal damage can also be caused by radiation, surgical procedures, and medical devices.

Obstruction caused by expanding tumors is fairly common. Bronchogenic carcinomas (or metastatic lesions) often cause partial airway obstruction, leading to the development of postobstructive pneumonia, bronchopleural fistula, and empyema. Biliary tract obstruction results in ascending cholangitis. Ureteral obstruction causing urinary tract infections occurs in patients with genitourinary and prostatic tumors.

Surgery, medical procedures, radiation, and catheters and other devices (shunts, stents, and prostheses) are often associated with infection. Vascular access catheters facilitate the drawing or administration of blood or blood products, as well as administration of chemotherapy, antimicrobial agents, or other supportive therapy. Infection is the most common complication associated with these catheters. Urinary catheters are frequently used when urinary obstruction or incontinence is present. Local involvement of the bladder or ureters with the malignancy often requires the creation of surgical diversions into ileal or colonic segments. Acute or chronic pyelonephritis progressing to abscess formation or bacteremia can also occur. Many patients with central nervous system tumors require cerebrospinal fluid shunts. Infection at the central nervous system end of the shunt produces symptoms consistent with ventriculitis or meningitis, whereas an infection at the distal end of the shunt produces symptoms consistent with pleuritis or peritonitis. Surgically implanted prosthetic devices are frequently used in patients with osteosarcoma and other bone tumors. Infection is the most common complication associated with these devices.

Table 23.3 Common sites of infection in patients with solid tumors

Tumor	Site or type of infection
Brain (central nervous system)	Wound infection; epidural or subdural infection; brain abscess; meningitis/ventriculitis; shunt-related infection; pneumonia (aspiration); urinary tract infection
Head and neck	Cellulitis; wound infection; deep facial space infection; mastoiditis; sinusitis; osteomyelitis; aspiration/nosocomial pneumonia; cavernous (or other) sinus thrombosis; meningitis; brain abscess; retropharyngeal and paravertebral abscess; percutaneous endoscopic gastrostomy tube-related infection
Gastrointestinal	Mediastinitis; tracheo-esophageal fistula with pneumonia/empyema; gastric perforation and abscess; percutaneous endoscopic gastrostomy tube-related infections; peritonitis; abdominal/pelvic abscesses
Breast	Wound infection; cellulitis and lymphangitis; mastitis; abscess; breast expander-related infections
Hepatobiliary and pancreatic	Wound infection; peritonitis; ascending cholangitis ± bacteremia; hepatic, pancreatic, or sub-diaphragmatic abscess
Genitourinary and prostate	Urinary tract infection; wound infection; prostatitis; pelvic or abdominal abscess
Bone, joint, cartilage	Wound infection; skin and skin structure infection; bursitis; septic arthritis; synovitis; osteomyelitis; infected prosthesis

Site and Spectrum of Infection

The site of infection depends on the location and size of the tumor or the site and nature of the medical device or surgical procedure (see Table 23.3). Most infections are caused by the patient's resident microflora (Wisplinghoff et al. 2003). Surgical wound infections and catheter-related infections are caused most often by organisms colonizing the skin, although certain opportunistic pathogens, such as *Pseudomonas aeruginosa*, are beginning to emerge. Most respiratory infections are caused by the oropharyngeal flora; *Staphylococcus* species and gram-positive bacilli are the predominant pathogens observed in various health care settings. Polymicrobial infections occur when the infection includes tissue involvement (Rolston et al. 2007). Examples include perirectal abscesses, neutropenic enterocolitis, pneumonia, and complicated skin–skin structure infections. Catheter-associated infections may also be polymicrobial. Fungal and viral infections are less common in patients with solid tumors. A breakdown of predominant pathogens according to the site of infection is provided in Table 23.4.

Diagnosis and Treatment

Because such a wide variety of infections occur in patients with solid tumors, a detailed discussion of diagnosis and treatment is beyond the scope of this chapter. As a general rule, patients with severe neutropenia and those receiving

Table 23.4 Common pathogens by site of infection

Infection site	Common pathogens
Bloodstream	Coagulase-negative staphylococci; *Staphylococcus aureus*; *Enterococcus* species; enteric gram-negative bacilli; *Candida* species
Central nervous system (including shunt-related and postsurgical infection)	Coagulase-negative staphylococci; *S. aureus*; enteric gram-negative bacilli; *Streptococcus pneumoniae*; *Haemophilus influenzae*; mouth anaerobes; *Listeria monocytogenes*; *Cryptococcus neoformans*
Respiratory tract (upper and lower)	*S. pneumoniae*; *H. influenzae*; *S. aureus*; Enterobacteriaceae; *Pseudomonas aeruginosa*; mouth anaerobes
Biliary tract	Enteric gram-negative bacilli; *Enterococcus* species (including VRE); enteric anaerobes; *Candida* species
Intra-abdominal/pelvic	Enteric gram-negative bacilli; *Enterococcus* species (including VRE); enteric anaerobes; *Candida* species
Skin/skin structure	*S. aureus*; *Streptococcus* species (Groups A, B, C, G, and F); *P. aeruginosa*; enteric gram-negative bacilli; anaerobes; *Candida* species
Central venous catheter-related	Coagulase-negative staphylococci; *S. aureus*; *Bacillus* species; *Corynebacterium* species; *P. aeruginosa*; *Stenotrophomonas maltophilia*; *Acinetobacter* species; *Candida* species

VRE indicates vancomycin-resistant *Enterococcus*

corticosteroids or other immunosuppressive agents have blunted inflammatory responses, leading to a paucity of clinical manifestations. In contrast, most patients with solid tumors have normal inflammatory responses, making clinical evaluation easier to accomplish. Therapy is usually based on knowledge of current local epidemiology and susceptibility patterns. There are few indications for empiric therapy in patients with solid tumors because documented infections are much more common. Surgical intervention for drainage or removal of devitalized tissue, as well as placement of drainage catheters or stents, is more common in patients with solid tumors. Many neutropenic patients with solid tumors are considered to have a low risk of developing severe infections and can safely be treated without hospitalization, or they can be discharged early, often after only a 24- to 48-hour period of hospital-based therapy, to complete therapy at home (Rolston 1999; Kern 2006; Klastersky and Paesmans 2007; Freifeld et al. 2011).

Antimicrobial Stewardship

Antimicrobial agents are used frequently and for a number of indications in patients with cancer. Heavy antimicrobial usage leads to the development of resistant pathogens (Rolston 2005). In addition, the pipeline for new drugs is relatively dry (Talbot et al. 2006; Boucher et al. 2009). Therefore, the judicious use of currently available antiinfective agents, usually referred to as antimicrobial stewardship, has become an important strategy in the overall management of infections, whether the patient has cancer or not (Dellit et al. 2007).

Key Practice Points

- Immunologic deficits are common in cancer patients and survivors.
- Specific deficits are associated with specific infections, although there is some overlap.
- Multiple deficits may be present, increasing the risk and severity of infection.
- Neutropenia is the most common immunologic deficit in patients with hematologic malignancies.
- Hematopoietic stem cell transplantation recipients develop almost global loss of immunity.
- Patients with solid tumors, in general, experience less immunosuppression than patients with hematologic malignancies or hematopoietic stem cell transplantation recipients.
- Infection management strategies include infection prevention, diagnosis, and treatment.
- Antimicrobial stewardship is important, especially considering that new antimicrobial drug development is minimal.

Suggested Readings

Boucher HW, Talbot GH, Bradley JS, et al. Bad bugs, no drugs: no ESKAPE! An update from the Infectious Diseases Society of America. *Clin Infect Dis* 2009;48:2–12.

Crawford J, Dale DC, Lyman GH. Chemotherapy-induced neutropenia. Risks, consequences, and new directions for its management. *Cancer* 2004;100:228–237.

Dellit TH, Owens RC, McGowan JE, et al. Infectious Diseases of America and the Society for Healthcare Epidemiology of America guidelines for developing an institutional program to enhance antimicrobial stewardship. *Clin Infect Dis* 2007;44:159–177.

Freifeld AG, Bow EJ, Sepkowitz KA, et al. Clinical practice guideline for the use of antimicrobial agents in neutropenic patients with cancer: 2010 update by the Infectious Diseases Society of America. *Clin Infect Dis* 2011;52:e56-e93.

Karlsson J, Andréasson B, Kondori N, et al. Comparative study of immune status to infectious agents in elderly patients with multiple myeloma, Waldenstrom's macroglobulinemia, and monoclonal gammopathy of undetermined significance. *Clin and Vaccine Immunol* 2011;18: 969–977.

Kern WV. Risk assessment and treatment of low-risk patients with febrile neutropenia. *Clin Infect Dis* 2006;42:533–540.

Klastersky J, Paesmans M. Risk-adapted strategy for the management of febrile neutropenia in cancer patients. *Support Care Cancer* 2007;15:487–482.

Klastersky J, Paesmans M, Rubenstein EB, et al. The Multinational Association for Supportive Care in Cancer risk index: a multinational scoring system for identifying low-risk febrile neutropenic cancer patients. *J Clin Oncol* 2000;18:3038–3051.

Martin SI, Marty FM, Fiumara K, Treon SP, Gribben JG, Baden LR. Infectious complications associated with alemtuzumab use for lymphoproliferative disorders. *Clin Infect Dis* 2006;43:16–24.

Mir MA, Battiwalla M. Immune deficits in allogeneic hematopoietic stem cell transplant (HSCT) recipients. *Mycopathologia* 2009;168:271–282.

Rolston KVI. New trends in patient management: risk-based therapy for febrile patients with neutropenia. *Clin Infect Dis* 1999;29(3):515–521.

Rolston KVI. Challenges in the treatment of infections caused by gram-positive and gram-negative bacteria in patients with cancer and neutropenia. *Clin Infect Dis* 2005;40:S246–S252.

Rolston KVI, Bodey GP. Infections in patients with cancer. In: Kufe DW, Bast RC Jr, Hait WN, Hong WK, Pollock RE, Weichselbaum RR, Holland JR, Frei E III, eds. *Cancer Medicine 8*. 8th ed. Hamilton, Ontario: BC Decker; 2010:1921–1940.

Rolston KVI, Bodey GP, Safdar A. Polymicrobial infections in patients with cancer: an underappreciated and underreported entity. *Clin Infect Dis* 2007;45:228–233.

Rubenstein EB, Rolston K, Benjamin RS, et al. Outpatient treatment of febrile episodes in low-risk neutropenic patients with cancer. *Cancer* 1993;71:3640–3646.

Samonis G, Kontoyiannis DP. Infectious complications of purine analog therapy. *Curr Opin Infect Dis* 2001;14:409–413.

Su YB, Sohn S, Krown E, et al. Selective CD4+ lymphopenia in melanoma patients treated with temozolomide: a toxicity with therapeutic implications. *J Clin Oncol* 2004;22:610–616.

Talbot GH, Bradley J, Edwards JE Jr, Gilbert D, Scheld M, Bartlett JG. Bad bugs need drugs: an update on the development pipeline from the Antimicrobial Availability Task Force of the Infectious Diseases Society of America. *Clin Infect Dis* 2006;42:657–668.

Tomblyn M, Chiller T, Einsele H, et al. Guidelines for preventing infectious complications among hematopoietic cell transplantation recipients: a global perspective. *Biol Blood Marrow Transplant* 2009;15:1143–1238.

Wisplinghoff H, Seifert H, Wenzel RP, Edmond MB. Current trends in the epidemiology of nosocomial bloodstream infections in patients with hematological malignancies and solid neoplasms in hospitals in the United States. *Clin Infect Dis* 2003;36:1103–1110.

Chapter 24
Rehabilitation

Jack Fu

Contents

Chapter Overview As the number of cancer survivors has increased owing to more effective treatment, more attention has been placed on quality of life for these individuals. Physiatry, or physical medicine and rehabilitation, emphasizes function. Physiatrists prevent, diagnose, and treat disorders of the nervous and musculoskeletal systems. Commonly addressed issues in the cancer survivor population include neurogenic bowel, neurogenic bladder, spasticity, lymphedema, pain, and return to work. Generalized weakness and fatigue are among the most common diagnoses in patients with cancer and the most commonly addressed by physiatrists.

L.E. Foxhall, M.A. Rodriguez (eds.), *Advances in Cancer Survivorship Management*,
MD Anderson Cancer Care Series, DOI 10.1007/978-1-4939-0986-5_24,
© The University of Texas M.D. Anderson Cancer Center 2015

Rehabilitation Issues in Cancer Survivors

According to the American Academy of Physical Medicine and Rehabilitation (2011), physical medicine and rehabilitation, or physiatry, is the branch of medicine emphasizing the prevention, diagnosis, and treatment of disorders, particularly those related to the nerves, muscles, bones, and brain. Physiatry is concerned with quality of life, with a focus on function. Rehabilitation physicians, or physiatrists, may also perform electromyograms and subspecialize in a number of areas, including pediatrics, sports medicine, palliative care, spinal cord injury, and pain management. Physiatry is a relatively new specialty; the American Board of Physical Medicine and Rehabilitation was formed in 1947.

Cancer rehabilitation has become increasingly important in the young field of physiatry. The major goal of cancer rehabilitation is to improve quality of life by minimizing the disability caused by cancer and its treatment and decreasing the "burden of care" needed by cancer patients and their caregivers (Fu and Shin 2011). Dietz (1980) classified cancer rehabilitation into four categories: preventive, restorative, supportive, and palliative.

Preventive rehabilitation occurs before or immediately after a treatment to prevent loss of function or disability. An example of preventive rehabilitation is teaching a patient with a lower-extremity sarcoma about stump care and walker ambulation prior to amputation. Courneya and Friedenreich (2001) described a concept called "buffering," in which a cancer patient performs exercises and undergoes therapies to increase physical and functional reserves before treatment. The concept of "prehabilitation" is similar to preventive rehabilitation.

Restorative rehabilitation occurs in patients who are believed to be disease-free or in whom a stable disease course is anticipated. An example of this is postamputation prosthetic rehabilitation in a patient with a lower-extremity sarcoma and no known metastatic disease. Preventive and restorative cancer rehabilitation are not substantially different from conventional nononcologic rehabilitation. However, as cancer survivorship has increased, restorative rehabilitation has become more prominent. Issues commonly addressed include disability, return to work, and lymphedema management.

Supportive and palliative rehabilitation occur in patients whose disease has not been fully cured. Supportive rehabilitation is performed in patients with persistent ongoing disease. Palliative rehabilitation is done to reduce discomfort and improve independence in patients with advanced disease (Dietz 1980).

Improvements in cancer survivorship over the past two decades have largely been due to improved detection, surgeries, chemotherapeutic agents, and radiation therapies (Kevorkian 2009). Improved survival has led to increasing attention to the quality-of-life implications of cancer and its treatment. Physiatry's emphasis on quality of life and return of function has made it an important piece of cancer survivorship care. The definition of a cancer survivor can include a broad range of patients; this chapter will focus on restorative rehabilitation in cancer survivors with no evidence of disease who are not undergoing active treatment. However, many of the concepts and topics discussed here are applicable to cancer survivors receiving ongoing treatment as well. We will discuss the issues that a physiatrist encounters in the cancer survivor population.

Pain

Chronic pain is a common symptom in the general population but it is very pervasive in the cancer population. Chronic pain is the third largest global health problem, the most common cause of disability in the United States, and the second most common reason for physician visits (Greenberg et al. 2003). Sixty percent to 85% of patients with advanced cancer and 40% of 5-year cancer survivors report pain (Caraceni 2001; Nelson et al. 2001). When assessing pain in this patient population, physiatrists should never overlook the possibility of cancer recurrence or metastasis. A conscientious physical examination is invaluable. Imaging studies such as x-rays can also often be useful to evaluate the possibility of bony metastasis.

Musculoskeletal Pain

Physiatrists frequently encounter patients with pain originating in the muscles, ligaments, tendons, and bones. These patients are often referred to physiatrists by their oncologists. Although musculoskeletal pain is quite common in patients who do not have cancer, cancer survivors may be at increased risk for musculoskeletal ailments. Many cancer survivors undergo substantial muscle loss (Mourtzakis and Bedbrook 2009) owing to the cancer, its treatment, and complications. Cachexia and significant weight loss are very common. Weight loss in cancer disproportionately favors muscle loss over fat loss.

Steroids are frequently used in cancer treatment, and prolonged use of steroids can lead to steroid myopathy. This condition typically favors proximal muscles, and patients often present with significant hip weakness. Sit-to-stand transfers and climbing stairs may be particularly difficult for these patients.

In addition, many surgical treatments for cancer involve muscle flaps, neurolysis of innervating motor nerves, damage to muscles in the body, and significant alterations in musculoskeletal anatomy. Changes to muscles and anatomy during the course of cancer treatment can suboptimally alter the body's biomechanics, often leading to chronic repetitive trauma injuries. The most common areas of repetitive trauma injury are the shoulder and back. Low back pain caused by loss of strength in the core musculature is common, as is patellofemoral knee pain caused by quadriceps weakness.

It is important for patients to maintain activity and nutrition during treatment for cancer. Early rehabilitation may help minimize deconditioning and muscle loss during treatment. A musculoskeletal treatment plan for a cancer survivor may be similar to that of a patient who does not have cancer. However, strengthening of muscles that were disproportionately affected by cancer and its treatment, special emphasis on nutrition, and rehabilitation focused on anatomic changes may be required.

Reduced range of motion in musculoskeletal joints can lead to painful symptoms. Debility and prolonged immobility from lengthy hospitalizations or stays in the intensive care unit can become problematic when soft tissue changes lead to decreased range of motion. Many patients with cancer experience adhesive capsulitis. Lack of consistent range of motion in the shoulder joint because of pain from a nearby tumor or lack of activity is common. Many patients also experience decreased passive or active range of motion in the bilateral ankles secondary to contracture formation and lack of daily movement.

Treatment for reduced range of motion often requires serial casting and aggressive range-of-motion exercises that are often painful. Joints with reduced range of motion can impair function, including gait and activities of daily living (e.g., upper extremity dressing). It is important for clinicians to maintain range of motion during acute hospitalizations through exercises or simply by applying pressure relief ankle foot orthosis boots. This often is overlooked by the acute care clinician when more pressing medical issues are being addressed. Prior radiation therapy or surgery and the effects of the cancer can also lead to chronic inflammation and scar tissue formation that can reduce range of motion.

The PRICE acronym describes protect, rest, ice, and elevation; this concept can be applied to acute musculoskeletal injury and pain. Treatment with nonsteroidal anti-inflammatory drugs as analgesia is helpful if not medically contraindicated. (Use of nonsteroidal anti-inflammatory drugs is not recommended in patients with thrombocytopenia, poorly controlled hypertension, renal insufficiency, or a history of gastrointestinal bleeding, or for those receiving treatment with anticoagulants.) This simple treatment plan leads to improvement in most musculoskeletal injuries. If the musculoskeletal pain continues despite PRICE, referral to a physiatrist, orthopedist, or sports medicine physician is warranted.

Therapists often request to use other treatment modalities as an adjunct to rehabilitation. Heat modalities include ultrasound, shortwave diathermy, microwave diathermy, heat packs, paraffin baths, and infrared lamps. Cold modalities include ice packs, cold baths, and vapocoolant sprays. Transcutaneous electrical nerve stimulation units and massage are also useful treatment modalities in rehabilitation. Unfortunately, the safety of these modalities in patients with cancer is not well defined. Patients theoretically increase their risk of developing metastasis when using the transcutaneous electrical nerve stimulation units and heat modalities, especially near the site of a known cancer lesion. Use of these modalities is often dependent on the prescribing clinician's viewpoint (Strax et al. 2004). A referral to an acupuncturist or a massage therapist may be useful.

Neuropathic Pain

Neuropathic pain is prevalent in cancer survivors. Peripheral neuropathy is caused by a number of chemotherapeutic agents. Radiation-induced plexopathy, neurolysis after surgery, phantom neuropathic pain after amputation, and central pain syndrome after brain surgery or stroke also occur.

At times patients with these symptoms present directly to the physiatrist for management of pain. However, many cancer survivors present to a physiatrist for functional impairments related to the neuropathic pain described above. Gait deviations are common in patients with neuropathy and in those who have undergone amputation or brain surgery. Controlling these neuropathic symptoms can improve function. Anticonvulsants and opiate pain medications are commonly used. Rehabilitation of these patients is focused on gait and activities of daily living. Desensitization techniques can be performed by therapists to reduce dysesthesia and paresthesia.

Chronic Fatigue and Deconditioning

Fatigue is the most common symptom in patients with cancer (Zeng et al. 2012), and physiatrists often encounter complaints of fatigue and deconditioning among cancer survivors. There are many causes of fatigue in cancer survivors, and workup is similar to that used for patients complaining of fatigue who do not have cancer. However, deconditioning, depression, inadequate nutrition, chronic pancytopenia, infection, hormonal changes (such as adrenal insufficiency after prolonged use of steroids or testosterone deficiency after treatment for testicular cancer), and medications are among the most common causes of fatigue in cancer survivors. The standard laboratory panel used to assess chronic fatigue at the MD Anderson fatigue clinic includes complete blood count, electrolytes, blood urea nitrogen, creatinine, calcium, magnesium, phosphorus, thyroid-stimulating hormone, free T4 cortisol, vitamin B12, vitamin D, and C-reactive protein. Testosterone and prostate-specific antigen levels are also tested in men.

A self-perpetuating cycle may develop in which fatigued patients avoid activity to reduce fatigue, but the reduced activity leads to worse deconditioning and fatigue (Winningham et al. 1994). An important step to combat this cycle is to encourage activity and use therapy to insure continued activity, especially during treatment for cancer. Educating patients and caregivers regarding the importance of staying active is just as valuable as therapy. Patients should be encouraged to sit in a chair whenever possible and avoid lying in bed for extended periods of time during the day. Keeping blinds open to help maintain sleep-wake cycles and avoiding excessive napping may also help.

Cessation of sedating medications should be considered. Stimulant medications may be an option, if a reversible cause for the fatigue is not found. Methylphenidate (Ritalin) and modafinil (Provigil) have been studied as treatments for fatigue, with mixed results (Portela et al. 2011). Other treatment strategies include brief steroid boluses and other neurostimulants such as amantadine and carbidopa/levodopa (Sinemet).

Rehabilitation of patients with fatigue should focus on improving patients' conditioning and activity. Motivation is often a difficult obstacle. Physical therapy may be useful to develop a home exercise program that the patient can maintain. Having the guidance of a therapist can be helpful, especially for a poorly motivated patient. It is important to emphasize that reconditioning takes time and persistence. Recovering from deconditioning can take up to two to three times longer than the period of deconditioning (Choi et al. 2006). Typically, the patient is advised to gradually increase the distance walked or time spent exercising. Often the analogy of training for a marathon is useful, describing the technique of gradually increasing distances, speed, and conditioning. Incorporating the patient's hobbies into the therapy can also help motivate the patient. The effectiveness of exercise for reducing fatigue and increasing physiologic conditioning has been well studied. Exercise leads to reduced body fat, improved lean mass, increased bone mass, and increased well-being in patients with cancer (Courneya and Friedenreich 2001; Irwin et al. 2009).

Common Conditions Treated by Physiatrists

Neurogenic Bowel

Physiatrists frequently encounter patients with neurogenic bowel. Managing this condition requires patience, persistence, and an understanding of the underlying neurologic innervation of the intestinal tract.

Neurogenic bowel can be caused by either an upper or a lower motor neuron lesion. With an upper motor neuron lesion, cortical innervation and thus external anal sphincter control is lost. This scenario, referred to as hyperreflexic bowel, can occur with a brain injury or a spinal cord injury at L1 or above (the conus medullaris). Without voluntary control, the sphincter cannot be relaxed and the pelvic floor muscles become spastic. However, reflexive activity between the colon and spinal cord remains intact, and these reflexes are utilized in the "bowel programs" to manage hyperreflexic bowel (see below).

A lower motor neuron lesion, which is below the level of the anterior horn cell, frequently occurs with nerve root damage or spinal cord injury below the level of the conus medullaris. In patients with cancer, these injuries are often found among those who have undergone a sacrectomy and sometimes among those who have undergone internal hemipelvectomy for chondrosarcoma. Lower motor neuron lesions result in an areflexic bowel, in which reflexive defecation is impeded. The Auerbach myenteric plexus coordinates peristalsis and movement of stool, but the movement is very slow, and the most common outcome is constipation. A flaccid external anal sphincter may lead to small releases of stool throughout the day.

Physiatrists prescribe "bowel programs" to help these patients regain some control of their bowel movements. The bowel program involves emptying the bowel at set consistent times so that if the colon does move at a socially embarrassing or inconvenient time, the colon is empty and therefore does not release any stool. Ideally bowel movements occur once per day, but an areflexic bowel may require 2–3 movements per day. Two reflexes in particular are exploited in bowel programs. The first is the gastrocolic reflex, which is stimulated 30–60 minutes after a meal. The second is the anorectal reflex (rectocolic reflex), in which colonic wall distension caused by stool buildup results in relaxation of the internal anal sphincter.

A bowel program consists of two basic phases. The first is the oral phase, which consists of a large meal, preferably with hot prune juice or hot coffee or tea, at the same time every day. The most commonly chosen meal is breakfast, but other meals can be used to fit with the patient's typical routine. If the patient typically had a bowel movement in the morning prior to the injury, then the patient is encouraged to use breakfast for the oral phase of the bowel program. Consistency is the key; patients are advised to always use the same meal for the bowel program. The oral phase stimulates the gastrocolic reflex. The patient should also take stool softeners or gentle laxatives such as sennosides daily, typically 8–12 hours prior to the planned bowel movement.

The second phase occurs approximately 35–55 minutes after the meal, at which point the patient inserts a rectal suppository and performs digital stimulation for at least 3–15 minutes. Digital stimulation consists of using a finger to press against the walls of the rectum. Patients may also disimpact any hard stools they may feel in the rectum. The rectal irritation from the suppository combined with rectal wall expansion from digital stimulation is meant to stimulate the anorectal reflex. In a patient with hyperreflexic bowel, a large bowel movement is often stimulated: because spinal cord injuries in cancer patients are rarely complete, some degree of these reflexes is preserved. However, in patients with lower motor neuron injury, these reflexes are typically muted significantly. The bowel movements stimulated by digital stimulation in a patient with lower motor neuron injury are typically much smaller, and multiple stimulations throughout the day may be required to empty the colon.

Patients begin training for bowel programs as soon as possible. Patients and their caregivers are educated about the basics of the bowel program. Patients are encouraged to perform the digital stimulation and suppository insertion themselves if they are physically capable. In the cancer population, special consideration should be addressed to those with neutropenia and thrombocytopenia. A safe blood count threshold for bowel programs has not been established. However, at MD Anderson, platelet counts of less than 70,000/μL and white blood cell counts of less than 2,000/μL are generally the thresholds to stop the rectal stimulation portion of the bowel program.

Neurogenic Bladder

Similar to neurogenic bowel, neurogenic bladder can be the result of a lower motor neuron injury (areflexic bladder) or an upper motor neuron injury (hyperreflexic bladder).

Upper motor neuron lesions are those that occur above the anterior horn cell. Typically, these lesions occur at L1 or above (conus medullaris) or within the cauda equine, with significant damage above the sacral micturition center (S2-S4). Hyperreflexic bladder is characterized by a spastic bladder, which results in frequent urination and inability to store significant amounts of urine. Treatment typically involves bladder relaxers such as anticholinergic medications (e.g., oxybutynin

[Ditropan], tolterodine [Detrol]). In some cases, a Foley catheter may be used. In men, a condom catheter may be useful to prevent wetting clothing without the infection risks of an indwelling Foley catheter.

With areflexic bladder, lesions are typically located at the sacral micturition center (S2 and below). The resultant flaccid bladder is unable to contract or empty, and the patient experiences overflow incontinence with frequent small drops of urine escaping. Treatment for areflexive bladder requires emptying the retained urine. The most preferred method is clean intermittent catheterization. Careful care should be taken to clean the catheter to prevent infection, and the patient and caregiver are instructed on how to accomplish this. At times, the assistance of an occupational therapist may be needed if the patient's neurologic weakness makes this challenging. If the patient is uncomfortable or unable to perform intermittent catheterization, an indwelling Foley catheter may be a more appealing alternative. Other less effective methods of emptying the bladder include the Valsalva and Crede maneuvers to "push out" urine by increasing intraabdominal pressure. Patients are typically encouraged to catheterize instead, but if they do use the Valsalva and Crede maneuvers, a urologic evaluation is indicated to ensure that retrograde travel of urine does not occur.

A postvoid bladder scan or catheterization may also be useful to determine the amount of retained urine. Generally, less than 200 mL of urine is considered acceptable. Cancer survivors typically present with some ability to void but are unable to empty the bladder adequately. If the patient can consistently maintain less than 200 mL of retained urine, the patient is permitted to urinate without catheters. However, if the patient is unable to consistently maintain retained volumes of less than 200 mL, the patient should use intermittent catheterization or an indwelling Foley catheter. A simple way to test the patient's ability to void is timed voluntary voids followed by a postvoid bladder ultrasound.

A combination type of neurogenic bladder may also occur in some patients. These patients typically have spinal cord lesions between the sacral micturition center and the brain. The resultant condition is called detrusor sphincter dyssynergia, in which both the bladder and sphincter are hyperactive. This creates a situation in which the bladder pushes urine against a closed sphincter, which increases intravesicular pressure and forces the urine to ascend through the ureters toward the kidneys. Urologic evaluation is highly recommended. A cystometrogram can confirm the diagnosis. Treatment typically involves anticholinergic bladder relaxants in combination with clean intermittent catheterization. At times, surgical interventions such as sphincterotomy or suprapubic tube insertion are indicated.

Spasticity

Spasticity forms in many patients with upper motor neuron or central nervous system damage. In clinical practice at MD Anderson, spasticity has been found to be particularly prevalent in patients with meningioma and survivors of stroke.

The Modified Ashworth Scale is used by clinicians to measure spasticity and hypertonia. The scale ranges from 0 to 4: 0 indicates no increase in tone; 1, a slight increase in tone with a "catch and release" accompanied by minimal resistance at the end of the range of motion; 2, a slight increase in resistance through less than half of the range of motion; 2+, an increase in resistance through more than half of the range of motion; 3, considerably increased resistance that makes passive movement difficult; and 4, a rigid joint that cannot be passively moved.

Spasticity can be treated in a variety of ways. One important method is daily stretching and range of motion exercises to stretch the muscles and prevent contracture formation. Contracture forms from the accumulation of scar tissue within the muscle when the muscle does not routinely go through its range of motion. Treatment modalities such as heat, cold, splinting, serial casts, relaxation techniques, biofeedback, and electrical stimulation may also help.

Oral medications can also be used to treat spasticity. Commonly used oral medications include baclofen, diazepam (Valium), dantrolene (Dantrium), clonidine (Catapres), and tizanidine (Zanaflex). Liver function should be monitored in patients treated with tizanidine and dantrolene. Blood pressure should be monitored in patients treated with clonidine and tizanidine in particular, although all of these medications can cause hypotension. A problematic and unfortunately common side effect of these oral agents is sedation. Many patients who have significant spasticity have brain injuries, and their arousal and cognition may already be impaired. Sedating them with oral medications can be problematic.

Injectable medications can be useful when oral medications are not tolerated. Phenol can be used to block a nerve by demyelination. The phenol is injected via ultrasound or electrical stimulation into the nerve that innervates affected muscles. Typically, the effect of the agent is almost immediate and the effects can linger for up to 6–12 months. Phenol is relatively inexpensive but it is more difficult to administer than botulinum toxin (see below). Phenol can also affect sensation and may cause paresthesia or dysesthesia. If these side effects become bothersome, treatment with a neuropathic pain agent can be attempted, or a repeated injection to further block the nerve may be helpful.

Botulinum toxin can also be injected into affected muscles to reduce muscle activity. Several types of botulinum toxin are available on the market. The most widely used is botulinum toxin A (under the brand names Dysport, Botox, and Xeomin). Botox, or onabotulinum toxin, is approved by the US Food and Drug Administration for the treatment of upper extremity spasticity. The toxin works at the neuromuscular junction and inhibits release of acetylcholine, thereby reducing muscle activity. Botulinum toxin is more expensive, does not produce a clinical effect immediately, and typically does not last as long as phenol. However, the botulinum toxin does not cause sensory problems and is easier to administer than phenol.

Another option is the intrathecal baclofen pump (produced by Medtronic), which delivers baclofen directly into the cerebrospinal fluid of the spinal cord. This device has several advantages, including the ability to fine-tune the level of baclofen delivered and maintain a steady level of baclofen and spasticity control.

The intrathecal baclofen pump also produces fewer cognitive side effects than those that occur with oral antispasmodic agents and requires fewer needle sticks than those required with injected agents. In addition, the baclofen can be mixed with opiate analgesics in the intrathecal pump if the patient has severe pain. Disadvantages of the intrathecal baclofen pump include high cost, the need for maintenance, the possibility of complications owing to malfunction and infection, and the fact that it is an implanted device. Refills must be placed before the reservoir is empty to prevent baclofen withdrawal. The pump battery typically lasts about 7 years, and the pump must be replaced when the battery runs out.

The intrathecal baclofen pump is usually pursued after more conservative treatments have failed. The patient undergoes a trial in which baclofen is administered intrathecally, typically by lumbar puncture. The patient's spasticity is measured by a physician or therapist both before and after the intrathecal infusion. A documented improvement is necessary to proceed with pump installation. Effects of the intrathecal baclofen pump tend to be more prominent in the lower extremities. However, placing the catheter slightly higher may improve upper extremity effects as well. It is not unusual for patients with an intrathecal baclofen pump to continue to require botulinum toxin injections in the upper extremities after pump placement. The rate of infusion is controlled by a wireless handheld computer and can be fine-tuned to prevent excessive or insufficient flow.

Lymphedema

Malignancy is the leading cause of lymphedema in the United States. Breast, gynecologic, and urologic cancer, as well as melanoma and lymphoma, are the most commonly implicated malignancies. Direct metastatic invasion of the lymphatic system, as well as radiation therapy and surgical treatments, can lead to damaged lymph nodes and lymphatic function. Breast cancer and associated upper extremity swelling is the most common lymphedema scenario that American physiatrists encounter. An estimated 24–49% of patients with breast cancer have lymphedema after mastectomy.

The lymphatic system has three main functions. The first is to transport or drain interstitial fluid from the limbs, the second is to move chyle fluid, and the third is to maintain immunity. Lymphedema can be divided into four distinct stages. In stage 0, no overt edema is present but lymphatic function is impaired. In stage 1, fluid high in protein begins to accumulate, but the accumulation subsides with limb elevation. In stage 2, fibrosis develops, and limb elevation alone rarely allows the swelling to subside. In stage 3, no pitting occurs and trophic skin changes develop.

Patients with lymphedema can suffer from complications such as recurrent cellulitis, lymphangitis, and skin changes, including hyperkeratosis, papillomatosis, skin breakdown, and cutaneous tumors. Peau d'orange occurs on the affected breast of patients with lymphedema; in this condition, the skin resembles an orange skin. Stemmer's sign is often a sign of late-stage lymphedema. The hallmark of Stemmer's sign is the inability to pinch the skin on a patient's affected toes.

The diagnosis of lymphedema is typically clinical. Known risk factors for lymphedema include cancer, recent lymph node dissection, and known lymph node tumor involvement with new-onset progressive swelling. Most patients with swelling of an extremity could benefit from lymphedema management. However, cardiac, renal, and hepatic malfunction, as well as malnutrition, venous insufficiency, and deep venous thrombosis should also be considered as possible causes of swelling. Ruling out other causes of swelling by laboratory or radiologic tests can be helpful. If the diagnosis is in question, a computed tomographic scan or magnetic resonance imaging may be helpful. However, the gold standard test is the lymphoscintigram, or lymphangiogram. This nuclear medicine test consists of injecting a radionucleotide dye into both the affected and unaffected limbs. The transit time for the dye and the amount of dye that has arrived at the torso are examined. This test is not done frequently but can be useful in certain cases.

If a patient has suspected lymphedema and other potential causes for swelling have been eliminated, a referral to a lymphedema-certified physical therapist is indicated. Patients with stage 0 lymphedema or those at high risk of developing lymphedema could also benefit from seeing a lymphedema therapist. The therapist teaches the patient and caregiver techniques of manual lymph drainage and educates them about the basics of lymphedema. A detailed description of manual lymph drainage is beyond the scope of this text; essentially, it incorporates massage, wrapping the limb with multilayered bandages, and using compression garments. The goal of manual lymph drainage is to increase lymph return, establish protein lysis by macrophages, and break down collagens. If successful, manual lymph drainage can improve the appearance of the affected limb, improve function by decreasing the weight and volume of the affected limb, and prevent progression of the lymphedema to higher stages. External pneumatic compression devices may also be used. These consist of multiple air-filled bladders that place pressure on the limb sequentially to assist with fluid return. In the event that conservative management through manual lymph drainage is unsuccessful, a number of surgical procedures can be considered.

Exercise and lymphedema has been a controversial topic. Recent research suggests that moderate exercise is acceptable for patients with lymphedema. Previously, many feared that exercise involving the affected limb may lead to further lymphatic damage and progression of lymphedema, and patients were told not to use the affected limbs. However, recent research has shown no change, and in some cases improvement, in swelling with moderate resistance exercise (Kim et al. 2010). Furthermore, depriving patients of the benefits of exercise is detrimental to quality of life. In light of recent research, the physiatrists at MD Anderson encourage patients to engage in aerobic exercise and allow them to participate in light to moderate weight resistance exercise, but no heavy weight exercises.

Resuming Life After Cancer Treatment

Independent Living

The patient's cognitive function after completion of treatment is an important consideration when determining the patient's level of independence. If the patient shows signs of or is at risk for cognitive impairment (e.g., after brain tumor removal or a stroke), an evaluation by a speech therapist, occupational therapist, or neuropsychologist can confirm and document these issues. Evaluations examining whether the patient's cognitive function is adequate for living in his or her environment are particularly useful. If independent living is not an option, living with relatives, in assisted living, or in a nursing home should be considered. Unfortunately, assisted living and nursing home facilities are often very costly for the patient.

Driving

Physiatrists assist patients with their return to normal life. After a major surgery, treatment, or hospitalization, the patient is primarily advised to focus on resuming household mobility and basic activities of daily living. However, once the patient has achieved these goals, the topic of driving often comes up. In many parts of the country, access to a car and the ability to drive can add convenience and independence to one's life.

Driving requires vision, motor coordination, proprioception, cognition, and vestibular function to some degree. Most states do not have a formal process for assessing a patient's ability to drive after a hospitalization or major disability. Physicians are often asked to "permit" patients to resume driving. However, the physician is rarely able to observe the patient driving in a vehicle or simulator. An examination of vision, motor function, proprioception (especially in the right leg), and cognitive reasoning are used to formulate a decision regarding driving.

If the patient's ability to drive safely is questionable, the assistance of a certified driving occupational therapist may be helpful. The Association of Driver Rehabilitation Specialists is a useful resource to find a certified driving occupational therapist in an area. Most occupational therapists are not certified or trained in this field. However, occupational therapists that are specially trained can evaluate the patient's driving ability by observing the patient behind the wheel or in a simulator. If the patient passes, the therapist typically issues a certificate. Sometimes, the therapist will recommend changes to the vehicle before allowing the patient to drive. Vehicle modifications can include changes to the pedals, steering wheel, and even the addition of extra mirrors. In other circumstances, the therapist may forbid the patient from driving. The certification by an occupational therapist, although not required by law in most states, can be useful for liability purposes and to reassure the family, patient, and physician.

Most patients who resume driving have not sat behind the wheel for months. They are encouraged to start off with small amounts of driving in low-traffic areas and gradually increase the time spent driving and level of traffic over time.

Return to Work and Disability

Returning to employment is important to cancer survivors. Cancer and its treatment are financially burdensome and a common cause of bankruptcy (Andrews 2007). Employment brings income and perhaps health insurance. Psychologically, employment is one more step toward a return to "normal life." Financial independence and identity can be tied to employment.

Studies reveal that cancer survivors are 1.4 times more likely to experience long-term unemployment than healthy controls (de Boer et al. 2009). Rates of unemployment among cancer survivors have been reported to range from 10% to 20% (Carlsen et al. 2008; Syse et al. 2008), with some variations on the basis of age, cancer type, cancer treatment, education, occupation, and work load (Taskila-Abrandt et al. 2005). A comparison of primary cancer types and time to return to work showed that patients with skin cancer returned to work the fastest (median 55 days) and those with lung cancer took the longest to return to work (median 377 days; Roelen et al. 2011).

Cancer survivors encounter a number of obstacles when resuming work. Physical limitations include fatigue, pain, and other chronic symptoms. Stress and anxiety related to having cancer and maintaining work performance can be psychologically challenging (Spelten et al. 2003). Verbeek (2006) described three ways for physicians to assist patients with the transition back to work. First, the physician and therapists should incorporate skills necessary to return to work in the rehabilitation process. If a patient must perform a specific physical task at work, the therapist can teach him or her how to perform it given their new disabilities. Second, the physician should advise the patient and employer regarding accommodations necessary at the workplace. The most common accommodations include changes to work times and even work tasks. Most employers have forms that are to be filled out by the physician describing specific limitations. Last, special attention should be paid to cognition and executive function. Radiation effects, chemotherapy, intracranial surgeries, and other cancer-related complications can affect cognition (Verbeek 2006).

The Americans with Disabilities Act, passed in 1990, prohibits discrimination based on disability. The Americans with Disabilities Act consists of multiple titles covering a variety of topics, including access to public facilities and telecommunications. Title I covers most nonfederal employers with more than 15 employees. These employers must make "reasonable accommodations" in the hiring and maintenance of qualified disabled persons unless those accommodations pose an "undue hardship." The accommodations must be requested by the employee or applicant; employers are not required to make accommodations that have not been requested.

In addition, employers are forbidden from asking about impairments unless they are specifically job-related. Pre-employment physical examinations can be performed if similar screenings are performed on all applicants (Choi et al. 2006). Most large corporations' human resources departments are keenly aware of the Americans with Disabilities Act.

If the patient has determined that he or she is incapable of returning to work, filing for disability may be necessary. Many employers offer short-term and long-term disability. The physiatrist is often involved in filling out forms necessary for maintaining the disability coverage.

Conclusion

Cancer survivors have endured the emotional, psychological, and physical gauntlet of cancer and its treatment and are ready to move on. Oncology helps save their life; physical medicine and rehabilitation helps them to live it.

Key Practice Points

- Because cancer survivorship is increasing, cancer rehabilitation is playing an increasingly greater role in the field of physiatry. Physiatrists must take into account the patient's prognosis, ongoing treatments, functional level, and discharge disposition.
- Deconditioning, fatigue, and asthenia are among the most common diagnoses encountered by cancer physiatrists.
- The treatment of lymphedema is important to prevent its progression and reduce limb volume, which makes function easier.
- Bowel incontinence is a significant problem in patients with central nervous system disease. A bowel program can help prevent unplanned bowel accidents.
- Returning to employment is important for patients for income, health insurance, and personal identity. Cancer survivors are more likely to be unemployed than the general population. The Americans with Disabilities Act ensures that employers make reasonable accommodations for their employees without undue hardship on the employer.

Suggested Readings

American Academy of Physical Medicine and Rehabilitation. What is a physiatrist? http://www.aapmr.org/patients/aboutpmr/pages/physiatrist.aspx. Published 2011. Accessed October 31, 2013.
Andrews M. Insured but not covered. *US News & World Report* 2007;143(10):65–66.

Caraceni A. Evaluation and assessment of cancer pain and cancer pain treatment. *Acta Anaesthesiol Scand* 2001;45(9):1067–1075.

Carlsen K, Dalton SO, Diderichsen F, Johansen C. Risk for unemployment of cancer survivors: a Danish cohort study. *Eur J Cancer* 2008;44(13):1866–1874.

Choi H, Sugar R, Fish D, Shatzer M, Krabak B. *Physical Medicine & Rehabilitation Pocketpedia*. Philadelphia: Lippincott Williams & Wilkins, 2006.

Courneya KS, Friedenreich CM. Framework PEACE: an organizational model for examining physical exercise across the cancer experience. *Ann Behav Med* 2001;23(4):263–272.

de Boer AGE, Taskila T, Ojajarvi A, van Dijk FJ, Verbeek JH. Cancer survivors and unemployment: a meta-analysis and meta-regression. *JAMA* 2009;301(7):753–762.

Dietz JH Jr. Adaptive rehabilitation of the cancer patient. *Curr Probl Cancer* 1980;5(5):1–56.

Fu J, Shin K. Rehabilitation. In: *The M.D. Anderson Manual of Medical Oncology*. 2nd ed. New York: McGraw Hill, 2011:1351–1365.

Greenberg PE, Leong SA, Birnbaum HG, Robinson RL. The economic burden of depression with painful symptoms. *J Clin Psychiatry* 2003;64(Suppl 7):17–23.

Irwin ML, Alvarez-Reeves M, Cadmus L, et al. Exercise improves body fat, lean mass, and bone mass in breast cancer survivors. *Obesity (Silver Spring)* 2009;17(8):1534–1541.

Kevorkian C. The history of cancer rehabilitation. In: Stubblefield M, O'Dell M, eds. *Cancer Rehabilitation: Principles and Practice*. New York: Demos Medical Publishing, 2009.

Kim DS, Sim Y-J, Jeong HJ, Kim GC. Effect of active resistive exercise on breast cancer-related lymphedema: a randomized controlled trial. *Arch Phys Med Rehabil* 2010;91(12):1844–1848.

Mourtzakis M, Bedbrook M. Muscle atrophy in cancer: a role for nutrition and exercise. *Appl Physiol Nutr Metab* 2009;34(5):950–956.

Nelson JE, Meier DE, Oei EJ, et al. Self-reported symptom experience of critically ill cancer patients receiving intensive care. *Crit Care Med* 2001;29(2):277–282.

Portela MA, Rubiales AS, Centeno C. The use of psychostimulants in cancer patients. *Curr Opin Support Palliat Care* 2011;5(2):164–168.

Roelen CAM, Koopmans PC, Schellart AJM, van der Beek AJ. Resuming work after cancer: a prospective study of occupational register data. *J Occup Rehabil* 2011;21(3):431–440.

Spelten ER, Verbeek JH, Uitterhoeve AL, et al. Cancer, fatigue and the return of patients to work—a prospective cohort study. *Eur J Cancer* 2003;39(11):1562–1567.

Strax T, Grabois M, Gonzalez P, Escaldi S, Cuccurullo S. Physical modalities, therapeutic exercise, extended bedrest, and aging effects. In: Cuccurullo S, ed. *Physical Medicine & Rehabilitation Board Review*. New York: Demos Medical Publishing, 2004:553–570.

Syse A, Tretli S, Kravdal O. Cancer's impact on employment and earnings—a population-based study from Norway. *J Cancer Surviv* 2008;2(3):149–158.

Taskila-Abrandt T, Pukkala E, Martikainen R, Karjalainen A, Hietanen P. Employment status of Finnish cancer patients in 1997. *Psychooncology* 2005;14(3):221–226.

Verbeek JH. How can doctors help their patients to return to work? *PLoS Med* 2006;3(3):e88.

Winningham ML, Nail LM, Burke MB, et al. Fatigue and the cancer experience: the state of the knowledge. *Oncol Nurs Forum* 1994;21(1):23–36.

Zeng L, Koo K, Zhang L, et al. Fatigue in advanced cancer patients attending an outpatient palliative radiotherapy clinic as screened by the Edmonton Symptom Assessment System. *Support Care Cancer* 2012;20(5):1037–1042.

Chapter 25
Sexuality

Leslie R. Schover

Contents

Chapter Overview Sexual dysfunction in men and women after treatment for cancer is one of the most common problems of survivorship, yet most survivors experiencing sexual dysfunction do not receive medical help. Left untreated, sexual dysfunction does not resolve, but instead persists over many years. Not all survivors are distressed about sexual dysfunction. Factors associated with distress include young age, being in a relationship, and having enjoyed sexuality before the cancer diagnosis. The most common problem for which men seek help is erectile dysfunction, although loss of desire for sex, difficulty reaching orgasm, and pain during sexual activity also occur after a number of treatments. Pelvic surgery and radiation are common causes of erectile dysfunction, but hypogonadism also sometimes occurs in survivors of intensive chemotherapy. In women, chemotherapy-induced ovarian failure is a major risk factor for vaginal dryness, dyspareunia, and consequent loss of interest in sex. Pelvic radiation therapy, surgery that changes vaginal or vulvar anatomy, or vaginal complications of graft-versus-host disease are also problematic. Oncology clinics should provide basic education, counseling, and

L.E. Foxhall, M.A. Rodriguez (eds.), *Advances in Cancer Survivorship Management*,
MD Anderson Cancer Care Series, DOI 10.1007/978-1-4939-0986-5_25,
© The University of Texas M.D. Anderson Cancer Center 2015

referrals. The optimal treatment for sexual dysfunction is multidisciplinary, with a medical specialist and a mental health professional working together to assess the problem and create a treatment plan.

How Many Cancer Survivors Have Sexual Problems?

A recent report by the Centers for Disease Control and Prevention noted that 69% of the estimated 14 million cancer survivors currently living in the United States have had prostate, breast, gynecologic, urinary tract, or colorectal malignancies (Rowland et al. 2011). A number of studies have suggested that at least half of survivors of these pelvic cancers end up with long-term sexual dysfunction that does not resolve without medical or psychological treatment (Sadovsky et al. 2010). Furthermore, these sexual problems tend to be severe, affecting desire, ability to become aroused, and ability to reach orgasm. Pain with sex is a major problem, particularly for women. A recent survey by the Livestrong Foundation of more than 2,300 cancer survivors who were younger than 55 years at diagnosis confirmed that 46% experienced sexual problems in the first few years after their treatment, and less than a quarter of this group sought professional help (Rechis and Boerner 2010). Survivors ranked sexual problems third among their concerns about physical health, behind energy and concentration.

At MD Anderson, a survey was used to estimate how many outpatients wanted help for sexual problems (Huyghe et al. 2009b). Respondents included 129 men and 124 women who either received the questionnaire in the mail or picked it up during a clinic visit. Although this survey had only a 29% return rate, the results were quite similar to those in reports from the literature. Most respondents had breast or prostate cancer. Eighty percent of men reported that they had been sexually active at diagnosis, but only 60% were active when completing the questionnaire. Among women, 73% were sexually active at diagnosis compared with 59% when completing the questionnaire. About half of men attributed a new problem with erectile function to their cancer treatment, and 30% said it was hard to reach an orgasm or their sensation of pleasure was weak. Forty-six percent of women developed a problem with vaginal dryness after cancer or treatment, and 45% experienced a loss of desire for sex. Given the conventional wisdom that negative changes to "body image" are a major factor in sexual problems in cancer survivors, it was interesting that only 18% of men and 16% of women believed that a partner would not find them attractive. Physiologic changes in ability to enjoy sex were much more common.

Respondents were also asked how likely they would be to make an appointment in the next year in a clinic that treated cancer-related sexual problems. Twenty-four percent of men and 21% of women said they would definitely make an appointment. In a phone survey of almost 1,500 Americans aged 40–80 years (not selected for health status), a very similar percentage of men and women reported seeking help for their sexual problem (Laumann et al. 2009).

Obviously, not all men and women with cancer are distressed about having a sexual problem. Risk factors for distress in both men and women include young age, having a sexual partner, and being in a relatively new relationship. For men, having a much younger partner often prompts them to seek help (Schover et al. 2002).

Types of Cancer-Related Sexual Problems

Despite the very large variety of cancer sites and treatments, most sexual problems among male and female cancer survivors fall into a few categories (Sadovsky et al. 2010). Typical complaints for women are loss of desire for sex and vaginal dryness that causes pain with sexual touching or intercourse. If a woman is not in the mood for sex and experiences pain with caressing, she is of course also unlikely to experience strong sexual pleasure or to reach an orgasm, but these tend to be secondary issues (Carter et al. 2011).

For men, difficulty getting or maintaining firm erections is the most common problem leading them to seek help. Some men lose interest in sex despite having normal erections, but more often, repeated erectile dysfunction leads to emotional distress and avoidance of sexual activity. Most men can still experience the sensation of orgasm, even without a firm erection, but many men stop sexual stimulation if an erection does not result, and thus no longer have orgasms either. Cancer treatment may also interfere with ejaculation of semen and with the subjective quality of orgasm, although either one may be impaired while the other remains intact. Most men who have dry orgasms report that the sensation is still satisfying and intense, but at least a third complain that their pleasure is weaker, and a few report that orgasms are more prolonged and pleasurable than normal (Barnas et al. 2004).

Although pain during sex is less common in male than in female cancer survivors, about 10% of male cancer survivors also notice pain after radical pelvic surgery, either upon getting an erection or at the moment of orgasm. Such problems are particularly common after surgery or radiation therapy for prostate cancer, although these symptoms tend to improve over time (Barnas et al. 2004; Huyghe et al. 2009a). Pain with erection is sometimes associated with inflammation and eventual fibrosis and plaque formation in the tunica albuginea, leading to penile curvature (Peyronie disease). Penile curvature has recently been noted to be more common than usual after radical prostatectomy (Tal et al. 2010).

How Cancer Treatment Interferes with Sexual Function

Physiologically, normal sexual function in men and women requires intact pathways in the brain and spinal cord, normally functioning autonomic nerves in the pelvis, and reasonably healthy cardiovascular systems in the genital area, as well as normal levels of the hormones involved in sexual desire and arousability. Cancer treatment may damage one or more of these systems.

Central Nervous System Malignancies

Little is known about the direct effects of tumors in the central nervous system on sexual function. The limited survival time for many patients with brain tumors is one barrier. Researchers have not attempted to correlate brain tumor location with specific sexual problems. Areas of the brain and neurotransmitters involved in sexual desire and arousal have only recently been identified (Pfaus 2009). However, changes in personality or motivation can also cause indirect damage to a couple's sex life. The caretaking partner may lose interest in sex if the person with a brain tumor develops dementia or is chronically angry and depressed. Patients with brain tumors often have decreased sexual desire, but hypersexuality also occasionally occurs. Tumors affecting the spine, either as a primary site (e.g., Ewing sarcoma) or as a metastatic site (as in leptomeningeal disease), can interrupt erotic sensation and orgasm or disrupt the reflexive increase in genital blood flow during sexual arousal.

Hematopoietic Cancer

For men and women treated for hematopoietic cancer, the stronger the intensity of the chemotherapy regimen, the more likely that sexual function will be damaged (Yi and Syrjala 2009). For women, alkylating chemotherapy drugs and combination chemotherapy administered at high doses (e.g., in preparation for stem cell or bone marrow transplantation) can cause permanent, premature ovarian failure. Menopausal symptoms are usually more severe after these abrupt hormonal changes than after natural menopause. Cancer survivors with ovarian failure often have severe hot flashes that disturb their sleep, adding to chronic fatigue and problems with concentration.

However, vaginal atrophy is most destructive to sexual function in women (Carter et al. 2011). Normally during female sexual arousal, the vagina deepens considerably and the upper vagina "balloons," rising from the pelvic floor. As blood flow increases dramatically in the clitoris, vulvar tissues, and vaginal walls, a slippery transudate appears as droplets of fluid on the vaginal mucosa, preparing the vagina for sexual intercourse. With estrogen deprivation, the vaginal mucosa and vulvar skin become thin and easily irritated or torn. Genital blood flow is decreased, so that these changes take place more slowly and are attenuated. The woman experiences vaginal dryness and tightness. Attempts at penetration often cause burning pain, with spotting of blood caused by small mucosal tears. The vaginal pH increases, leaving women vulnerable to repeated bacterial or yeast infections. Postcoital urinary tract infections also may become chronic.

If women end up with permanent ovarian failure, systemic hormonal replacement therapy can reverse vaginal atrophy as well as protect bone density and reduce hot flashes. However, the genital symptoms are better controlled with vaginal estrogen, whether in the form of a cream, suppository, or vaginal ring (Suckling et al. 2006). Low-dose rings and suppositories can treat vaginal atrophy without elevating serum estrogen above the usual postmenopausal levels.

Women who develop graft-versus-host disease (GVHD) after an allogeneic hematopoietic transplantation are at risk of developing vaginal symptoms (Stratton et al. 2007). The granulocyte colony-stimulating factors used in stem cell rescue appear to elevate genital GVHD rates even more than bone marrow transplantation, affecting at least 25% of women with systemic GVHD. Women should be warned to watch for early signs of genital GVHD, which include pain and redness on the vulva, similar to symptoms of vulvar vestibulitis. If untreated, genital GVHD can lead to vaginal adhesions and stenosis, making intercourse very painful or even impossible. Most centers treat women with a combination of medication for the systemic GVHD and topical ointments for the genital area that combine estrogen with a strong corticosteroid or other immunosuppressant medication. Adhesions can often be gently stretched and eventually eliminated by frequent use of vaginal dilators.

Intensive chemotherapy is not as destructive to male sexual function but can sometimes damage the Leydig cells in the testicles, leading to a hypogonadal state (Yi and Syrjala 2009). If a man experiences decreased desire for sex, often accompanied by difficulties with erection, hot flashes at night, and severe fatigue, it is important to check serum testosterone levels. Testosterone replacement restores sexual function for most men. Injections often produce high initial hormone tests but cannot maintain normal levels even when given every 2 weeks. Patches or gels can provide a more stable level of testosterone.

It is unclear whether genital GVHD in men contributes to the high rates of male sexual problems that occur after hematopoietic transplantation, but chronic skin irritation on the glans of the penis can make sexual stimulation painful in some survivors. Topical creams similar to those used in women (but without the estrogen) may be used to treat these problems in men.

Breast Cancer

Chemotherapy is the treatment most likely to cause sexual dysfunction in women treated for breast cancer (Schover 2008a). Early research was focused on the psychological impact of breast loss, but now that most women can choose either breast reconstruction or conservation, the type of localized treatment with surgery and radiation is not correlated with sexual outcomes. Women treated with tamoxifen or raloxifene notice few changes in sexual desire or vaginal dryness. Some problems attributed to tamoxifen in women diagnosed with breast cancer before menopause actually are related to ovarian failure caused by the chemotherapy preceding treatment with tamoxifen. A number of young women experience temporary ovarian failure during and after adjuvant chemotherapy for breast cancer. It is unclear whether their levels of sexual function return to normal if their menstrual cycles return.

With the advent of aromatase inhibitors as the treatment of choice for postmenopausal women with hormone-sensitive breast cancer, rates of sexual problems have increased greatly (Baumgart et al. 2011). Aromatase inhibitors prevent estrogen from being produced in peripheral tissue, further reducing the estrogen available in the genital area, even in women who already had mild vaginal atrophy. Vaginal dryness and pain with sex are problems for as many as two-thirds of women treated with aromatase inhibitors. However, even a low-dose vaginal estrogen therapy may elevate serum estrogen levels enough to interfere with the beneficial effects of aromatase inhibitors in some women, making breast oncologists very reluctant to prescribe hormonal therapies.

Pelvic Radiation Therapy

In both men and women, radiation to the pelvic area causes high rates of sexual dysfunction. The timing of these changes is important in designing follow-up research, which often does not assess patients for a long enough period to detect the damage. At the end of treatment, acute genital pain can be a problem. Sexual function may then seem to normalize, only to get worse again beginning several months after the end of radiation therapy (Sadovsky et al. 2010). Sexual function may worsen for at least 3–5 years after completion of treatment. Inflammation in the target zones leads to a gradual process of fibrosis that can reduce blood flow in the genital area.

In premenopausal women, pelvic radiation therapy in the doses used to treat localized, invasive cervical or anal cancer, or included as part of treatment for Hodgkin lymphoma, usually damages the ovaries enough to cause permanent ovarian failure, leading to all of the symptoms of vaginal atrophy and hot flashes described above. In addition, women are at risk to have the vagina agglutinate and close off if they do not have intercourse or use a vaginal dilator during the healing period. Some women also struggle with painful radiation ulcers that take a long time to heal. Vaginal stenosis—a narrowing of the canal in one area—can limit penetrative sex and may need correction with dilation under anesthesia or with vaginal reconstructive surgery.

In men, erectile dysfunction is the most common problem caused by pelvic radiation therapy. Radiation for prostate cancer is the most typical example (van der Wielen et al. 2007), but preoperative radiation therapy worsens rates of erectile dysfunction in men who have colorectal cancer as well. Many attempts have been made to decrease the impact of radiation for prostate cancer on erectile function, including use of brachytherapy, intensity-modulated radiation therapy, and proton or photon beams. Although using computers and imaging to target the prostate while sparing the surrounding tissues has reduced the rate of erectile dysfunction somewhat, longer-term follow-up studies have been disappointing (van der Wielen et al. 2007). Some men choose definitive radiation therapy in an attempt to avoid a radical cystectomy for bladder cancer, but the sexual and urinary morbidity can be considerable. Recent protocols using chemoradiation are more promising (Sandler and Mirhadi 2010).

Radiation targeting the prostate also usually reduces semen volume sharply, sometimes to the point of a totally dry orgasm. If men are not told to expect such changes, the changes may cause a great deal of anxiety. Pain with orgasm is also common after brachytherapy for prostate cancer (Huyghe et al. 2009a).

Radical Pelvic Surgery and Male Sexual Dysfunction

For men, radical surgery to treat prostate, bladder, or colorectal cancer remains a major cause of sexual dysfunction. Because the autonomic nerves that direct blood flow into the penis during sexual arousal are located between the prostate and rectum, coursing along the left and right sides of the prostate and then along the urethra, surgery in this central area often damages the neurologic system needed for a healthy erection (Sadovsky et al. 2010). Although nerve-sparing techniques were introduced in the 1980s, the number of men who regain reliable and firm erections, even after a bilateral nerve-sparing procedure, is far lower than suggested in early studies (Schover et al. 2002; Tal et al. 2009). Much of the recovery takes place in the first 12 months after surgery, but some men continue to experience improvement in their erections after 2 or even 3 years. Men most likely to recover erections are those who had firm erections before surgery, those younger than 60 years, and those who underwent a bilateral nerve-sparing procedure (Tal et al. 2009). Loss of penile blood flow also contributes to erection problems. Although the main penile arteries are spared, the surgeon may tie off small, accessory arteries. After radical prostatectomy, most men have some fibrosis of the spongy tissue in the cavernous bodies of the penis, resulting in loss of length and thickness of erections (Gontero et al. 2007). In addition to no longer ejaculating semen, many men leak urine during orgasm after radical prostatectomy, which can be emotionally upsetting for them and their partners (Choi et al. 2007).

Sparing the prostatic nerves is even more difficult with radical cystectomy. Often a bilateral nerve-sparing procedure with adequate margins is not possible (Sadovsky et al. 2010). Erectile dysfunction remains common after surgery for rectal cancer, even with improved surgical techniques, such as total mesorectal excision. Men who undergo abdominoperineal resection or adjuvant preoperative radiation therapy have the poorest sexual outcomes.

Surgeries That Interfere with Ejaculation of Semen

Radical prostatectomy and cystectomy include removal of the prostate and seminal vesicles so that semen manufacture no longer occurs. Emotional reactions to the loss of ejaculation, as well as the impact of loss of ejaculation on pleasurable sensations with orgasm, vary quite a bit (Barnas et al. 2004; Schover et al. 2002). Men with testicular cancer who have surgery to remove lymph nodes in the retroperitoneum or men who have surgery to remove sigmoid colon cancer sometimes have dry orgasm because of sympathetic nerve damage that prevents the prostate and seminal vesicles from contracting and releasing seminal fluid during emission, the first stage of male orgasm (Sadovsky et al. 2010). Although techniques to spare nerves near the aorta have been shown to reduce orgasmic dysfunction after retroperitoneal node dissection, nerve-sparing procedures are not always possible when surgery is performed after chemotherapy to remove residual disease (Winter et al. 2009), a common scenario in recent years. Less severe nerve damage can result in retrograde ejaculation, in which semen spurts backwards into the bladder because the bladder neck does not close completely during orgasm. In either case, men experience a "dry orgasm" with pleasurable sensation but no semen.

Radical Pelvic Surgery and Female Sexual Dysfunction

Radical pelvic surgery in women, in contrast with men, often leaves sexual function relatively intact. Although premenopausal women who undergo bilateral oophorectomy experience hormonal effects (Schover 2008a), women report normal sensation and ability to reach orgasm after radical hysterectomy (Frumovitz et al. 2005). Autonomic nerve-sparing surgical techniques have been described, but their major impact may be in preserving bladder function rather than sexual function. The main function of autonomic nerves in women is to direct blood flow to the genital area during sexual arousal. Even with reduced blood flow, women can often compensate for the reduction in vaginal expansion and lubrication by using moisturizers, lubricants, and extra sexual stimulation. The sensory nerves that mediate female orgasm are located close to the pelvic sidewalls, protected under fascia. They are unlikely to be damaged in pelvic cancer surgeries.

Radical cystectomy in women has traditionally included removing the entire anterior vaginal wall. Recent modifications that preserve this tissue are associated with reduced sexual dysfunction (Sadovsky et al. 2010). Female sexuality after rectal cancer surgery has been difficult to study because of poor response rates in elderly women and small sample sizes (Sadovsky et al. 2010), but it appears that problems with pain during sex and loss of desire are prevalent, even in women who do not undergo adjuvant chemoradiation or a change in their hormonal status from oophorectomy. As in men, abdominoperineal resection appears to have the most severe sexual side effects.

Facilitating Sexual Rehabilitation

Barriers to resolving sexual problems in patients with cancer include the lack of practice guidelines to encourage oncology professionals to bring up the topic of sexual problems, decreased time with patients in busy clinics, and discomfort in discussing this very personal topic. Yet, for many men and women, some practical suggestions and brief medical interventions can make the difference in staying sexually active (Schover 2008b). In site-specific clinics or private practice oncology offices, an allied health care professional (e.g., an oncology nurse or social worker) can be trained in basic knowledge of cancer-related sexual problems and counseling strategies. Workshops on sexual function and cancer are often provided at annual meetings of oncology nurses, social workers, or psychosocial professionals. When a new patient is going to receive a treatment that carries a risk of sexual dysfunction, that member of the team can provide education about what to expect, as well as hope of recovery of sexual pleasure and intimacy. If a patient is in a committed relationship, it helps to include the partner in this discussion. Otherwise, the patient is left at a difficult time to disclose complex and upsetting news that could disrupt their relationship.

At follow-up visits, the same professional can assess a range of quality-of-life issues, including sexual function, concerns about fertility, return to work, and emotional distress. If a sexual problem occurs, information about self-help strategies as well as referrals for appropriate medical care should be provided.

The sexuality specialist should keep a "library" of patient education materials such as books, pamphlets, or videos, as well as a list of web sites providing reliable and accurate information. A referral network of local specialists should be available, including a urologist comfortable with providing a range of treatments for erectile dysfunction as well as for problems with desire and orgasm; a gynecologist with the patience and expertise to help women with dyspareunia and menopausal symptoms; an endocrinologist who can assess and treat hormonal abnormalities; and mental health professionals with training in cognitive-behavioral sex therapy (and hopefully also experience with oncology patients). Outside of urban areas or large cancer centers, the oncology team may need to actually train some local practitioners to enhance the quality of care available. A research team at MD Anderson is currently creating and testing computerized, multimedia educational and counseling tools on sexuality and cancer for men and women (Schover et al. 2013). These tools may soon be available to the general public. Each intervention includes a "therapist manual" for medical and mental health professionals who can help patients use the educational information and cognitive-behavioral exercises more effectively.

Issues in Male Sexual Rehabilitation

Despite the impressive array of medical and surgical treatments for erectile dysfunction, most male cancer survivors do not find a satisfactory solution (Schover 2008b). Phosphodiesterase-5-inhibitors such as sildenafil, vardenafil, or tadalafil are not powerful enough to produce firm and reliable erections in men who have severe problems after pelvic surgery or radiation therapy. Men are given high expectations of these drugs both by commercial advertisements and often by their physician, and when the results are disappointing, patients may blame themselves or feel ashamed to reveal the drugs' failure to the prescribing physician. Many fewer men are motivated to try more invasive treatments, such as a vacuum erection device, penile injections, or surgery to implant an inflatable penile prosthesis. Dropout rates from pumps and injections are very high, particularly if the man is single or has a partner who has lost interest in sexual activity.

Sexual satisfaction in both partners in a couple, as well as adherence to an effective treatment for erectile dysfunction, can be boosted significantly by just a few sessions of sex therapy, delivered in person or over the internet (Schover et al. 2012). Treatment focuses on the partners making a joint decision about the treatment for erectile dysfunction that they want to try, ensuring that sexual communication skills are good and that the couple focuses on sharing sexual pleasure and intimacy rather than on sexual performance.

Men who are single often believe that they should not attempt to date if they have erectile dysfunction. Reassurance about the shortage of unattached men compared with women older than 40 years can be helpful, because most men are in that age group. In addition, suggestions about how to meet new partners through hobbies, mutual friends, or dating organizations can be helpful.

Issues in Female Sexual Rehabilitation

For women who have vaginal dryness and pain, a simple treatment algorithm can often help resolve the problems (Carter et al. 2011). Ideally, a gynecologist and a sex therapist can consult together, providing both a pelvic examination and instructions for behavioral change. The first step is to advise the woman to use a vaginal moisturizer two to three times per week at bedtime. Products on the market include polycarbophil gels or gels containing a mild solution of hyaluronic acid. These moisturizers hydrate the vaginal mucosa. Another type of moisturizer is a prebiotic that restores a premenopausal pH to the vagina and creates an environment in which lactobacilli can grow. In addition, women are counseled to use either a water- or silicone-based lubricant during sexual activity. Lubricants should not contain perfumes, flavors, parabens, or glycerine and should help maintain a low pH in the vagina. Both partners should spread the lubricant on their genital area before trying penetrative sex. It is best to keep the lubricant nearby during sex in case more needs to be applied.

If the woman has become anxious or avoidant of sex because of repeated experiences of painful sex, it is also helpful to teach her to be aware of pelvic floor muscle tension. Women can learn to control the muscles around the vaginal entrance by practicing Kegel squeezes. The goal is to be able to keep the muscles relaxed during vaginal penetration. Performing Kegel exercises while inserting vaginal dilators of graduated size can be helpful to women with more severe muscle tension problems. In some health care settings, a physical therapist who works with pelvic pain may conduct similar training using biofeedback equipment.

If dyspareunia persists despite all of these interventions, women may want to consider using a low-dose vaginal estrogen, particularly if they have not had a hormone-sensitive type of cancer. Women prefer rings or suppositories to creams, but creams may be helpful if the vulvar skin is dry and sensitive because the estrogen from other types of products may not reach that part of the genitals.

Loss of desire for sex in female cancer survivors is often multifactorial. Each contributing factor should be identified and treated either medically or with psychosocial care. These factors include fear that sex will hurt; feeling unattractive because of the impact of cancer treatment on appearance; depressed mood; use of psychotropic medications such as antidepressants, anxiolytics, and opiate pain medications that can blunt sexual desire; chronic fatigue in the months after cancer treatment; chronic tensions between partners; or difficulty getting into the mood for sex because of distraction from fear of cancer recurrence. In some subcultures or communities, women may be rejected by a partner because cancer is stigmatizing. In these situations, the counsel of a community opinion leader or religious figure may be helpful.

Key Practice Points

- Sexual dysfunction is very common and persistent after treatment for cancer.
- Most sexual dysfunction after treatment is caused, at least in part, by neurologic, vascular, or hormonal damage to the reproductive system.
- Although erectile dysfunction is the most common problem in men, loss of desire for sex, difficulty with orgasm, and pain during sex are also important problems.
- In women, abrupt ovarian failure can lead to vaginal dryness, pain with sexual activity, and, consequently, loss of desire. Sexual dysfunction may be exacerbated by damage to the vulvar or vaginal anatomy after pelvic surgery or radiation therapy, or by complications from genital GVHD.
- An oncology clinic should train an allied health care professional to assess sexual problems and provide education and brief counseling.
- Optimal assessment and treatment of sexual dysfunction after cancer is multidisciplinary, with a medical specialist collaborating with a mental health professional.
- Couples may need counseling to integrate a medical treatment into their sex lives and to resume sex comfortably after a period of illness-related abstinence.

Suggested Readings

Barnas JL, Pierpaoli S, Ladd P, et al. The prevalence and nature of orgasmic dysfunction after radical prostatectomy. *BJU Int* 2004;94:603–605.
Baumgart J, Nilsson K, Stavreus-Evers A, et al. Urogenital disorders in women with adjuvant endocrine therapy after early breast cancer. *Am J Obstet Gynecol* 2011;204:e1–e7.
Bhatt A, Nandipati K, Dhar N, et al. Neurovascular preservation in orthotopic cystectomy: impact on female sexual function. *Urology* 2006;67:742–745.

Carter J, Goldfrank D, Schover LR. Simple strategies for vaginal health promotion in cancer survivors. *J Sex Med* 2011;8:549–559.

Choi JM, Nelson CJ, Stasi J, Mulhall JP. Orgasm associated incontinence (climacturia) following radical pelvic surgery: rates of occurrence and predictors. *J Urol* 2007;177:2223–2226.

Frumovitz M, Sun CC, Schover LR, et al. Quality of life and sexual functioning in cervical cancer survivors. *J Clin Oncol* 2005;23:7428–7436.

Gontero P, Galzerano M, Bartoletti R, et al. New insights into the pathogenesis of penile shortening after radical prostatectomy and the role of postoperative sexual function. *J Urol* 2007;178: 602–607.

Huyghe E, Delannes M, Wagner F, et al. Ejaculatory function after permanent ^{125}I prostate brachytherapy for localized prostate cancer. *Int J Radiat Oncol Biol Phys* 2009a;74:126–132.

Huyghe E, Sui D, Odensky E, Schover LR. Needs assessment survey to justify establishing a reproductive health clinic at a comprehensive cancer center. *J Sex Med* 2009b;6:149–163.

Laumann EO, Glasser DB, Neves RC, Moreira ED Jr; GSSAB Investigators' Group. A population-based survey of sexual activity, sexual problems and associated help-seeking behavior patterns in mature adults in the United States of America. *Int J Impot Res* 2009;21:171–178.

Müller A, Parker M, Waters BW, Flanigan RC, Mulhall JP. Penile rehabilitation following radical prostatectomy: predicting success. *J Sex Med* 2009;6:2806–2812.

Pfaus JG. Pathways of sexual desire. *J Sex Med* 2009;6:1506–1533.

Rechis R, Boerner L. How cancer has affected post-treatment survivors: a Livestrong report, June 2010. http://www.livestrong.org/What-We-Do/Our-Approach/Reports-Findings/LIVESTRONG-Survey-Report. Accessed November 5, 2013.

Rowland JH, Mariotto A, Alfano CM, Pollack LA, Weir HK, White A. Cancer Survivors—United States, 2007. *MMWR* 2011;60:269–272.

Sadovsky R, Basson R, Krychman M, et al. Cancer and sexual problems *J Sex Med* 2010;7: 349–373.

Sandler HM, Mirhadi AJ. Current status of radiation therapy for bladder cancer. *Expert Rev Anticancer Ther* 2010;10:895–901.

Schover LR. Premature ovarian failure and its consequences: vasomotor symptoms, sexuality, and fertility. *J Clin Oncol* 2008a;26:753–758.

Schover LR. Reduction of psychosexual dysfunction in cancer patients. In: Miller SM, Bowen DJ, Croyle RT, Rowland, JH, eds. *Handbook of Cancer Control and Behavioral Science.* Washington, DC: American Psychological Association Press; 2008b:379–390.

Schover LR, Canada AL, Yuan Y, et al. A randomized trial of internet-based versus traditional sexual counseling for couples after localized prostate cancer treatment. *Cancer* 2012;118: 500–509.

Schover LR, Fouladi RT, Warnecke CL, et al. Defining sexual outcomes after treatment for localized prostate carcinoma. *Cancer* 2002;95:1773–1785.

Schover LR, Ying Y, Fellman BM, Odensky E, Lewis PE, Martinetti P. Efficacy trial of an internet-based intervention for cancer-related female sexual dysfunction. *J Natl Comp Cancer Network* 2013;in press.

Stratton P, Turner ML, Childs R, et al. Vulvovaginal chronic graft-versus-host disease with allogeneic hematopoietic stem cell transplantation. *Obstet Gynecol* 2007;110:1041–1049.

Suckling J, Lethaby A, Kennedy R. Local oestrogen for vaginal atrophy in postmenopausal women. *Cochrane Database Syst Rev* 2006;4:CD001500.

Tal R, Alphs HH, Krebs P, Nelson CJ, Mulhall JP. Erectile function recovery rate after radical prostatectomy: a meta-analysis. *J Sex Med* 2009;6:2538–2546.

Tal R, Heck M, Teloken P, Siegrist T, Nelson CJ, Mulhall JP. Peyronie's disease following radical prostatectomy: incidence and predictors. *J Sex Med* 2010;7:1254–1261.

van der Wielen GJ, Mulhall JP, Incrocci L. Erectile dysfunction after radiotherapy for prostate cancer and radiation dose to the penile structures: a critical review. *Radiother Oncol* 2007;84: 107–113.

Winter C, Raman JD, Sheinfeld J, Albers P. Retroperitoneal lymph node dissection after chemotherapy. *BJU Int* 2009;104:1404–1412.

Yi JC, Syrjala KL. Sexuality after hematopoietic stem cell transplantation. *Cancer J* 2009;15: 57–64.

Part V
Other Crosscutting Issues

Chapter 26
Legal Issues

Laurel R. Hyle

Contents

Chapter Overview This chapter explores a number of important legal issues that cancer survivors may encounter. Issues explored include health and other insurance coverage; labor law issues, including the Americans with Disabilities Act; travel and leisure; financial estate and advance care planning, including different types of advance directives commonly used in the health care setting; and genetic testing, research study participation, and intellectual property. This chapter is intended to provide a brief, cursory overview and is not an in-depth or exhaustive analysis. Following review of this chapter, the reader will hopefully be better informed regarding certain general concerns that may arise in the legal arena related to cancer survivorship.

Introduction

Cancer survivors may encounter a number of legal issues. These issues might be initially encountered early in the cancer experience or might appear only during the survivorship phase. This chapter attempts to provide insight into an array of legal

L.E. Foxhall, M.A. Rodriguez (eds.), *Advances in Cancer Survivorship Management*,
MD Anderson Cancer Care Series, DOI 10.1007/978-1-4939-0986-5_26,
© The University of Texas M.D. Anderson Cancer Center 2015

issues that cancer survivors may encounter, but it must be emphasized that nothing in this chapter is legal advice; any legal questions or concerns should be addressed with a competent professional legal advisor.

Insurance Issues

One of the foremost concerns experienced by cancer patients and cancer survivors is access to comprehensive, affordable health insurance. Health insurance can be difficult to find and cost-prohibitive for cancer survivors. Health insurance "risk pools" have been established to deal with this issue, and although these risk pools appear to increase access to insurance for certain individuals, they do not necessarily always address other, related issues, such as lifetime or yearly benefit caps, the high cost of co-pays and deductibles, or lack of coverage for certain services. The Patient Protection and Affordable Care Act may help ameliorate this situation because the new law seeks to define the minimum coverage required by insurance plans, eliminate certain caps on coverage, abolish the exclusion of coverage for preexisting conditions, provide subsidies to help make insurance coverage more affordable, and set up health insurance exchanges intended to increase access and reduce costs. However, gaining access to appropriate health care services through an affordable health insurance plan continues to be one of the primary issues of concern for cancer survivors.

Additionally, cancer survivors may encounter issues with other types of insurance products. For instance, life insurance policies may have increased premiums, short- and long-term disability policies may be more difficult or more expensive to obtain, and specialized health insurance policies, such as for vision or dental care, may also be more difficult to obtain or more costly.

Employment Issues

Cancer survivors may also encounter a variety of employment-related issues. Survivors often have concerns related to access to group insurance benefits that may restrict their employment options. Additionally, survivors may encounter issues related to posttreatment needs and abilities that may or may not fall within the purview of the Americans with Disabilities Act (ADA). For instance, survivors may encounter physical or mental limitations after treatment that they did not experience before. These limitations may be related to surgical changes, such as amputation or reconstruction; general physical function, such as how long or how far the individual is comfortable walking or traveling or the need for assistive devices such as a cane, walker, or wheelchair; or a diverse range of mental functioning and neurologic issues, such as anxiety or changes in cognitive function.

Although the ADA requires employers to make reasonable accommodations in certain circumstances, employers may not necessarily be obligated to permit survivors to continue with their former jobs if the survivors' abilities with regard to essential job functions have changed. Employers also are not necessarily obligated to provide additional time for breaks, travel, or medical appointments. ADA law is a specialized area of legal practice and some survivors may need to consult an attorney with expertise in this area to fully understand the legal rights and responsibilities of employers and employees in this context. Also, because the ADA is a federal law, the United States Department of Justice maintains an ADA webpage (http://www.ada.gov) that may be of benefit to survivors with questions regarding this area of the law.

Travel and Leisure Issues

Survivors may encounter changed circumstances related to travel and leisure as well. Some of these circumstances may pertain to transportation and access to health care while traveling, and others may pertain to the signing of waivers and disclaimers associated with certain leisure activities both at home and abroad. Travelers may be asked to sign waivers indicating that they have no preexisting conditions that would increase their risk of injury from participating in certain activities, and cancer survivors may be unsure of how to approach this because the exact parameters for such waivers are often unclear.

As with almost any traveler, cancer survivors should be aware of issues relating to access to care when they travel and they may want to be especially aware of emergency evacuation options and their ability to get back home or to a particular level of care quickly should an emergency or unexpected medical situation occur. Numerous emergency evacuation and international health care plans are available on the market and are well worth exploring.

Financial, Estate, and Advance Care Planning

Advance care planning is an important aspect of health care planning, including and perhaps especially for cancer survivors. Cancer survivors may find themselves with changed perspectives, altered financial circumstances, new or different relationships with loved ones, clearer visions of preferences regarding medical interventions, or a general renewed awareness of the importance of advance care planning. Individuals often mistakenly think of advance care planning as end-of-life planning, when in fact advance care plans can be engaged to assist individuals any time they are unable to communicate their wishes to the health care team; this can happen at any stage of life and may be transient or permanent.

Many advance care planning tools are available to assist patients in communicating their health care choices to their current and future health care providers. Financial and estate plans should be considered and revised as appropriate. A variety of resources are available for setting up and revising such plans, including financial planners; tax, estate, and financial planning attorneys; and numerous online resources of widely varying quality and reliability.

Advance care planning tools can take a variety of forms, especially if they are drafted by competent professional advisors. For example, professionals consulted about advance care planning may draft documents that allow for a greater variety of customization than standardized forms would otherwise allow. However, the advance care planning tools most commonly encountered in a standardized environment are the medical power of attorney and living will. These documents may go by different names in different jurisdictions and can be drafted in a variety of ways, with various effects and consequences. However, in general, a medical power of attorney allows an individual to name someone to serve as a surrogate medical decision-maker should the individual become unable to make his or her own medical decisions or unable to communicate with health care providers. A living will typically allows an individual to comment prospectively on health care interventions that the individual would want or not want in a variety of circumstances. Sometimes elements of the medical power of attorney and living will are combined, either in standardized or customized forms. Although efforts have been made to standardize these and other advance care planning tools across jurisdictional lines, substantial variations remain among countries and states. It is important for individuals to understand the rules of advance care planning in any place(s) where they live and where they are receiving or may plan to receive health care services.

The most important element of advance care planning is communication. Using communication tools appropriate to individual circumstances can help empower an individual to contribute to his or her own health care decision-making prospectively and can help ensure that an individual's wishes are known even if the individual becomes unable to communicate these wishes to loved ones or health care providers. Advance care planning is typically discussed in terms of official legal documentation, but more everyday human communications can also be an important part of effective advance care planning. For instance, it may be quite helpful for loved ones to understand the decisions an individual has made regarding health care, because if the loved ones understand such decisions, they may be better prepared to support them. Toward this end, it may be helpful to write a letter to loved ones explaining the reasons for health care choices and preferences; such a communication can serve multiple purposes, including personalizing what can be, for some, a fairly difficult conversation, and providing a written record of the individual's wishes that others can refer back to in a time of need or concern. Such a letter can become a personalized touchstone that reflects the patient's wishes and can be returned to as often as needed.

Genetic Testing, Research Study Participation, and Intellectual Property

Cancer patients and survivors may experience a variety of circumstances in which very specific legal rules and regulations apply. Three of these areas are highlighted here: genetic testing, research study participation, and intellectual property. These are not the only areas of concern, merely some common ones.

Highly specific laws apply to the areas of genetic testing, research study participation, and intellectual property. Some of these laws pertain to matters of confidentiality and some pertain to the division of legal rights and responsibilities. For instance, research study participants may be asked to surrender all property rights to any research sample that is collected from them as part of a study. And genetic information, including genetic testing results and residual tissue or blood samples, may sometimes be available to a patient's family members, with or without the patient's consent, either while the patient is alive or after death. It is important for individuals providing such information to be aware of the implications of such disclosures, understanding that such material might survive well beyond any individual patient's lifetime, and there is no reliable way to know for certain what future laws or regulations might be enacted or altered with regard to such information.

Because of this, in addition to exploring specific legal questions or concerns they might have about these or other areas of the law with appropriate advisors, survivors should remember that laws can change, sometimes quite quickly. In general, in the law, as in life, there are no guarantees. Thus, to the extent that a survivor is interested in a particular course of action only with, for instance, a guarantee of absolute confidentiality, caution is likely warranted.

Resources

Many resources are available to assist cancer survivors in understanding various concerns they may encounter as part of their journey through cancer. A few of these resources are listed in the Suggested Readings section below. The author is not responsible for maintaining any of these sources of information and cannot ensure their accuracy or helpfulness or make any warranties or representations about these resources, but some individuals might find that these resources provide additional information on topics of interest related to survivorship.

Key Practice Points

- When in doubt, ask.
- Communication is essential.
- Advance care planning is an important patient advocacy tool.
- Expertise is a valuable commodity.
- Knowledge is power.

Suggested Readings

American Bar Association. Public resources. http://www.americanbar.org/portals/public_resources.html. Accessed April 26, 2013.

Centers for Disease Control and Prevention. Cancer prevention and control: cancer survivorship. http://www.cdc.gov/cancer/survivorship/. Updated April 24, 2013. Accessed April 26, 2013.

Cornell University Law School. Legal Information Institute. http://www.law.cornell.edu/. Accessed April 26, 2013.

Library of Congress. Thomas home. http://thomas.loc.gov/home/thomas.php. Accessed April 26, 2013.

MedlinePlus. Advance directives. http://www.nlm.nih.gov/medlineplus/advancedirectives.html. Updated April 11, 2013. Accessed April 26, 2013.

Medline Plus. Consumer rights and responsibilities. http://www.nlm.nih.gov/medlineplus/ency/article/001947.htm. Updated March 22, 2013. Accessed April 26, 2013.

National Cancer Institute. Cancer survivorship research. http://dccps.nci.nih.gov/ocs/. Updated April 22, 2013. Accessed April 26, 2013.

National Cancer Institute. Survivorship—living with and beyond cancer. http://www.cancer.gov/cancertopics/coping/survivorship. Accessed April 26, 2013.

National Institutes of Health. Certificates of confidentiality: background information. http://grants.nih.gov/grants/policy/coc/background.htm. Updated January 20, 2011. Accessed April 26, 2013.

United States Department of Justice. ADA home page. http://www.ada.gov/. Accessed April 26, 2013.

United States Department of State. Tips for traveling abroad. http://travel.state.gov/travel/tips/tips_1232.html. Accessed April 26, 2013.

World Health Organization. Cancer information. http://www.who.int/cancer/en/. Accessed April 26, 2013.

Chapter 27
Communication Between Patients and Health Care Providers

Daniel E. Epner

Contents

Chapter Overview Cancer survivors face many challenges resulting from the side effects of treatment, the effects of the cancer itself, and the many emotions that accompany their illness. Cancer survivors often fear recurrence, suffering, or death and feel sad or angry when bad things happen. Discussing emotional issues with patients is challenging. One reason that emotional conversations are so uncomfortable is that formal communication skills training is underemphasized during medical education and training, which primarily focuses on biomedical issues. Discussing difficult questions or concerns takes health care providers out of the familiar biomedical realm and thrusts them into the less comfortable psychosocial realm. However, these challenging conversations can be turned into opportunities to establish trust and rapport with a few key communication strategies. These strategies include exploring patients' concerns; listening actively; seizing empathic opportunities when emotions arise; engaging in natural, free-flowing conversations; and allowing space (silence) in the conversation. These key strategies can be applied to discussions of a variety of clinical scenarios, including recurrence or fear of recurrence, prognosis, and other difficult conversations.

L.E. Foxhall, M.A. Rodriguez (eds.), *Advances in Cancer Survivorship Management*,
MD Anderson Cancer Care Series, DOI 10.1007/978-1-4939-0986-5_27,
© The University of Texas M.D. Anderson Cancer Center 2015

Introduction

> The pessimist sees difficulty in every opportunity. The optimist sees opportunity in every difficulty. –Winston Churchill

Clinic visits with cancer survivors are often joyful reunions to celebrate life and health, or an opportunity to catch up and share recent photos of family and friends. Such visits are very gratifying for health care providers and patients. Unfortunately, many survivorship visits are not so joyful. Many cancer survivors experience tremendous fear and uncertainty over the prospect of recurrence. For some, this fear is so strong that they no longer enjoy life, sleep well, eat well, or even go to follow-up visits (National Cancer Institute 2010). Worse yet, many cancer survivors actually experience recurrence. Other survivors feel stress from losing the emotional support provided by the cancer treatment team. Many others experience long-term side effects of cancer or its treatment, such as lymphedema, altered cognition ("chemobrain"), or altered body image. Survivorship clinic visits therefore often quickly evolve from joyful reunions to emotional heart-to-heart conversations. What should a provider say, for example, to a patient who cries and says, "I live in constant fear my cancer will come back"? How does a provider tell a patient that her worst fear has been realized: her breast cancer has spread to lungs, liver, and bones? What does the provider say when that patient asks, "How long do I have?"

One reason that conversations such as these are so uncomfortable is that formal communication skills training is underemphasized during medical education, which primarily focuses on biomedical issues. Discussing difficult questions or concerns takes providers out of the familiar biomedical realm and thrusts them into the less comfortable psychosocial realm. Success in this domain requires key communication skills that can be taught and learned. Furthermore, these skills require constant practice. No matter how skilled providers become at handling difficult conversations, such conversations are never easy. Nonetheless, with sound communication skills, providers can view every challenge as an opportunity to build trust and rapport with patients and to support patients' psychosocial needs. This chapter presents a series of clinical vignettes that illustrate difficult conversations that commonly arise as providers care for cancer survivors, as well as strategies for successfully engaging in these difficult conversations.

Addressing Feelings Before Facts

"A weight on my shoulders": fear of recurrent cancer

Mr. S is a 61-year-old man who was diagnosed with T3N1 colon cancer 18 months ago. He underwent hemicolectomy and adjuvant chemotherapy. Surveillance studies remain normal, but he nonetheless fears his cancer will recur. "I have a hard time focusing at work, because it seems like every day someone reminds me about my cancer. They mean well by asking how I am doing, but I wish I could just forget about it. I constantly worry about my cancer coming back. I feel like I have a weight on my shoulders."

Acknowledging Emotions

Many providers try to "fix" patients' fears by offering reassurance in the form of factual statements, such as "your chances of long-term remission are greater than 50%." However, this factual approach can make patients feel that their fears are being trivialized and that they are not being heard. Another common strategy is to be a cheerleader, telling patients to "focus on the positive," or "be tough—you have to think positive." This approach can leave patients feeling guilty, as though their negative thoughts or lack of strength caused their illness or will increase the likelihood of recurrence. Addressing feelings before facts is a key strategy for dealing with emotions.

Addressing feelings before facts requires recognizing and naming emotions. Empathic opportunities emerge when patients express negative emotions. Empathy means putting yourself in the other person's shoes and imagining what his or her life is like (Back et al. 2009). Patients have less anxiety and depression and report greater satisfaction and adherence to therapy when oncologists seize empathic opportunities by responding with "continuer" statements that encourage patients to continue expressing emotions rather than with "terminator" statements that discourage disclosure (Pollak et al. 2007). An example of a continuer statement is, "I can imagine how scary it must be for you to wonder whether your cancer will come back." An example of a terminator statement is, "We are doing everything we can to monitor your situation, so if your cancer recurs, we will catch it early." This statement may seem reassuring, but it is likely to cut off further expression. Continuer statements can be categorized into five groups represented by the mnemonic "NURSE," as detailed in Table 27.1 (Pollak et al. 2007).

When Patients Cry

Emotional expression often takes the form of crying. According to Dr. David Spiegel, a psychiatrist well known for his work with support groups, "We physicians are trained to treat crying as bleeding, to apply direct pressure to stop it" (Spiegel et al. 1989; Hope 2005). However, crying is often very therapeutic, so providers should let it happen. When patients cry, it does not mean that the provider has been cruel to them; in fact, just the opposite. Patients are most likely to open up emotionally and cry when they know that the provider cares about them. Crying is often a sign of trust and rapport. When patients cry, providers should give them space by sitting with them silently, offering a tissue, and perhaps touching them gently on the forearm. Providers should resist the temptation to immediately reassure or offer factual information. If the provider says anything when a patient cries, it should be something empathic, such as, "I can see how difficult this is for you. I wish things were different." Responding to patients' emotions with empathic statements may seem very time consuming, but it extends the length of consultations by

Table 27.1 Empathic opportunities in patient-provider communication

Opportunity	Definition	Examples
Type of empathic opportunity		
Direct	Explicit verbal expression of emotion	"I have been really depressed lately."
Indirect	Implicit verbal expression of emotion	"Does this mean I am going to die?"
"Continuer" statements (NURSE)		
Name	State the patient's emotion	"I wonder if you're feeling sad about the test result."
		"I can see this is making you angry."
Understand	Empathize with and legitimize the patient's emotion	"I can imagine how scary this must be for you."
		"Many of my patients feel discouraged when they aren't seeing the response they want, so it makes sense that you feel this way."
Respect	Praise the patient for strength	"You've done a great job at keeping everything in perspective."
		"I applaud you for your courage in all of this."
Support	Show support	"I will be with you until the end."
		"No matter what happens, I will always be your doctor."
Explore	Ask the patient to elaborate on the emotion	"Tell me more about what is upsetting you."
		"What do you mean when you say this is not going to happen to me?"

Adapted from Pollak et al. (2007)

an average of only 21 seconds (Kennifer et al. 2009). The more attentive and empathic providers are, the less emotional distress their patients experience (Zachariae et al. 2003).

Empathy is very powerful "medicine" for just about any negative emotion, including the grieving or sadness that patients feel when they experience permanent side effects of cancer or its treatment, such as lymphedema following mastectomy and radiation, altered cognition related to chemotherapy or radiation therapy, and neuropathy. Providers can refer patients to lymphedema specialists, physical therapists, neurologists, occupational therapists, and psychiatrists, but they cannot "fix" these problems. These challenges therefore represent opportunities for providers to show how much they care by simply listening and offering empathy.

Respectful and supportive statements are most effective after patients have had the opportunity to express their emotions. Examples of supportive statements are listed in Table 27.2. These are often most useful at the end of a clinic visit, so that the visit ends on a positive note. These statements also make it clear to patients that the provider will not abandon them in their time of greatest need (Epner et al. 2011).

Table 27.2 Examples of respectful and supportive statements

You've been through so much already.
I respect you for being so brave in the face of adversity.
I am inspired by your courage and fighting attitude.
Don't worry; we'll be here to help you if your cancer comes back, heaven forbid.
We are here for you no matter what.
We are here to help you meet any challenge you encounter, no matter how daunting.
I think your chances of (being cured, benefitting) are good (or X%).
I am optimistic about your situation.
I respect your religious faith. Your faith is very powerful medicine.

Delivering Difficult News

I am afraid I have some bad news for you. Your CT showed…

Mrs. Taylor is a married 45-year-old mother of an 8-year-old son and 12-year-old daughter. She underwent surgery, chemotherapy, and radiation for T2N2, poorly differentiated, invasive ductal breast cancer 3 years ago. Surveillance studies remained normal until 1 month ago, when blood work revealed elevated liver transaminases and alkaline phosphatase. She also noticed left hip pain for the first time a few weeks ago, but she attributed the pain to her new exercise regimen. CT and bone scans yesterday revealed new liver and bone metastases. She returns to the clinic to discuss test results.

This scenario is unfortunately all too common in the survivorship clinic. Recurrent, incurable cancer not only creates an existential crisis for the patient, but also forces everyone involved to face their own mortality. Discussing recurrence is therefore stressful for everyone involved, and it never becomes easy.

The "SPIKES" mnemonic represents an established strategy for discussing serious news (Baile et al. 2011). The first step is to create the proper **setting**, represented by the "S" in SPIKES. Serious conversations should be held in a quiet, private space, with the provider sitting at eye-level at a comfortable distance from the patient, close enough to touch him on the forearm and offer tissues if necessary. At least one close family member or friend should accompany the patient for moral support if possible, but no more than about four or five people should be in the room.

The next step in SPIKES is to assess the patient's understanding, or **perception**, of his illness, symbolized by the "P." This involves "asking before telling." The idea is to use open-ended questions to elicit a reasonably accurate picture of how the patient perceives the medical situation—what it is and whether it is serious. A good patient-centered conversation of this type involves *reciprocal* information exchange, rather than unidirectional flow of information from provider to patient.

The language should be simple and free of technical jargon to keep the message clear. A good starting point is for the provider to ask, "What is your understanding of your illness?" or, for the patient described above, "What is your understanding of why we did the CT and bone scan?" On the basis of this information, providers can correct misinformation and tailor the serious news to the patient's level of understanding. This approach can also accomplish the important task of determining whether the patient is in denial. The patient may respond, "I know I had the CT and bone scan to see if my cancer came back. Please don't tell me it has!" The provider and patient then respond to each other's comments in a free-flowing manner.

The next step in the SPIKES protocol involves obtaining the patient's permission, or "**invitation**," to discuss the serious news, symbolized by the "I." This means negotiating how the news will be handled, which may involve asking the patient how much detail she wants, whether she wants other family members present for the discussion, or whether she wants to delegate others to receive information on her behalf.

Making a warning statement, such as "I am afraid I have bad news…" immediately before disclosing the news (K for "**knowledge**") allows her to brace herself. Knowledge should be offered in nontechnical, clear language in small aliquots. Providers should avoid blunt language, such as, "You are going to die."

The "E" in SPIKES represents responding to **emotions** with **empathic** responses, as described above. Providers should continue to respond to strong emotions empathically rather than factually until the patient has calmed down enough to hear cognitive information about what is next. The patient may signal readiness by asking, "What comes next?" (Back et al. 2009).

The final "S" in SPIKES represents **summarize**. Ideally, the patient should summarize the conversation so that the provider knows that the patient understood. This can be accomplished by the provider saying, "Please tell me what you take away from this conversation and where we go from here."

Tell Me More: The Healing Power of Listening

The "E" in SPIKES represents emotions and empathy, but it can also represent **exploration**. The "E" in the NURSE acronym, previously discussed, also represents "exploration," which refers to letting the patient be heard. The idea is to get patients talking about whatever is most important to them. Most people have a profound need to discuss their fears and concerns, especially when those concerns pertain to life-threatening issues. Nonetheless, providers should get permission by asking, "Do you want to talk more about ….?" and continue with a series of open-ended questions until the patient calms down and is able to refocus on other topics, such as treatment options. Table 27.3 lists additional examples of exploratory statements. Table 27.4 lists examples of emotional statements and three strategies for responding to them: with a factual response (not usually helpful), an empathic response, and an exploratory response.

Table 27.3 Examples of exploratory statements and questions for a provider to use

Tell me more.
Tell me more about …
What worries you most about taking chemotherapy again?
What worries you most about dying of your cancer?
Heaven forbid, if your cancer recurs, how will your family be affected?

Table 27.4 Three strategies for responding to emotional statements from patients

Emotional patient statement	Typical factual response (usually not very effective)	Empathic response	Exploratory response
I constantly worry about my cancer returning.	Don't worry—I'm optimistic. Your chances of staying in remission are good.	I can't imagine how difficult it must be to live with the uncertainty.	Tell me more about what worries you.
I can't believe this is happening! The cancer is back after only 6 months. I have two kids to raise!	We have great treatments for this cancer; better treatments are coming all the time.	I can't imagine how scary this must be for you. I know this is not what you wanted to hear.	What do you worry about most about the cancer coming back?
	We have to deal with the results we have.	I know it has been difficult, and this must be a shock.	
I'm sorry to cry.		It's okay to cry. Crying is completely normal under these difficult circumstances.	[No response needed. Just sit in silence with the patient for a while until she stops crying and refocuses on the issues at hand. Let the patient resume the conversation if possible.]
I can't believe I need more surgery!	It's not that major of a procedure. You will get through it just fine.	I know you weren't expecting to hear this. I can imagine having surgery must be very scary.	Tell me more about what worries you most about surgery.

Listening Is Hard Work

The process of listening carefully to patients may seem passive, but it is actually a very active process that requires a great deal of practice. Mindful and attentive listening is arguably the most critical skill for effective communication, despite the fact that many people equate effective communication with speaking rather than listening. Truly patient-centered conversations involve patients sharing their illness experience by doing the vast majority of the talking, while providers gently guide and stimulate discussion with strategic interludes. Showing sincere interest in the patient helps establish rapport, relieve tension, and facilitate assessment of the patient's level of understanding. Encouraging the patient to narrate his illness also validates the importance of his perspective, provides the clinician with useful information, and encourages additional discussion. Establishing eye contact, nodding, and leaning forward are nonverbal methods that also demonstrate genuine interest (Stetten 1981; Epstein 1999; Bendapudi et al. 2006).

This process of reciprocal information exchange should be as free flowing and natural as possible. Sometimes the patient or provider needs to redirect the natural flow of information to accomplish specific communication goals, such as discussing logistics of treatment, informed consent, or code status. Regardless, providers should minimize interruptions and respond to nonverbal and verbal cues that signal the patient's desire to say something. Listening to family members, understanding who the patient is as a person by asking open-ended questions, listening carefully to the responses, and eliciting questions from the family is more effective than simply asking, "Any questions?" (Curtis et al. 2001; Lilly and Daly 2007). Silence is often very useful because it lets both participants reflect on what was just said and respond appropriately. When silence continues for what seems like an uncomfortably long time, it is often useful for the provider to re-engage the patient by asking, "What's on your mind?"

Dr. Jeff Kane noted in *How to Heal: A Guide for Caregivers* that individuals who are ill have a particularly great need for attention. All people need to be heard, especially those who are ill. Silence is golden; however, eventually patients want to know that providers hear them.

Many therapists and communication professionals recommend "mirroring," or reflecting back to the person what they just said, not word for word, but by paraphrasing, just to show that you are listening. For instance, if someone tells you that he is afraid, rather than urging him not to be fearful, you can simply acknowledge his feelings by saying something like, "it is scary," or "that sounds frightening." You can also listen well by clarifying what the speaker has said to you. In other words, if he says, "I don't want to go back to the doctor tomorrow," you might respond, "It sounds like you need some down time to focus on things other than your illness." This approach opens the door and encourages the person to express rather than repress his feelings.

Active, compassionate listening involves riding the rough road with a patient without trying to "fix" his problem. In *Let me Live*, by Lori Hope (2005), Father Siciliano explains: "Compassion is when you feel the pain but don't come up with easy answers. It's what I'd want, someone to feel the pain with me, sit with me and not come up with easy answers." Patient support groups are particularly powerful, because they serve the profound human need to be heard (Golant and Taylor-Ford 2010).

"How Long Do I Have, Doc?": Responding to Difficult Questions or Comments

Exploratory questions, such as those listed in Table 27.3, are also useful for responding to other difficult or uncomfortable questions or comments. For instance, patients often ask, "How long do I have (to live)?" Many providers respond with facts, such as survival statistics. However, it is often more useful to take an exploratory approach. The provider should first validate the question by saying, "You pose a very difficult and important question," and then say, "I will answer it to the best of my ability. But first help me understand why you ask about prognosis. What's on your mind?" (Baile et al. 2011).

An exploratory approach such as this may feel evasive to providers, but patients almost never see it that way. They value the opportunity to express themselves. Listening to their responses creates opportunities for providers to respond empathically. Many people express specific reasons for asking about prognosis, some of which are very practical. For instance, some patients want to know whether they are likely to be alive to attend a landmark family event, such as a wedding. If not, they can take the opportunity to prepare a video tribute or otherwise commemorate the occasion ahead of time. Other patients discuss prognosis to become emotionally prepared for the worst. Many patients have no "practical" reason for asking about prognosis but nonetheless appreciate the opportunity to discuss their concerns. After doing so, some patients are no longer interested in discussing survival estimates, which were ironically never the point of the prognostic question. Other patients still want to discuss time frames. If so, providers should answer as honestly, but sensitively, as possible. When offering numerical estimates, it is often useful to give a range of times, such as "days to weeks," "weeks to months," or "several months to a few years." Making an empathic statement after the time estimate shows compassion and sensitivity. For instance, "I wish I could say you will live a normal lifespan," effectively says, "I care, but the reality is…"

Key Practice Points

- Discussing emotional topics with cancer patients requires key communication skills that can be taught and learned.
- Everyone has a fundamental need to be heard, especially vulnerable cancer patients and survivors. Providers should spend most of their time with patients listening to patients' concerns, fears, hopes, dreams, and perspectives rather than "educating" them. Patients' perspectives should be elicited by asking open-ended questions, such as "What is your understanding of your illness?" or by simply saying, "Tell me more" or some variation thereof.

- Providers should address emotions with empathy rather than reverting back to biomedical or factual responses. For instance, when a patient says, "I am afraid of leaving my children without a mother. Who will care for them?", providers should resist the temptation to provide premature reassurance and instead reply: "I can't imagine how difficult this is for you" or "That must be a scary thought."
- Silence should be allowed in every conversation. Sometimes the most profound, meaningful statements arise after periods of reflection.
- Providers should avoid technical jargon and use clear language and simple phrases when explaining something to a patient.

Suggested Readings

Back A, Arnold R, Tulsky JA. *Mastering Communication With Seriously Ill Patients: Balancing Honesty With Empathy and Hope*. Cambridge: Cambridge University Press; 2009.

Baile WF, Brown R, Epner DE. Communicating prognosis. http://university.asco.org/communicating-prognosis. Published 2011. Accessed October 15, 2013.

Baile WF, Buckman R, Lenzi R, Glober G, Beale EA, Kudelka AP. SPIKES—a six-step protocol for delivering bad news: application to the patient with cancer. *Oncologist* 2000;5:302–311.

Bendapudi NM, Berry LL, Frey KA, Parish JT, Rayburn WL. Patients' perspectives on ideal physician behaviors. *Mayo Clin Proc* 2006;81;338–344.

Cororve Fingeret M. Body image and disfigurement. In: Duffy JD and Valentine AD, eds. *MD Anderson Manual of Psychosocial Oncology*. New York: McGraw Hill; 2011:271–288.

Curtis JR, Patrick DL, Shannon SE, Treece PD, Engelberg RA, Rubenfeld GD. The family conference as a focus to improve communication about end-of-life care in the intensive care unit: opportunities for improvement. *Crit Care Med* 2001:29;N26–N33.

Diefenbach MA, Turner GA, Bar-Chama N. Male sexuality and fertility after cancer. In: Miller KD, ed. *Medical and Psychosocial Care of the Cancer Survivor*. Boston: Jones and Bartlett; 2010:73–88.

Epner DE, Ravi V, Baile WF. When patients and families feel abandoned. *Support Care Cancer* 2011;19:1713–1717.

Epstein RM. Mindful practice. *JAMA* 1999;282:833–839.

Epstein RM and Street RL Jr. *Patient-Centered Communication in Cancer Care: Promoting Healing and Reducing Suffering*. Bethesda: National Cancer Institute; 2007.

Golant M, Taylor-Ford M. Post-traumatic stress in cancer survivors. In: Miller KD, ed. *Medical and Psychosocial Care of the Cancer Survivor*. Boston: Jones and Bartlett; 2010:31–42.

Haidet P. Jazz and the "art" of medicine: improvisation in the medical encounter. *Ann Fam Med* 2007;5:164–169.

Haidet P and Paterniti DA. "Building" a history rather than "taking" one: a perspective on information sharing during the medical interview. *Arch Intern Med* 2003;163:1134–1140.

Hope L. *Help Me Live: 20 Things People With Cancer Want You to Know*. Berkeley: Celestial Arts; 2005.

Hughes MK. Sexuality and cancer. In: Duffy JD, Valentine AD, eds. *MD Anderson Manual of Psychosocial Oncology*. New York: McGraw Hill; 2011:125–137.

Kane J. How to Deal: A Guide for Caregivers. New York: Allworth Press, 2003.

Kennifer SL, Alexander SC, Pollak KI, et al. Negative emotions in cancer care: do oncologists' responses depend on severity and type of emotion? *Patient Educ Couns* 2009;76:51–56.

Lilly CM, Daly BJ. The healing power of listening in the ICU. *N Engl J Med* 2007;356:513–515.

Pollak KI, Arnold RM, Jeffreys AS, et al. Oncologist communication about emotion during visits with patients with advanced cancer. *J Clin Oncol* 2007;25:5748–5752.

Rashid A. Anxiety in cancer patients. In: Duffy JD, Valentine AD, eds. *MD Anderson Manual of Psychosocial Oncology*. New York: McGraw Hill; 2011:71–85.

Rollnick S, Mason P, Butler C. *Health Behavior Change: A Guide for Practitioners*. Edinburgh: Churchill Livingston; 1999.

Spiegel D, Bloom JR, Kraemer HC, Gottheil E. Effect of psychosocial treatment on survival of patients with metastatic breast cancer. *Lancet* 1989;2:888–891.

Stetten D Jr. Coping with blindness. *N Engl J Med* 1981;305:458–460.

Suchman AL. A new theoretical foundation for relationship-centered care. Complex responsive processes of relating. *J Gen Intern Med* 2006;21:S40–S44.

National Cancer Institute. Facing forward: life after cancer treatment [pamphlet]. http://www.cancer.gov/cancertopics/coping/life-after-treatment.pdf. Published 2010. Revised August 2012. Accessed September 30, 2013.

Zachariae R, Pederson CG, Jensen AB, Ehrnrooth E, Rossen PB, von der Maase H. Association of perceived physician communication style with patient satisfaction, distress, cancer-related self-efficacy, and perceived control over the disease. *Br J Cancer* 2003;88:658–665.

Chapter 28
Integrative Oncology

Gabriel Lopez, Richard Lee, M. Kay Garcia, Alejandro Chaoul, and Lorenzo Cohen

Contents

L.E. Foxhall, M.A. Rodriguez (eds.), *Advances in Cancer Survivorship Management*,
MD Anderson Cancer Care Series, DOI 10.1007/978-1-4939-0986-5_28,
© The University of Texas M.D. Anderson Cancer Center 2015

Chapter Overview Integrative oncology is an expanding discipline holding tremendous promise for additional treatment and symptom control options. An integrative approach provides patients with a comprehensive system of care to help meet their needs, from diagnosis through survivorship. Most patients with cancer are either using complementary medicines or want to know more about them, so it is incumbent on the conventional medical system to provide appropriate education and evidenced-based clinical services. The clinical model for integrative care requires a patient-centered approach with attention to patient concerns and enhanced communication skills. In addition, it is essential that conventional and nonconventional practitioners work together to develop a comprehensive, integrative care plan. In this way, patients with cancer will receive the best medical care making use of all appropriate treatment modalities in a safe manner to achieve optimal clinical outcomes.

Introduction

Integrative medicine seeks to merge conventional medicine and complementary therapies in a manner that is comprehensive, personalized, evidence-based, and safe to achieve optimal health and healing. Although applying the concept of integrative medicine to cancer care is still in its formative years, a number of comprehensive cancer centers in the United States are putting this concept into practice under the term *integrative oncology*. This chapter will review the role of integrative oncology in cancer survivorship, with an emphasis on a comprehensive approach, an overview of the evidence, educational resources to guide health care providers and patients, and guidelines for creating a comprehensive, integrative treatment plan for cancer survivors.

Definitions

In the United States, *complementary and alternative medicine* (CAM) is defined by the National Center for Complementary and Alternative Medicine (NCCAM) as a group of diverse medical and health care systems, practices, and products that are not normally considered to be part of conventional medicine. NCCAM classifies CAM therapies into four broad categories: natural products, mind and body medicine, manipulative and body-based practices, and other CAM practices (see Table 28.1).

CAM includes nonconventional modalities that may or may not have high-quality evidence or financial incentives to support their intended use in the conventional medicine setting. *Alternative* medicine is when a patient makes use of a CAM modality for which there is no evidence for its efficacy in place of conventional medicine. *Complementary* medicine is when a patient makes use of a CAM modality

Table 28.1 Categories of complementary and alternative medicine, as defined by the National Center for Complementary and Alternative Medicine

Categories	Examples
Natural products	Herbal medicines (botanicals)
	Vitamins
	Minerals
	Probiotics
Mind and body medicine	Meditation
	Yoga
	Acupuncture
	Qigong
	Tai chi
Manipulative and body-based practices	Massage
	Spinal manipulation
	Chiropractic
	Osteopathic
	Physical therapy
Other complementary and alternative medicine practices	Whole medical systems
	Ayurvedic medicine
	Traditional Chinese medicine
	Homeopathy
	Naturopathy
	Energy therapies
	Magnet therapy
	Reiki
	Healing touch
	Movement therapies
	Feldenkrais method

for which there may or may not be evidence for its efficacy in combination with conventional medicine.

Integrative medicine, or complementary and integrative medicine (CIM), is becoming more prevalent in medical settings. *Integrative medicine* describes a philosophy of practice using an evidence-based approach to merge conventional and nonconventional therapies. The Consortium of Academic Health Centers for Integrative Medicine has defined this term as "the practice of medicine that reaffirms the importance of the relationship between practitioner and patient, focuses on the whole person, is informed by evidence, and makes use of all appropriate therapeutic approaches, healthcare professionals and disciplines to achieve optimal health and healing" (Consortium of Academic Health Centers for Integrative Medicine 2009). Integrative medicine uses an interdisciplinary approach to evaluate the risks and benefits of individual therapies. Practitioners of all disciplines should be aware of all treatment options and openly communicate with each other. The opportunity exits to optimize outcomes through a coordinated, comprehensive treatment plan. Throughout this chapter, we will use the term CIM in favor of CAM or other terms.

Prevalence

The World Health Organization estimates that up to 80% of people in developing countries rely on nonconventional traditional medicines for primary health care. People in more developed countries also seek out complementary medicine and practices. A 1997 survey of adults in the United States showed that CIM use (excluding self-prayer) varied from 32% to 54%. A 2007 survey by the US Centers for Disease Control and Prevention showed that 38% of adults had used CIM therapies during the past 12 months (Barnes et al. 2008).

Among patients with cancer and cancer survivors, the use of CIM is higher than in the general population. An estimated 40–69% of patients with cancer in the United States use CIM therapies (Navo et al. 2004; Richardson et al. 2000). A survey of five clinics within a United States comprehensive cancer care center found that CIM therapies (excluding psychotherapy and spiritual practices) were used by 68.7% of patients (Richardson et al. 2000). In a survey of cancer survivors, 43.3% reported using CIM in the past year. Patients with breast cancer use CIM more often than patients with other types of cancer; the overall prevalence of CIM use among patients with cancer ranges from 17% to 87%, with a mean of 45%. This range of prevalence reflects differences in patient populations studied.

In most cases, people who use CIM are not disappointed or dissatisfied with conventional medicine. Patients with cancer use CIM to reduce side effects (such as organ injury), to improve quality of life, to protect and stimulate immunity, or to prevent second primary cancers or recurrences. Whether or not patients use CIM therapies to treat cancer or its effects, they may use CIM to treat other chronic conditions such as arthritis, heart disease, diabetes, and chronic pain.

Comprehensive and Integrative Care Planning: Patient-Clinician Communication

Research indicates that neither adult nor pediatric patients with cancer receive sufficient information or discuss CIM therapies with physicians, pharmacists, nurses, or CIM practitioners. Most patients do not bring up the topic of CIM because no one asks; thus, patients may believe it is unimportant. It is estimated that 38–60% of patients with cancer use complementary medicines without informing their health care team (Navo et al 2004; Richardson et al. 2000). This lack of discussion is of concern because biologically based therapies (such as herbs) may interact with cancer treatments. Patients are commonly unaware of differences between medicines approved by the US Food and Drug Administration and supplements defined by the Dietary Supplement Health and Education Act of 1994. Supplements defined under this legislation are exempt from the same scrutiny that the US Food and Drug Administration imposes on medications; these supplements are not intended to treat, prevent, or cure diseases. The common belief among patients that "natural" means safe needs to be addressed with education. Some herbs and supplements have been associated with drug interactions (Ulbricht et al. 2008), increased cancer risk, and organ injury. These concerns are addressed later in this chapter.

Table 28.2 Recommended websites for evidence-based resources

Organization/website (alphabetical order)	URL
Cochrane Review Organization	http://www.cochrane.org
Consumer Lab	http://www.consumerlab.com
Memorial Sloan-Kettering Cancer Center Integrative Medicine Service	http://www.mskcc.org/aboutherbs
National Center for Complementary and Alternative Medicine	http://nccam.nih.gov/
Natural Medicines Comprehensive Database	http://www.naturaldatabase.com/
Natural Standard	http://www.naturalstandard.com/
National Cancer Institute Office of Cancer Complementary and Alternative Medicine	http://www.cancer.gov/cam
The University of Texas MD Anderson Cancer Center Complementary/Integrative Medicine Education Resources	http://www.mdanderson.org/integrativemedicine

Existing research suggests that most patients with cancer desire communication with their doctors about CIM (Verhoef et al. 1999). To provide optimal patient care, oncologists must be willing and able to discuss all therapeutic approaches, including CIM, with their patients. It is the health care professional's responsibility to ask patients about their use of complementary medicines. The discussion should ideally take place before the patient starts using a complementary treatment—whether it is a nutritional supplement, mind-body therapy, or other CIM approach.

A number of strategies can be used to address CIM use during a health care encounter. One approach is to include the topic of CIM as part of a new patient assessment. For example, when asking about medications, physicians should inquire about herb and supplement use. Physicians may consider having the patients bring in the actual bottles of herbs and supplements for evaluation. When asking about a patient's medical history, physicians may ask if the patient has visited with naturopathic or chiropractic practitioners. If the issue of CIM arises, clinicians need to develop an empathic communication strategy. The strategy needs to balance clinical objectivity with creation of a therapeutic alliance, benefitting both patient and health care provider. Patients need reliable information on CIM from reliable resources, with adequate time to discuss this information with their oncologists. Table 28.2 provides a list of websites useful for health care professionals seeking information on CIM therapies.

Safety Concerns

CIM therapies have the potential to lead to adverse outcomes (Palmer et al. 2003). With adequate precautions, yoga, massage, or acupuncture can be used safely during treatment and throughout survivorship. Herbs and supplements, however, should be considered more similar to prescription medications and therefore may be useful but can also lead to harm. The pathways by which biologically based CIM therapies may lead to negative clinical outcomes include metabolic interactions, treatment interactions, organ toxicity, cancer promotion, and lack of quality control standards.

Metabolic Interactions

Vitamins, supplements, or herbal products have the potential to interact with pathways of prescription drug metabolism. Increasing interest in these potential interactions has led to expanding literature in the area (Ulbricht et al. 2008; Palmer et al. 2003). These interactions should be carefully reviewed prior to integrating herbs, vitamins, or nutritional supplements during or after the completion of cancer-directed therapies.

The clinical efficacy of chemotherapeutic or chemopreventive agents metabolized through the hepatic cytochrome P450 (CYP) system may be compromised by herbs or supplements acting as inducers or inhibitors. As an example, St John's wort (*Hypericum perforatum*), an inducer of CYP 3A4 and 2C9, may reduce the clinical efficacy of irinotecan or imatinib (Smith et al. 2004). Although tamoxifen is also metabolized through CYP 2C9, CYP 2C9 is only a minor enzyme system involved in the metabolism of tamoxifen.

Treatment Interactions (Antioxidants)

The use of antioxidants has been proposed for cancer prevention and treatment. Examples include vitamins A, C, and E, selenium, and green tea extract. However, antioxidant supplementation may interfere with radiation and chemotherapeutic agents that depend on oxidative damage to exert their cytotoxic effects (e.g., alkylating agents, anthracyclines, or platinum-based agents; Lawenda et al. 2008). A randomized trial of head and neck cancer patients evaluated the use of beta-carotene and vitamin E for the reduction of radiation side effects and improvement in quality of life (Bairati et al. 2005a, b). Although side effects were reduced, results also demonstrated increased local recurrence and incidence of second primary cancers in patients in the supplement arm (Bairati et al. 2005a, b).

Antioxidant supplements require further study to determine when they are safe to use during active therapy or as chemoprevention (Lawenda et al. 2008; Block et al. 2007). Our current recommendation is to obtain antioxidants through whole food sources until more evidence becomes available regarding the use of antioxidant supplements.

Organ Toxicity

Hepatic and Renal Toxicity

Prolonged use of concentrated natural products may lead to organ damage. Although short-term exposure to hepatotoxins or nephrotoxins present in natural products may lead to transient and reversible organ injury, prolonged exposure can lead to organ failure. A thorough review of potential organ toxicities of natural products is warranted when combining prescription drugs with natural products. Early recognition of potentially hepatotoxic or nephrotoxic herbs or supplements can lead to timely discontinuation of potentially dangerous preparations.

Hematologic Toxicity

Certain herbs and supplements result in an increased risk of bleeding. The suspected mechanism is interference with platelet function. *Ginkgo biloba*, saw palmetto, fish oil, and garlic have all been associated with increased bleeding risk (Ulbricht et al. 2008). These agents should be discontinued before surgical procedures and should be used cautiously with other agents that increase bleeding risk.

Cancer Promotion (Phytoestrogens)

A common concern is the potential for herbs and supplements to stimulate cancer growth, leading to the development of new primary cancers or recurrences. One example comes from Dr. Sidney Farber of Harvard University, who discovered that antifolate agents can be used for cancer therapy after he observed that folic acid supplementation promoted disease progression. Until appropriate clinical trials have been conducted with herbs and supplements for individual cancer types, it is best to exercise caution with their use.

Phytoestrogens are plant-based compounds structurally similar to estradiol that are able to bind to estrogen receptors as agonists or antagonists. Products such as black cohosh, Essiac herbal tea, and soy contain phytoestrogens. Randomized clinical trials are needed before a definitive recommendation can be made regarding their safe use in patients with hormone-positive cancers. However, consumption of phytoestrogens such as soy as part of a healthy diet and as a whole food (i.e., not as supplements, powders, or processed soy products) has been shown in multiple observational studies in the United States and China to pose no risk for breast cancer survivors and may be beneficial.

Lack of Quality Control Standards

Herbal products and supplements from different manufacturers, or even from the same manufacturer, may vary considerably because of the lack of standardization and inconsistent quality control. Harmful contaminants, such as heavy metals, may be present in these preparations and pose a risk to patient health. Consumer Lab, accessible at http://www.consumerlab.com, is a useful resource that independently evaluates various natural product companies.

Role of Integrative Medicine in Cancer Survivorship: Clinical Model

An integrative treatment approach for cancer survivors should be comprehensive, personalized, evidence-based, and safe. The traditional model of cancer therapy involves three different approaches: surgery, radiation therapy, and chemotherapy. Integrative oncology aims to expand the interdisciplinary approach to include acupuncture, massage, yoga, meditation, diet, exercise, and other modalities. Engel's biopsychosocial model of health care, first published in *Science* more than 30 years ago, describes three domains of patient care and their importance in the treatment of all patients (Engel 1977). Our goal is to respond to patient needs in all three of these domains: social, psychological, and biological.

We propose an integrative oncology model as a framework to assist in creating comprehensive integrative care plans from diagnosis through survivorship (Fig. 28.1). Such a comprehensive care plan will address all of patients' needs with the greatest potential for improving their overall health and well-being. The concept of overall health and well-being is analogous to performance status. Assessment of performance status remains one of the most consistent prognostic factors for cancer. Similarly, quality of life has also been shown to predict survival in cancer patients. A meta-analysis of 30 randomized clinical trials demonstrated the benefit of including health-related quality of life in a model for predicting survival (Quinten et al. 2009). A basic comprehensive evaluation, addressing areas of psychosocial and physical well-being, will help improve patient performance throughout the continuum of care.

Psychosocial Well-Being

The mind-body connection is an important aspect of integrative oncology, as emphasized in the Institute of Medicine report entitled "Cancer Care for the Whole Patient." This comprehensive report mentions that "cancer care today often provides state-of-the-science biomedical treatment, but fails to address the psychological and social (psychosocial) problems associated with the illness. Psychological or social problems created or exacerbated by cancer…cause additional suffering, weaken adherence to prescribed treatments, and threaten patients' return to health" (Adler and Page 2008). Extensive research has shown that mind-body interventions appear to address many of the issues mentioned in the Institute of Medicine report.

The belief that what we think and feel can influence our health and healing dates back thousands of years. The importance of the role of the mind, emotions, and behaviors in health and well-being has been a part of various medical traditions of the world, such as Chinese, Tibetan, and Ayurvedic medicine. Many cancer patients turn to CIM therapies as a way to reduce stress; substantial

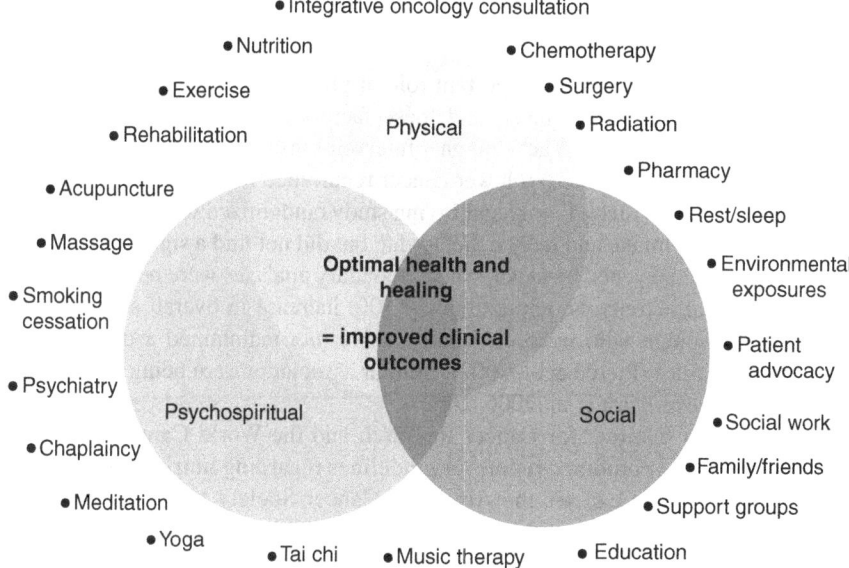

Fig. 28.1 Integrative medicine center model

evidence now demonstrates the negative health consequences of sustained stress on health and well-being. The profound psychological and behavioral effects of stress may include posttraumatic stress disorder, increased health-impairing behaviors (e.g., poor diet, lack of exercise, or substance abuse), poor sleep, and decreased quality of life. Research has shown that stress can also decrease regular health screening.

Many stress-induced physiological changes can have direct effects on health, such as persistent increases in sympathetic nervous system activity and the hypothalamic-pituitary axis that can cause increased blood pressure, heart rate, catecholamine secretion, and platelet aggregation. Furthermore, research has shown that stress is associated with increased latent viral reactivation, upper respiratory tract infections, and wound-healing time. Stress also deregulates a variety of immune indices, as shown in both healthy individuals and patients with cancer (Glaser and Kiecolt-Glaser 2005). Such stress-induced physiological changes may affect cancer progression, treatment, recovery, recurrence, and survival (Antoni et al. 2006; Lutgendorf et al. 2010). Andersen et al. (2010) demonstrated a survival advantage among patients with breast cancer who received a psychological intervention that included comprehensive education for stress management, maintaining a healthy diet, and engaging in regular physical activity; patients were followed for more than 10 years, including after they had a recurrence of disease. These studies underscore the importance of psychosocial intervention in cancer treatment.

Physical Well-Being

Growing evidence supports the important role of physical activity and nutrition in the health of patients with cancer, and these factors have been correlated with improved clinical outcomes. The Women's Intervention Study reported that a 24% reduction in fat intake resulted in lower cancer recurrence rates (Chlebowski et al. 2006). The Women's Health Eating and Living study randomized women to increase fruit and vegetable intake and reduce dietary fat, but did not find a significant reduction in breast cancer events; however, when secondary analyses were performed that included physical activity, an approximately 50% increase in overall survival was found among women who were physically active *and* maintained a diet high in fruits and vegetables (Pierce et al. 2007). Similar associations are being reported in colon cancer (Meyerhardt et al. 2006, 2007).

The American Institute for Cancer Research and the World Cancer Research Fund have created a combined report for guidelines regarding nutrition and physical activity to prevent cancer; the American Cancer Society has also published guidelines for those with cancer (Kushi et al. 2012). Additionally, a study examining obesity during neoadjuvant chemotherapy for breast cancer found that obesity was associated with decreased overall survival (Litton et al. 2008). Patients need to be encouraged to follow the American Cancer Society guidelines or the American Institute for Cancer Research/World Cancer Research Fund guidelines for cancer prevention; patients should also be encouraged to adopt healthful behaviors in regard to physical activity and diet. Details on the role of diet and physical activity can be found in Chaps. 15, 16, 17, and 18 on cancer prevention and screening.

Evidence-Based Approach

The field of integrative oncology is a constantly evolving set of disciplines and has experienced a dramatic increase in research. Below we list some of the key findings to date in integrative oncology in the main areas of CIM in which there is sufficient evidence to recommend the therapies as part of the standard of care: acupuncture, massage, and mind-body practices. These CIM therapies should be considered in conjunction with physical activity and nutrition, which are discussed in separate chapters. Although research is ongoing in many other areas, such as healing touch, homeopathy, natural products, and special diets, there is insufficient evidence to recommend these within the standard of care. Until there is evidence for the safety and efficacy of specific natural products (e.g., lycopene), these products should not be used as alternatives to the standard of care. Patients should be encouraged to seek whole food sources in moderation, avoiding extracts or purified formulations with purported "active" ingredients. The Society for Integrative Oncology's Integrative Oncology Practice Guidelines provides comprehensive, detailed, up-to-date evidence in these areas and is an excellent resource (Deng et al. 2009).

Acupuncture

Background

As part of traditional Chinese medicine, acupuncture has been practiced in China for thousands of years. It is one of the most popular traditional Chinese medicine thera- pies used outside of China, practiced in at least 78 countries. The traditional theory behind the benefits of acupuncture is that the placement of needles, heat, or pressure at specific places on the body can help to regulate the flow of qi (vital energy).

The most common form of acupuncture involves the placement of solid, sterile, stainless steel needles into various points on the body that are believed to have reduced bioelectrical resistance and increased conductance. Different techniques can be used to stimulate the needles, including manual manipulation or electrical stimulation (Helms 1995). For some patients, acupressure may be used, which involves applying heat or pressure to acupoints instead of puncturing the skin. Small stainless steel or gold (semipermanent) needles are also sometimes placed at spe- cific points on the ears and left in place for several days.

Clinical Studies

In 1997, a National Institutes of Health consensus statement supported the use of acupuncture for the treatment of postoperative and chemotherapy-related nausea and vomiting and some types of pain. Further research has substantiated this claim, and the American Cancer Society now states that clinical studies have found that acupuncture may help treat nausea caused by chemotherapy drugs and surgical anesthesia. In addition, specific neuroimaging research of patients while undergoing acupuncture treatments has helped to delineate the neural mechanisms of action. The mechanisms involved are believed to include enhanced conduction of bioelec- tromagnetic signals, activation of opioid systems, and activation of the autonomic and central nervous systems, causing the release of various neurotransmitters and neurohormones.

Several studies have investigated the use of acupuncture for symptom manage- ment in patients with cancer. A recent systematic review evaluated 42 randomized, controlled trials involving the use of acupuncture to help manage eight symptoms (nausea, pain, hot flashes, fatigue, radiation-induced xerostomia, prolonged postop- erative ileus, anxiety/mood disorders, and sleep disturbance) in patients with cancer (Garcia et al. 2013). This study showed that the strongest evidence to date is in sup- port of the use of acupuncture for the treatment of pain, nausea, and vomiting.

Although nausea and vomiting are among the top three most commonly reported side effects of cancer treatment, pain is the most common reason cancer survivors use acupuncture. One randomized, blinded, placebo-controlled trial investigating the use of acupuncture for the treatment of chronic pain among patients with cancer compared active auricular acupuncture with two placebo groups (Alimi et al. 2003). Pain scores were significantly lower in the active treatment group ($P < 0.001$).

Crew et al. (2010) also evaluated the use of acupuncture for the management of aromatase inhibitor-associated joint pain in women with breast cancer. In a small pilot crossover study (N=21), the authors concluded that acupuncture reduced joint symptoms and improved functional ability (Crew et al. 2010).

Although methodological rigor in acupuncture trials is improving, large definitive randomized clinical trials are still needed. Initial research suggests that acupuncture can be beneficial for symptom management, and in some cases can have a lasting effect. A recent study randomized women to receive acupuncture or venlafaxine and reported similar reductions in hot flash severity and frequency after 12 weeks of treatment (Walker et al. 2010). Preliminary studies also suggest that acupuncture may be a reasonable option for radiation-induced xerostomia, a common and often debilitating sequela to treatment in head and neck cancer survivors (Meng et al. 2012). For the management of other treatment- or cancer-related symptoms, emerging evidence suggests that acupuncture could be useful for the treatment of anxiety, depression, fatigue, constipation, loss of appetite, peripheral neuropathy, insomnia, dyspnea, and leukopenia (Garcia et al. 2013).

Safety

When performed correctly, acupuncture has been shown to be a safe, minimally invasive procedure with few side effects. The most commonly reported complications are fainting, bruising, and mild pain. Infection is also a potential risk, although very uncommon. Acupuncture should be performed only by a health care professional with an appropriate license and preferably one who has had experience in treating patients with malignant diseases.

If patients are experiencing uncontrolled symptoms despite conventional treatment, it is not unreasonable to accept a patient's choice to try acupuncture for symptom reduction, even in the absence of definitive data to support its use. The lack of conclusive human evidence for efficacy is balanced by the favorable safety record and the lack of other viable treatment options. Patients should be fully informed so that they know the potential risks, have realistic expectations, and know the financial implications.

Massage

Background

Massage has been used for thousands of years for relaxation and management of pain and discomfort. There are various forms of massage, and all typically apply some degree of pressure to muscle and connective tissue, in some cases working with specific pressure points. A clinical form of massage known as manual lymphatic drainage has been shown to decrease lymphedema when combined with elastic sleeves or bandaging for patients with arm edema after breast cancer surgery. Self-massage with this technique has not been shown to be as effective as massage done by either a trained therapist or a specially designed pump.

Clinical Studies

Research to date suggests that massage is helpful for relieving pain, anxiety, fatigue, and distress and increasing relaxation (Russell et al. 2008). Anecdotal and case report evidence has suggested a benefit from massage for relief of chemotherapy-induced peripheral neuropathy. A massage to the feet, hands, and head can provide therapeutic benefit because these areas are especially sensitive to tactile stimulation, and massage to these areas can result in relaxation and increased well-being. A challenge in conducting massage therapy research is having a placebo control group. It is therefore not clear what the exact mechanisms are for the benefits of massage in an oncology setting. Despite some of the imperfections in research design, the current findings are encouraging.

Safety

Massage is generally safe when it is conducted by a licensed practitioner who has had training in working with cancer patients. Graduated pressure of massage is reported as ranging from Level 1 (light touch) to Level 5 (deep tissue); these terms serve as descriptors to help adjust the level of massage to maximize safety. In general, cancer patients undergoing active treatment should not receive Level 5 massage and patients with bleeding tendencies should receive only Level 1 massage. Areas of the body that have recently undergone surgery or radiation therapy should be avoided. In patients with extremities subject to lymphedema, therapists will need to adjust their technique to maximize safety.

Mind-Body Practices

Background

Mind-body practices are defined by NCCAM as "a variety of techniques designed to enhance the mind's capacity to affect bodily function and symptoms." Mind-body techniques include relaxation, hypnosis, visual imagery, meditation, biofeedback, cognitive-behavioral therapies, group support, autogenic training, and spirituality, as well as expressive arts therapies such as art, music, or dance. Therapies such as yoga, tai chi, and qigong often fall into the CIM category of energy medicine because they are intended to work with bodily "energetic fields." However, these therapies are also likely to exert strong effects through a mind-body connection and as such also fall into the mind-body medicine category. Hypnosis, biofeedback, group support, and cognitive-behavioral therapy, once considered "alternative," are now integrated into most conventional medicine settings. As research continues, treatments found to be beneficial will continue to be integrated into conventional medical care.

Clinical Studies

Research has shown that after a cancer diagnosis, patients try to bring about positive changes in their lifestyles, often seeking to take control of their health. Stress management techniques that have proven helpful include progressive muscle relaxation, diaphragmatic breathing, guided imagery, social support, and meditation. Participating in stress management programs prior to treatment has enabled patients to tolerate therapy with fewer reported side effects. Supportive expressive group therapy has also been found to be useful for patients with cancer. Psychosocial interventions have been shown to specifically decrease depression and anxiety and to increase self-esteem and active-approach coping strategies (Syrjala and Chapko 1995).

Newell et al. (2002) reviewed psychological therapies for cancer patients and concluded that interventions involving self-practice and hypnosis for managing nausea and vomiting could be recommended, but further research was suggested to examine the benefits of relaxation training and guided imagery. Further research was also warranted to examine the benefits of relaxation and guided imagery for managing general nausea, anxiety, quality of life, and overall physical symptoms.

Research examining yoga, tai chi, and meditation incorporated into cancer care suggests that these mind-body practices help improve quality of life through improved mood, sleep quality, physical functioning, and overall well-being (Cohen et al. 2004). Hypnosis, especially self-hypnosis, helps reduce distress and discomfort during difficult medical procedures. A National Institutes of Health Technology Assessment Panel found strong evidence hypnosis can alleviate cancer-related pain.

Safety

Mind-body practices have an excellent safety profile, with some practices requiring more physical activity than others. Mind-body practitioners with experience working with cancer patient populations can provide guidance to help patients safely engage in practices such as meditation, yoga, and tai chi.

Key Practice Points

- Integrative medicine seeks to merge conventional medicine and complementary therapies in a manner that is comprehensive, personalized, evidence-based, and safe to achieve optimal health and healing.

- Early, open, and empathic patient-physician communication regarding CIM therapies can contribute to enhanced trust and empower patients from diagnosis through survivorship.
- Knowledge of herb and supplement interactions with cancer-directed and chemopreventive therapies is critical to minimize toxic effects and achieve optimal clinical outcomes.
- An evidence-based approach for recommendation of modalities such as acupuncture, massage, and mind-body practices can help better meet survivor needs.
- Growing evidence supports the importance of weight reduction, increased physical activity, and improved nutrition to decrease the risk of cancer development and recurrence.

Suggested Readings

Adler NE, Page AEK. *Cancer Care for the Whole Patient: Meeting Psychosocial Health Needs.* Washington, DC: National Academy Press; 2008.

Alimi D, Rubino C, Pichard L, et al. Analgesic effect of auricular acupuncture for cancer pain: a randomized, blinded, controlled trial. *J Clin Oncol* 2003;21:4120–4126.

Andersen BL, Thornton LM, Shapiro CL, et al. Biobehavioral, immune, and health benefits following recurrence for psychological intervention participants. *Clin Cancer Res* 2010;16:3270–3278.

Antoni MH, Lutgendorf SK, Cole SW, et al. The influence of bio-behavioural factors on tumour biology: pathways and mechanisms. *Nat Rev Cancer* 2006;6:240–248.

Bairati I, Meyer F, Gélinas M, et al. A randomized trial of antioxidant vitamins to prevent second primary cancers in head and neck cancer patients. *J Natl Cancer Inst* 2005a;97:481–488.

Bairati I, Meyer F, Gélinas M, et al. Randomized trial of antioxidant vitamins to prevent acute adverse effects of radiation therapy in head and neck cancer patients. *J Clin Oncol* 2005b;23:5805–5813.

Barnes PM, Bloom B, Nahin RL. Complementary and alternative medicine use among adults and children: United States, 2007. *Natl Health Stat Report* 2008;12:1–23.

Block KI, Koch AC, Mead MN, et al. Impact of antioxidant supplementation on chemotherapeutic efficacy: a systematic review of the evidence from randomized controlled trials. *Cancer Treat Rev* 2007;33:407–418.

Chlebowski RT, Blackburn GL, Thomson CA, et al. Dietary fat reduction and breast cancer outcome: interim efficacy results from the Women's Intervention Nutrition Study. *J Natl Cancer Inst* 2006;98:1767–1776.

Cohen L, Warneke C, Fouladi RT, Rodriguez MA, Chaoul-Reich A. Psychological adjustment and sleep quality in a randomized trial of the effects of a Tibetan yoga intervention in patients with lymphoma. *Cancer* 2004;100:2253–2260.

Consortium of Academic Health Centers for Integrative Medicine. About CAHCIM. http://www.imconsortium.org/about/home.html. Updated November 2009. Accessed September 26, 2013.

Crew KD, Capodice JL, Greenlee H, et al. Randomized, blinded, sham-controlled trial of acupuncture for the management of aromatase inhibitor-associated joint symptoms in women with early-stage breast cancer. *J Clin Oncol* 2010;28:1154–1160.

Deng GE, Frenkel M, Cohen L, et al. Evidence-based clinical practice guidelines for integrative oncology: complementary therapies and botanicals. *J Soc Integr Oncol* 2009;7:85–120.

Engel GL. The need for a new medical model: a challenge for biomedicine. *Science* 1977;196:129–136.

Garcia MK, McQuade J, Haddad R, et al. Systematic review of acupuncture in cancer care: a synthesis of the evidence. *J Clin Oncol* 2013;31:952–960.

Glaser R, Kiecolt-Glaser JK. Stress-induced immune dysfunction: implications for health. *Nat Rev Immunol* 2005;5:243–251.

Helms JM. *Acupuncture Energetics: A Clinical Approach for Physicians.* Berkeley, CA: Medical Acupuncture Publishers; 1995.

Kushi LH, Doyle C, McCullough M, et al. American Cancer Society Guidelines on nutrition and physical activity for cancer prevention: reducing the risk of cancer with healthy food choices and physical activity. *CA Cancer J Clin* 2012;62:30–67.

Lawenda BD, Kelly KM, Ladas EJ, Sagar SM, Vickers A, Blumberg JB. Should supplemental antioxidant administration be avoided during chemotherapy and radiation therapy? *J Natl Cancer Inst* 2008;100:773–783.

Litton JK, Gonzalez-Angulo AM, Warneke CL, et al. Relationship between obesity and pathologic response to neoadjuvant chemotherapy among women with operable breast cancer. *J Clin Oncol* 2008;26:4072–4077.

Lutgendorf SK, Sood AK, Antoni MH. Host factors and cancer progression: biobehavioral signaling pathways and interventions. *J Clin Oncol* 2010;28:4094–4099.

Meng Z, Garcia MK, Hu C, et al. Randomized controlled trial of acupuncture for prevention of radiation-induced xerostomia among patients with nasopharyngeal carcinoma. *Cancer* 2012;118:3337–3344.

Meyerhardt JA, Heseltine D, Niedzwiecki D, et al. Impact of physical activity on cancer recurrence and survival in patients with stage III colon cancer: findings from CALGB 89803. *J Clin Oncol* 2006;24:3535–3541.

Meyerhardt JA, Niedzwiecki D, Hollis D, et al. Association of dietary patterns with cancer recurrence and survival in patients with stage III colon cancer. *JAMA* 2007;298:754–764.

Navo MA, Phan J, Vaughan C, et al. An assessment of the utilization of complementary and alternative medication in women with gynecologic or breast malignancies. *J Clin Oncol* 2004;22:671–677.

Newell SA, Sanson-Fisher W, Savolainen NJ. Systematic review of psychological therapies for cancer patients: overview and recommendations for future research. *J Natl Cancer Inst* 2002;94:558–584.

Palmer ME, Haller C, McKinney PE, et al. Adverse events associated with dietary supplements: an observational study. *Lancet* 2003;361:101–106.

Pierce JP, Stefanick ML, Flatt SW, et al. Greater survival after breast cancer in physically active women with high vegetable-fruit intake regardless of obesity. *J Clin Oncol* 2007;25:2345–2351.

Quinten C, Coens C, Mauer M, et al. Baseline quality of life as a prognostic indicator of survival: a meta-analysis of individual patient data from EORTC clinical trials. *Lancet Oncol* 2009;10:865–871.

Richardson MA, Sanders T, Palmer JL, Greisinger A, Singletary SE. Complementary/alternative medicine use in a comprehensive cancer center and the implications for oncology. *J Clin Oncol* 2000;18:2505–2514.

Russell NC, Sumler SS, Beinhorn CM, Frenkel MA. Role of massage therapy in cancer care. *J Altern Complement Med* 2008;14:209–214.

Smith P, Bullock JM, Booker BM, Haas CE, Berenson CS, Jusko WJ. The influence of St. John's wort on the pharmacokinetics and protein binding of imatinib mesylate. *Pharmacotherapy* 2004;24:1508–1514.

Syrjala KL, Chapko ME. Evidence for a biopsychosocial model of cancer treatment-related pain. *Pain* 1995;61:69–79.

Ulbricht C, Chao W, Costa D, Rusie-Seamon E, Weissner W, Woods J. Clinical evidence of herb-drug interactions: a systematic review by the natural standard research collaboration. *Curr Drug Metab* 2008;9:1063–1120.

Verhoef MJ, White MA, Doll R. Cancer patients' expectations of the role of family physicians in communication about complementary therapies. *Cancer Prev Control* 1999;3:181–187.

Walker EM, Rodriguez AI, Kohn B, et al. Acupuncture versus venlafaxine for the management of vasomotor symptoms in patients with hormone receptor-positive breast cancer: a randomized controlled trial. *J Clin Oncol* 2010;28:634–640.

Index